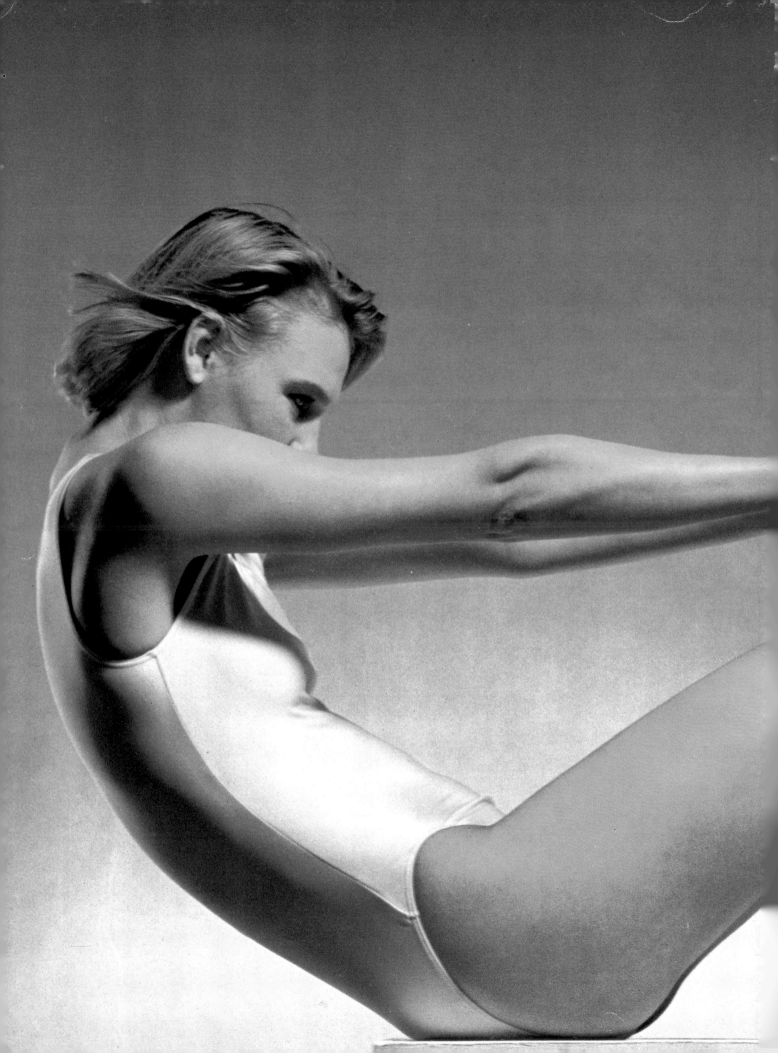

VOGUE
COMPLETE DIET AND EXERCISE

General Editor
Deborah Hutton

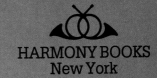

HARMONY BOOKS
New York

The contributors

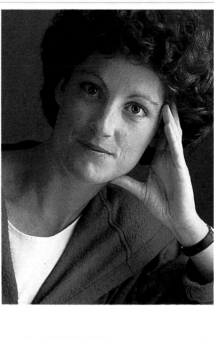
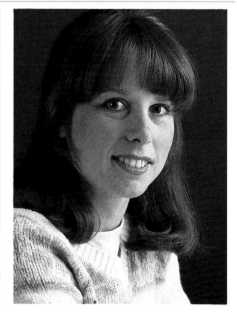

DEBORAH HUTTON devised the concept for the book, wrote and edited it. She has an honours degree in English from York University and gained a job on *Vogue* after entering their annual talent competition in 1979. She has been writing health features for the magazine for 5 years and is the author of *Vogue Complete Beauty* (Octopus).

DR SHEILA BINGHAM devised the special diets and some of the recipes. She is a nutritionist and has practised as a therapeutic dietician at several London hospitals, and is presently engaged in nutritional research. Her thirty papers and publications include a dictionary of nutrition for the consumer, *Nutrition: Better through Eating* (Corgi).

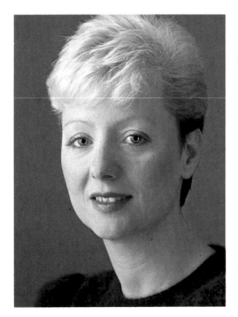
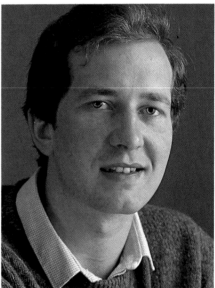

EILEEN FAIRBANE devised most of the exercise programme, the jazz pre-ski and therapeutic sections. A jazz dancer by training, she is also interested in many other forms of movement. She is a qualified beauty therapist, trained aromatherapist and has studied shiatsu (acupressure), macrobiotics and Feldenkrais work. She teaches in London and has produced her own exercise tape.

TONY LYCHOLAT acted as exercise consultant on the book and helped to check the text. He has an honours degree in Human Movement, specializing in sports science, and is currently completing an MSc degree. He is an athletics coach who regularly lectures on exercise and training theory, and he also works as Fitness Advisor at Barbara Dale's studio in London.

Illustrations copyright © 1985 by Octopus Books Limited
Text copyright © 1985 by the Condé Nast Publications Limited

Published in the United States in 1985 by Harmony Books, a division of Crown Publishers, Inc., One Park Avenue, New York, New York 10016.

Originally published in Great Britain by Octopus Books Limited

HARMONY and colophon are trademarks of Crown Publishers, Inc.

Manufactured in Spain

Library of Congress Cataloging in Publication Data

Hutton, Deborah.
   Vogue complete diet and exercise.

   1. Women–Health and hygiene.
   2. Physical fitness for women.
   3. Reducing diets–Recipes.
   4. Exercise for women.   I. Vogue.
   II. Title.
RA778.H9827   1985
613'.04244   84-12808

ISBN: 0-517-55581-6

10 9 8 7 6 5 4 3 2 1

First American Edition

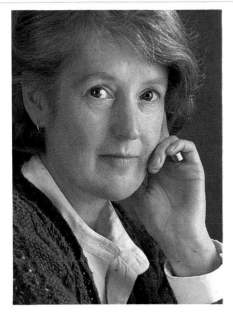
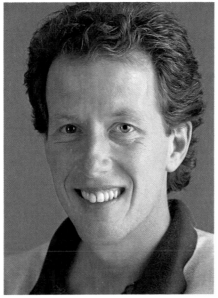
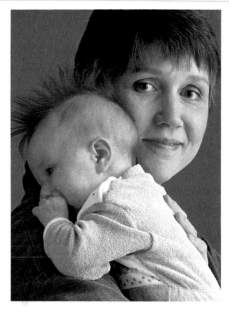

ARABELLA BOXER devised the dinner party menus and juice diet recipes for the Special Diets section. She has written many highly successful recipe books, and has been *Vogue* Food Editor since 1974. She works regularly for the *Sunday Times Magazine* and has twice won the Glenfiddich Award for Food Writer of the Year.

CHRISTOPHER CONNOLLY produced most of the Feldenkrais-based awareness movements for the programme, plus many of the therapeutic exercises, and helped to check the text. He is the only qualified teacher of the Feldenkrais method in the UK. He is co-author of *Sporting Body/Sporting Mind*, (Cambridge University Press), and has contributed to *Vogue*.

BARBARA DALE devised the pre- and post-natal exercise programme. She has trained in all aspects of dance and movement, and has devised her own method of exercise which she teaches at her studio in London. She has contributed to many books and magazines, including *Vogue Complete Beauty* (Octopus).

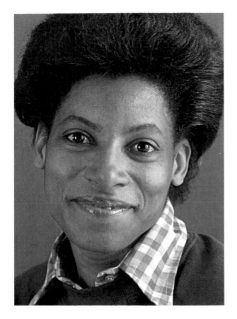
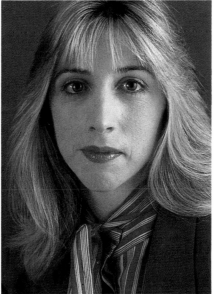
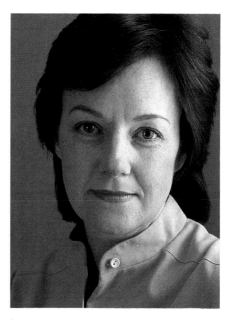

CYLE POLLARD devised the Rock and Roll section and the special preparatory exercises which appear in week 19 of the exercise programme. She was born in Chicago and has taught and performed in the Middle East, West Germany, Holland and Paris. She is the new Director of the Footwork Dance Studio in London, and her particular interest is in American jazz dance.

DR BARBARA JACQUELYN SAHAKIAN contributed to the self-assessment pages and to the notes running through the diet section, and has also acted in a consultative capacity. A psychologist by training, she is particularly interested in eating disorders. She is Co-Editor of *Psychopathology Today* (Peacock Press) and has published over forty articles.

JENNY SALMON devised the 24-week diet programme and compiled many of the recipes. She is a trained Home Economist, Nutritionist and Dietician and has worked for several London hospitals. She has contributed to a number of magazines and books, including the highly successful *F-Plan Diet* (Penguin), and has written four recipe books of her own.

CONTENTS

Introduction 7

The diet
  programme 10

Special diets 56

Entertaining 80

Recipe index 94

The exercise
  programme 126

Rock and roll 208

Jazz 212

Sports days 218

Pre-ski
  programme 224

Exercising
  for childbirth 226

Therapeutics 238

Index 246

INTRODUCTION

These exercise and diet programmes are based on the holistic philosophy that the whole always adds up to more than the sum of its parts. Follow them both and you will find them more than twice as effective as exercising or dieting alone. You get fitter quicker and have more energy if you eat in a healthy way; slim faster, shape up better if you exercise while losing weight.

Both programmes are concerned with health in its most positive sense – not the type of health that is merely about absence of illness, but the type of health that is about *thriving* – feeling alert, sharp, confident, full of mental and physical energy. And the changes that you make should not only take you towards this new, more positive level of health, but should make you feel better too.

These programmes challenge the widely held assumption that the cultivation of good health has to hurt, that something that feels good cannot possibly be doing you good at the same time. You will not be forced to run, heave, sweat or stretch further than you feel able, nor to gulp down foods you do not like because they are supposed to be 'good' for you. The focus is on enjoyment, not effort. Moving and eating may be two of life's necessities, but they should be two of life's pleasures too.

Discover what you enjoy and what works well for you by listening to your body, respecting it and acting accordingly. Fine-tune your awareness by following the programmes. There, you will find the information you need to interpret the information your body sends. Complete the programmes and you should be so attuned to your better interests that you won't need anyone – or any book – to tell you what you should be eating and how you should be exercising.

The programmes are longer than most diet and keep-fit schemes because, if permanent changes in weight and shape are to be had and if fitness is to be more than just a passing enthusiasm, a long-term structured programme is called for – one that takes you through your paces gradually and changes as you progress. The essence of all successful change is gradualness. Think how long it has taken to establish the habits that have spoiled our shape and undermined our health, and you will see why it takes months, not weeks, to change them permanently for the better.

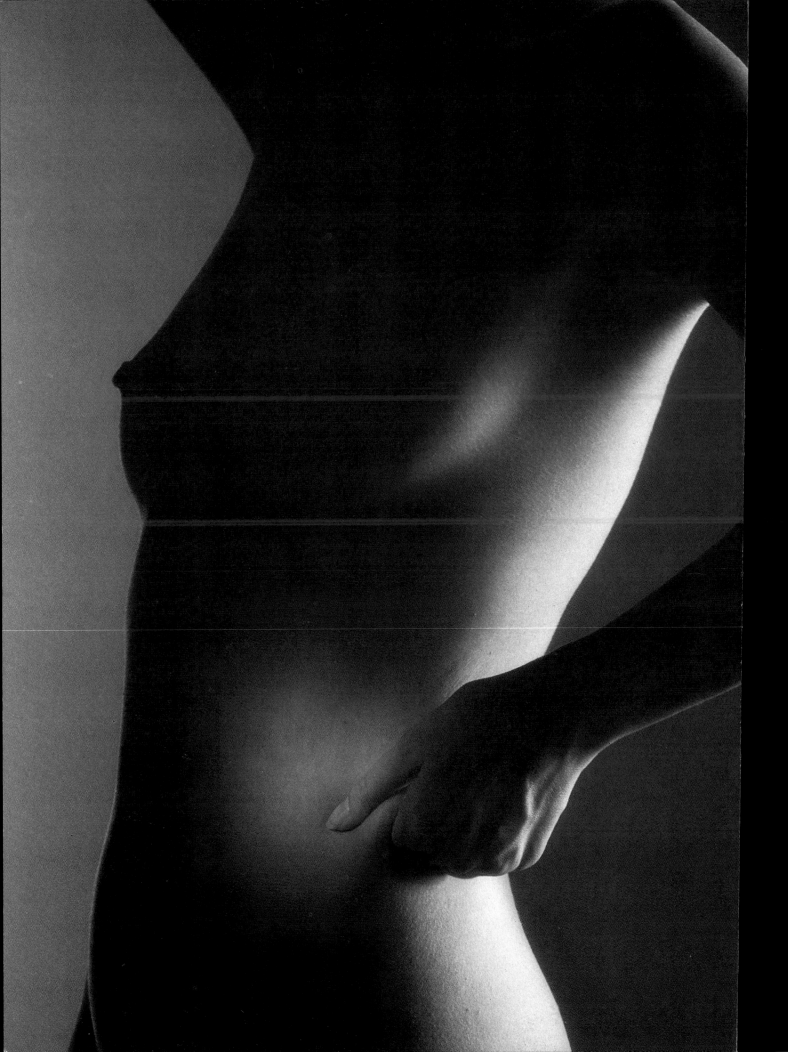

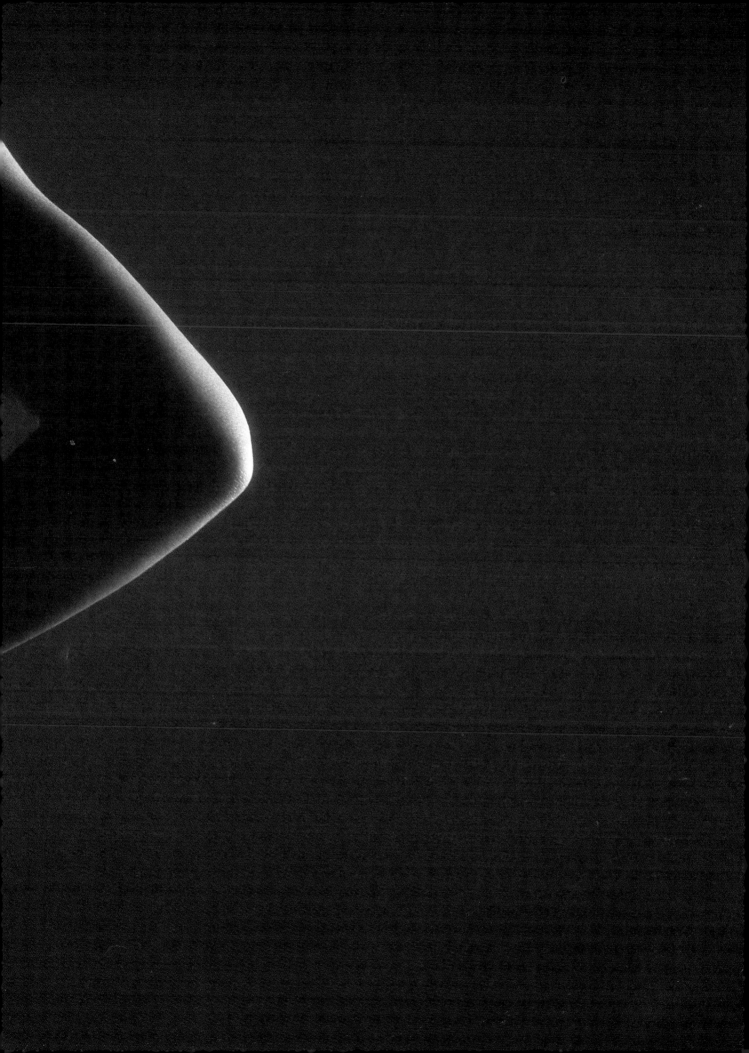

The diet programme

Diets have fallen into disfavour. They are now said to be dangerous, self-defeating, to damage your health and to make you fat[1]; they are described as 'low grade popular infections'[2] which cause widespread misery by perpetuating an ideal of slimness that can often only be achieved at tremendous personal cost. As diets have come to be associated with fads that don't work, so the meaning of the word itself has changed. Diet as good nutrition, as a healthy and enjoyable way of eating, has come to seem like a contradiction in terms...

And it's not just the value of dieting, but the ideal of slimness itself that has been called into question. Feminist writers see it as part of the cultural/sexist conspiracy, 'a much larger coercion against the full and natural development of women'[3], in which to diet is to collude and to grow fat is to rebel ('Fat offends Western ideals of female beauty and, as such, every 'overweight' woman creates a crack in the popular culture's ability to make us mere products'[4]). And an increasing number of people, men as well as women, are challenging the concept that being slim is any more desirable, or indeed any better for you, than being fat.

In place of the diet books of recent years, with their unappetizingly monotonous regimens of cottage cheese and yogurt, and promises of ever more rapid weight loss, we now have a string of anti-diet books advising us to drop the subject altogether, to eat whatever we like, to make friends with food, to take up vigorous exercise, to be happy with the way we are.

But the way we are, when left to the all-too-common excesses of rich, over-refined food and an inactive sedentary lifestyle, is often rather larger than we would like. Thinness may no longer be fashionable but fitness most certainly is. Being in shape is more important than ever. The 80s message is an encouraging one – first that *anyone* can get into shape, can become fit, firm, lithe, well-muscled and effective and second that this personal best is to be achieved not through months of deprivation and undernutrition but through an active lifestyle and a healthy diet.

But how many of us are in shape? How many of us do have an active lifestyle and a healthy diet? As a nation, we are fatter and unfitter than ever before. The average weight of every man, woman and child in the West has risen alarmingly over the last 20 years, *and* we are putting the weight on at an increasingly early age. In a recent study[5] conducted in the United Kingdom, half of all 20-year-olds were found to be already too heavy, so much so that one in four was 'incurring a health risk'. The figure rises to one in two by the mid-50s.

The anti-dieting league recognizes the problem but tells us to

'The 80's message is an encouraging one – first that anyone can get into shape, can become fit, firm, lithe, well-muscled and effective and second that this personal best is to be achieved not through months of deprivation and under-nutrition but through an active lifestyle and a healthy diet'..

stop counting the calories, to start eating nutritiously, and to take to the running track – where fat and flab will magically metamorphose into muscle. But is such transformation possible without restricting the amount you eat? The top nutritionists say no. Exercise alone is not enough just as diet alone is not enough. Exercise will help transform shape more effectively than many diets but it will not help shift those extra pounds nearly as swiftly. A combined approach is needed; exercise with diet and diet with exercise and both with an increased awareness of what they can do for you. You need to be attuned to what your body needs before you can hope to give it what it wants . . .

Because the way we eat and the way we move are so fundamental to our wellbeing, the aim of this programme is as much to promote positive health as to change shape or improve fitness. The 24-week programme, for example, is not just about losing weight but about gaining new insights, about discovering how much better you feel for eating in a healthy way. Food can make you fat, full, indigested, sick, headachey, bloated and guilty, but it can also make you feel fit, inspired, vital, full of life and energy. . . The way we feel depends, to a much greater degree than most of us realize, on the way we eat.

But what type of diet will produce long-term changes in shape and wellbeing? The choice is bewildering, the claims conflicting. Ironically, much can be learned from the books telling us not to diet at all, because these books justly expose the pointlessness as well as the dangers of life spent on or between diets – the misery of not being able to trust your appetite because it seems to 'make you gain weight' as soon as you start eating in anything approaching a normal way, the futility of trying to reach and maintain an impossible goal, the self-defeating process whereby diets deplete 'energy-expensive' lean tissue, sapping vitality and lowering metabolic rate, making weight regain not just likely but inevitable. . .

The news is that there is no easy, quick and effective way of losing weight permanently, no short cuts to real changes in shape and size. *Short-term losses always lead to long-term gains.* There are no wonder foods and formulae, no miraculous combinations that by some wondrous quirk of biochemistry will balance each other out so enabling you 'to eat all 'you like and still lose weight'. There is nothing magical about grapefruit and eggs or bananas and milk or bunches of grapes for every meal. If you were expecting to find them here, you will be disappointed.

The only way to lose weight is to lose weight slowly AND in conjunction with an exercise programme. The new-generation diets, compiled in the light of all available evidence, place as much emphasis on what you eat as how much, on how you feel as on what you weigh. In place of limited foods to be eaten at specific times and in specific quantities, these diets encourage you to widen the variety of foods you eat, to listen to your body and to trust your own instincts, hunger and appetite included. This twenty-four week programme has been produced for people who are fatter and unfitter than they would like to be, who suspect that they could be enjoying a much enhanced level of health and vitality but understand that high-level health demands high-level motivation; who would like to gain weight and lose weight relatively swiftly but realize that there are penalties to be paid for doing it too fast. It takes time to change the habits of a lifetime.

A long-term diet, designed to promote gradual weight loss helps avoid frustrating problems with plunging metabolic rates, keeps energy high and helps instil new awareness of all the positive things that food can do for you. All you need to do right now is to start. . .

1. *Claims contained in 'Dieting Makes You Fat' by Geoffrey Cannon and Hetty Einzig (Century, London, 1983)*
2. *'Breaking the Diet Habit' by C. Peter Herman and Janet Polivy (Basic Books, New York, 1983)*
3. *'Womansize' by Kim Chernin (The Women's Press, London 1981)*
4. *'Fat is a Feminist Issue' by Susie Orbach (Hamlyn, London, 1978)*
5. *'Obesity,' a Report by the Royal College of Physicians (London, 1983)*

Self assessment

How can you get into shape for good? Dieting starts with a question, because if putting on weight is easy and taking it off is harder, keeping it off is harder still. Any diet can work in the short term, but only you can make those results last permanently. Use the questionnaires and charts on the following pages to enhance awareness and gain insight. Self-knowledge is the key to success.

It is no secret that few diets work. The usual pattern is to lose weight for a while, and then to regain it...often with interest. Most of us lose and gain hundreds of pounds in this way (well over our own body weight) over the course of our dieting lives.

In one New York survey, 100 people advised by their doctors to take off weight were monitored for 2 years. Only 12 lost a significant amount of weight after a year and just 2 managed to sustain it by the end of the next. This depressing result is probably rather better than average because research shows that diets are generally *more* successful when accompanied by advice and encouragement from an authoritarian figure.

Faced with these figures, the obvious conclusion is that most diets are self-defeating and over 80 per cent of people following them are wasting their time – especially if they carry exactly the same expectations and eating habits into the new diet as the one before (and the one before that...and the one before that...)

A new approach is clearly needed. It may mean settling for a goal weight a few pounds above the 'ideal' or trying a different style of dieting or radically reassessing your present eating patterns – very possibly all three.

We believe that if you want to lose weight permanently, *and are realistic in the goal you set yourself*, you can lose weight permanently. But first you must question your attitudes and examine your eating patterns. Use this chapter to help determine the right approach. Make losing weight as easy as possible by picking a diet that suits you, and avoid regaining the weight you lose by making some lasting changes to your diet and by being sensitive to those factors which have led to overeating in the past.

Ensure your future success by analysing past failures. Was the diet at fault or were you? Recognize that diets do not only fail through weakness and lack of willpower, but through their own shortcomings. Diets that severely restrict the types of food allowed, for example, can rarely be followed for more than a few days simply because the nutrients necessary for good health can only be found in a wide range of foods. So respect the instinct that rebels and bear in mind that the diets that are hardest to follow are generally the most unsound. Reproach yourself for embarking on such diets by all means, but refuse to take the blame when you break them.

Even balanced diets can have their pitfalls if unsuited to your tastes and lifestyle. Despite the promises that are often made, no diet works for everyone. Some people require absolute rigidity with foods measured out to the ounce, while others need more flexibility; some do better on short sharp blitzes but most benefit from a longer-term eating programme; some like certain foods while others detest them. We are all different.

What is necessary, then, is to have the insight to pick a diet that works for you – and a diet that works for you is one that makes you feel good for being on it. Awareness of how you feel and enjoyment of what you eat is where the new nutritional emphasis lies. A diet that enhances wellbeing while promoting weight loss is much more likely to be successful in the long-term than one which asks you to rely on feelings of virtuous deprivation to carry you through. If you feel better on the diet than you did off it, sticking to it will not be a problem – and neither will carrying its healthy principles over to your everyday way of eating once you have reached your goal.

Real awareness of how you feel on what you eat may nevertheless be rather subtler than you realize. If your reaction to reading this is to say, 'Aha, but I enjoy cream cakes and gooey chocolates', ask yourself whether that's really true. Even if you enjoy eating them at the time, how do you feel for having eaten them? Light, refreshed and full of energy or stodgy, indigested and guilty? Explore your responses to food, and become more attuned to the crucial connection between what you eat and the way you feel, by filling out the diary pages at the end of this section.

Now read on...

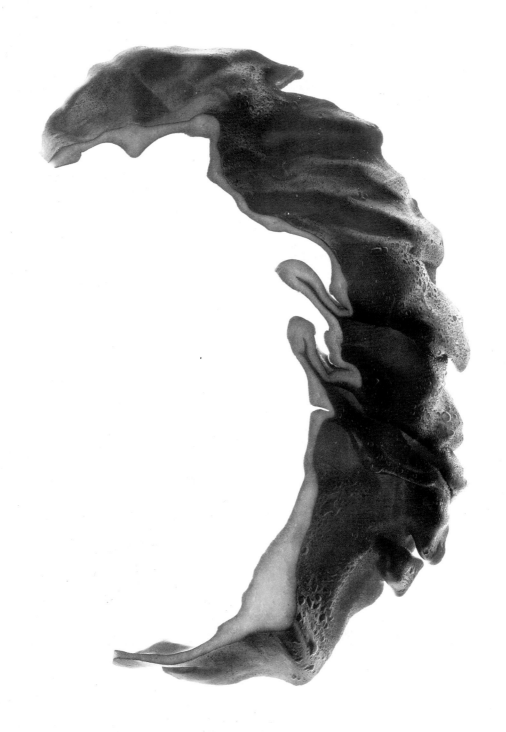
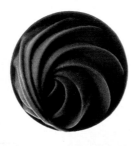

HOW MUCH SHOULD YOU WEIGH?

Desirable weight ranges are determined by insurance companies for the soundest business reason – they need to know how long their clients are likely to live. Their records show that, while normal-weight people have a normal life expectancy (all other things being equal), overweight people die young.

A survey compiled by the US Metropolitan Life Insurance Company over a period of 25 years has shown that people who are 10 per cent or more above the upper limit of 'acceptable' have a 50 per cent higher mortality. That means they are half as likely again to die before their time. In addition to falling prey to the killer diseases such as coronary heart disease and cancer, overweight people are more susceptible to disabling ones, such as diabetes.

But it is important to keep a sense of perspective. For, although no-one would contest that being very fat is very bad for you, being a little larger than you might like does not constitute a health hazard. In fact, being a few pounds overweight may actually be *better* for you than being a few pounds under. The 'fat equals unhealthy therefore thin equals healthy' equation flies in the face of available evidence. One major survey, carried out on the population of the town of Framingham in Massachusetts, USA, found no evidence to suggest that people who are *mildly* overweight are prejudicing their health. In fact, this group had the *best* survival record of the population – much better than the thinnest group, who were found to be more seriously at risk than the fattest . . .

Guidelines for women

Height without shoes (m)	Women Weight without clothes (kg)		
	Acceptable average	Acceptable weight range	Obese
1.45	46.0	42–53	64
1.48	46.5	42–54	65
1.50	47.0	43–55	66
1.52	48.5	44–57	68
1.54	49.5	44–58	70
1.56	50.4	45–58	70
1.58	51.3	46–59	71
1.60	52.6	48–61	73
1.62	54.0	49–62	74
1.64	55.4	50–64	77
1.66	56.8	51–65	78
1.68	58.1	52–66	79
1.70	60.0	53–67	80
1.72	61.3	55–69	83
1.74	62.6	56–70	84
1.76	64.0	58–72	86
1.78	65.3	59–74	89

Height without shoes (ft,in)	Women Weight without clothes (lb)		
	Acceptable average	Acceptable weight range	Obese
4 10	102	92–119	143
4 11	104	94–122	146
5 0	107	96–125	150
5 1	110	99–128	154
5 2	113	102–131	152
5 3	116	105–134	161
5 4	120	108–138	166
5 5	123	111–142	170
5 6	128	114–146	175
5 7	132	118–150	180
5 8	136	122–154	185
5 9	140	126–158	190
5 10	144	130–163	196
5 11	148	134–168	202
6 0	152	138–173	208

Bray, 1979; based on Metropolitan Life Insurance tables

ARE YOU TOO FAT?

Weight tables have been criticized for several reasons. One is that they make no assessment of fat. People come in all shapes and sizes as well as heights. You can be fit, firm and not a fraction too fat, yet be considerably heavier than someone of similar height but slighter build. It's proportion that counts.

Unfortunately, there is no easy, accurate and objective way of assessing proportion. Precise measurements of body fat require calipers and expertise. The pinch test, however, gives a rough guide. Reduce error by taking two 'pinches', one from the underside of your upper arm and the other from your hip. Add them together and divide by two to get an average and check it against the graph*, below.

Fat situated directly beneath the skin constitutes about 50 per cent of the total, so you can estimate how 'fat' you are by pinching your flesh. But make sure it is fat you are grasping, not muscle, which feels much firmer. Measure the distance between inner edges of thumb and forefinger.

WHAT IS YOUR 'BODY MASS INDEX'?

A third indication of excess weight is known as the Body Mass Index. This allows for increasing weight with increasing height and, very roughly, for differences in frame. It is expressed as follows:

$$\text{Body Mass Index} = \frac{\text{weight in kilogrammes}}{\text{height in metres}^2}$$

Check the tables, overleaf, to find the correct index for your weight and height. If the figure is under 19, you are definitely underweight and if the figure is over 24.4 you are definitely overweight – regardless of what build you are. If the figure comes within these two extreme ends of the range, however, things become more complicated because you may still be under- or overweight, depending on your build. To date, there is no completely reliable way of determining build (frame size) or its appropriate range, but the approximate ranges, given below, provide a rough guide. Assess frame size by taking two measurements – one from the tip of one shoulder to the tip of the other shoulder and the other from the tip of one shoulder to the tip (bony point) of the elbow. If these are roughly the same, assume frame size to be medium; if width is greater than length, assume frame size to be between medium and large; if the length is greater than the width, assume frame size to be between medium and small. If all this is too confusing, simply use your personal judgement and, if in doubt, choose medium.

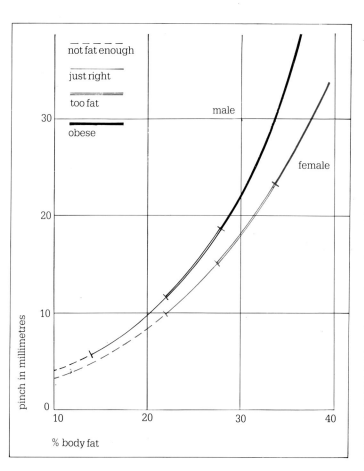

Weight ranges for adult women*

Frame	Desirable	Borderline	Overweight	Obese
Large	21.4–24	24.5–25.7	25.8–29	more than 29
Medium	20.1–22.3	22.4–23.7	23.8–26.7	more than 26.7
Small	19–20.5	20.6–22.5	22.6–24.4	more than 24.4

*devised from figures produced by J.V.G.A. Durnin and J. Wormersley in 'Body fat assessed from total body density and its estimation from skinfold thickness: measurements in 481 men and women aged 16 to 72 years' in the 'British Journal of Nutrition', 1974, 32, pp 77–99.

*approximate ranges estimated using 'Slimdicator' designed by T.J. Cole and W.P.T. James.

A GUIDE TO BODY MASS INDEX

Height in metres

Weight in kilogrammes

	1·46	1·48	1·50	1·52	1·54	1·56	1·58	1·60	1·62	1·64	1·66	1·68	1·70	1·72	1·74	1·76	1·78	1·80
45	21·1	20·5	20	19·5	19	18·5	18	17·6	17	16·7	16·3	15·9	15·6	15·2	14·9	14·5	14·2	13·9
46	21·6	21	20·4	19·9	19·4	18·9	18·4	18	17·5	17	16·7	16·3	15·9	15·5	15·2	14·8	14·5	14·2
47	22	21·5	20·9	20·3	19·8	19·3	18·8	18·4	17·9	17·5	17·1	16·6	16·3	15·9	15·5	15·2	14·8	14·5
48	22·5	22	21·3	20·8	20·2	19·7	19·2	18·7	18·3	17·8	17·4	17	16·6	16·2	15·8	15·5	15·1	14·8
49	23	22·4	21·8	21·2	20·1	20·2	19·6	19·1	18·7	18·2	17·8	17·4	17	16·6	16·2	15·8	15·5	15·1
50	23·5	22·8	22·2	21·6	21·1	20·5	20	19·5	19·1	18·6	18·1	17·7	17·3	16·9	16·5	16·1	15·8	15·4
51	23·9	23·3	22·7	22·1	21·5	21	20·4	19·9	19·4	19	18·5	18·1	17·6	17·2	16·8	16·5	16·1	15·7
52	24·4	23·7	23·1	22·5	21·9	21·4	20·8	20·3	19·8	19·3	18·8	18·4	18	17·6	17·2	16·8	16·4	16
53	24·9	24·2	23·6	22·9	22·3	21·8	21·2	20·7	20·2	19·7	19·2	18·8	18·3	17·9	17·5	17·1	16·7	16·4
54	25·3	24·7	24	23·4	22·8	22·2	21·6	21·1	20·6	20·1	19·6	19·1	18·7	18·3	17·8	17·4	17	16·7
55	25·8	25·1	24·4	23·8	23·2	22·6	22	21·5	21	20·4	20	19·5	19	18·6	18·2	17·8	17·4	17
56	26·3	25·6	24·9	24·2	23·6	23	22·4	21·9	21·3	20·8	20·3	19·8	19·4	18·9	18·5	18·1	17·7	17·3
57	26·7	26	25·3	24·7	24	23·4	22·8	22·3	21·7	21·2	20·7	20·2	19·7	19·3	18·8	18·4	18	17·6
58	27·2	26·5	25·8	25·1	24·5	23·8	23·2	22·7	22·1	21·6	21	20·5	20·1	19·6	19·2	18·7	18·3	17·9
59	27·7	26·9	26·2	25·5	24·9	24·2	23·6	23	22·5	21·9	21·4	20·9	20·4	19·9	19·5	19	18·6	18·2
60	28·1	27·4	26·7	26	25·3	24·7	24	23·4	22·9	22·3	21·8	21·3	20·8	20·3	19·8	19·4	18·9	18·5
61	28·7	27·8	27·1	26·4	25·7	25·1	24·4	23·8	23·2	22·7	22·1	21·6	21·1	20·6	20·1	19·7	19·3	18·8
62	29	28·3	27·6	26·8	26·1	25·5	24·8	24·2	23·6	23·1	22·5	22	21·5	21	20·5	20	19·6	19·1
63	29·6	28·7	28	27·3	26·6	25·9	25·2	24·6	24	23·4	22·9	22·3	21·8	21·3	20·8	20·3	19·9	19·4
64	30	29·2	28·4	27·7	27	26·3	25·6	25	24·4	23·8	23·2	22·7	22·1	21·6	21·1	20·7	20·2	19·8
65	30·5	29·7	28·9	28·1	27·4	26·7	26	25·4	24·8	24·2	23·6	23	22·5	22	21·5	21	20·5	20·1
66	31	30·1	29·3	28·6	27·8	27·1	26·4	25·8	25·1	24·5	24	23·4	22·8	22·3	21·8	21·3	20·8	20·4
67	31·4	30·6	29·8	29	28·3	27·5	26·8	26·2	25·5	24·9	24·3	23·7	23·2	22·6	22·1	21·6	21·1	20·7
68	31·9	31	30·2	29·4	28·7	27·9	27·2	26·6	25·9	25·3	24·7	24·1	23·5	22·9	22·5	22	21·5	21
69	32·4	31·5	30·7	29·9	29·1	28·4	27·6	26·9	26·3	25·7	25	24·4	23·8	23·3	22·8	22·3	21·8	21·2
70	32·8	31·9	31·1	30·3	29·5	28·8	28·1	27·3	26·7	26·1	25·4	24·8	24·2	23·7	23·1	22·6	22·1	21·6
71	33·3	32·4	31·5	30·7	29·9	29·2	28·5	27·7	27	26·4	25·8	25·1	24·5	24	23·5	22·9	22·4	21·9
72	33·8	32·8	32	31·1	30·3	29·6	28·9	28·1	27·4	26·8	26·1	25·5	24·9	24·4	23·8	23·3	22·7	22·2
73	34·2	33·3	32·4	31·6	30·8	30	29·3	28·5	27·8	27·2	26·5	25·8	25·2	24·7	24·1	23·6	23·1	22·5
74	34·7	33·7	32·8	32	31·2	30·4	29·7	28·9	28·2	27·6	26·9	26·2	25·6	25	24·5	23·9	23·4	22·8
75	35·2	34·2	33·3	32·4	31·6	30·8	30·1	29·2	28·6	27·9	27·2	26·5	25·9	25·4	24·8	24·2	23·7	23·1
76	35·6	34·7	33·7	32·9	32	31·2	30·5	29·6	29	28·3	27·6	26·9	26·2	25·7	25·1	24·5	24	23·4
77	36·1	35·1	34·2	33·3	32·4	31·6	30·9	30	29·3	28·7	28	27·3	26·6	26·1	25·4	24·9	24·3	23·7
78	36·6	35·6	34·6	33·7	32·9	32	31·3	30·4	29·7	29·1	28·3	27·6	26·9	26·4	25·8	25·2	24·6	24
79	37	36	35·1	34·1	33·3	32·5	31·7	30·8	30·1	29·4	28·7	28	27·3	26·7	26·1	25·5	25	24·3
80	37·5	36·5	35·5	34·6	33·7	32·9	32·1	31·2	30·5	29·8	29	28·3	27·6	27·1	26·4	25·8	25·3	24·6
81	38	36·9	36	35	34·1	33·3	32·5	31·6	30·9	30·2	29·4	28·7	28	27·4	26·8	26·2	25·6	25
82	38·4	37·4	36·4	35·4	34·5	33·7	32·9	32	31·2	30·5	29·8	29	28·3	27·7	27·1	26·5	25·9	25·3
83	38·9	37·8	36·8	35·9	35	34·1	33·3	32·4	31·6	30·9	30·1	29·4	28·7	28·1	27·4	26·8	26·2	25·6
84	39·4	38·3	37·3	36·3	35·4	34·5	33·7	32·8	32	31·3	30·5	29·7	29	28·4	27·8	27·1	26·5	25·9
85	39·9	38·8	37·7	36·7	35·8	34·9	34·1	33·2	32·4	31·7	30·9	30·1	29·4	28·8	28·1	27·5	26·8	26·2
86	40·3	39·2	38·2	37·2	36·2	35·3	34·5	33·5	32·8	32	31·2	30·4	29·7	29·1	28·4	27·8	27·2	26·5
87	40·8	39·7	38·6	37·6	36·7	35·8	34·9	33·9	33·2	32·4	31·6	30·8	30·1	29·4	28·8	28·1	27·5	26·8
88	41·3	40·1	39·1	38	37·1	36·2	35·3	34·3	33·5	32·8	32	31·2	30·4	29·8	29·1	28·4	27·8	27·1
89	41·7	40·6	39·5	38·5	37·5	36·6	35·7	34·7	33·9	33·2	32·3	31·5	30·7	30·1	29·4	28·8	28·1	27·4
90	42·2	41	40	38·9	37·9	37	36·1	35·1	34·3	33·5	32·7	31·9	31·1	30·5	29·8	29·1	28·4	27·8

THE SET RANGE THEORY AND WHY IT MATTERS

Statistics are great levellers. They allow only for differences in height and frame, and give 'acceptable' ranges which are often broad to a fault – over 12.5 kg (28 lb) in some cases. You may come well within them but still feel dissatisfied with your shape and no closer to knowing what your optimal weight should be.

There may be a second problem if what you feel to be your optimal weight does not coincide with the weight you naturally incline towards when eating well, but not excessively, and exercising regularly. When the weight at which you feel physiologically happiest, your 'natural' weight, is at odds with the weight at which you feel psychologically happiest, your 'ideal' weight, the seeds of an intractable weight problem are sown and a miserable life-long struggle can ensue, because every diet you pick simply pits you against yourself.

Scientists call the weight at which you feel physiologically happiest the 'set point' – a misleading term because it is more likely to be a range than any one particular weight. Whether your set range is small (as little as 1 kilo/2 pounds) or large (6 kilos/13 pounds or more) mostly depends on the genes you inherit and to a lesser, but nevertheless still appreciable, extent on your previous dieting history.

Just as some set ranges are broader than others, so some are lower or higher. This distinguishes people who put weight on very easily from those who don't. Two people of similar height can have very dissimilar set ranges – the lowest point of each representing that point beyond which they will each find it very difficult to lose weight. But even here there are differences. While some set ranges are controlled very tightly, making it difficult to dip even a kilo or so below them, others are more loosely defended. Defence takes two forms: *physiological/metabolic*, by using up energy-expensive lean tissue, reducing metabolic rate and slowing you down (see page 34) and *psychological/behavioural* by making you irritable, depressed, discontented and increasing your appetite and interest in food, especially deliciously fattening foods...

Set ranges may not be as 'set' as all that. Repeated dieting, and large weight fluctuations especially, appear to reset them upwards, possibly to create a 'safety margin' that will help protect against similar rash drops in weight in the future. So people who complain that they never had a weight problem until they started dieting may actually have a point! More positively, there are indications that regular vigorous exercise has a *lowering* effect on the set range.

Is your ideal weight within your set range or should you modify your goals?

1 What do you weigh?

2 What would/do you weigh without restriction or excessive binges?

3 What would you like to weigh?

4 Have you ever managed to get down to this weight?...

more than once/once only/never

5 ...and to stay there comfortably for at least 3 months?   *yes/no*

Fortunate individuals giving the same answer to the first 3 questions have no need for this book or, indeed, for any diet book, but anyone giving very different answers to these questions, and particularly to 2 and 3, should carefully examine their reasons for wanting to be the weight they gave and should, perhaps, modify their goals.

If your answer to question 2 was very much higher than your answer to question 3, your ideal weight is likely to be some way outside your set range.

Answers to questions 4 and 5 will indicate by how much. If you have never managed to get down to this ideal weight or only with extreme difficulty, and found staying there virtually impossible, you should set yourself a more realistic goal. Use the charts given earlier and the guidelines that follow to determine this.

If your answers to 2 and 3 are some way apart, but your answer to question 4 is 'more than once' and you managed to stay there comfortably, your ideal weight is probably within your set range – just – even if your present weight is some way above it and has been for a time. Follow the long-term eating plan, losing weight steadily at a rate of no more than 1 kg (2 lb) a week, to reattain it.

ASSESS YOUR SET RANGE

Think back over past diets. How did you feel at the weights you were?

Above set range	*able to eat quite substantially without gaining very much more weight.*
Within set range	*able to maintain weight fairly easily without great deprivation; able to diet down to the lowest point of the range quite easily but further weight loss significantly harder once past it.*
Below set range	*great effort, vigilance and deprivation required to keep weight stable; growing sense of frustration; obsessive preoccupation with food even to the point of dreaming about it; high susceptibility to hunger in general and high-calorie foods in particular.*

If the above is not guide enough, there are other ways of telling whether your weight lies inside or outside your set range – and these all refer to the way you *feel*.

Life below the set range, and the sort of dieting designed to get you there, is highly stressful. The conflict between you, trying to get your weight down, and your body, trying to push your weight up, produces measurable biochemical changes, such as raised levels of stress hormones (catecholamines) in the blood. These changes are accompanied by changes in mood. As weight drops, concentration falters, sense of humour diminishes, emotions become much more highly charged and irritability and agitation increase.

Keep stress down by keeping food intake at a reasonable level and expectations realistic. If your present weight is within your set range and you are still dissatisfied with your general shape, combine diet aimed for the lower point of the range (the point at which it *begins* to become hard to lose weight and to keep it off) with a structured exercise programme to firm specific problem areas. You will be amazed by the transformation.

WHAT KIND OF EATER ARE YOU?

(To convert pounds to kilogrammes, multiply by 0.45)

1. How often do you diet? (Circle one)

Never	Rarely	Sometimes	Usually	Always

2. What is the maximum amount of weight (in pounds) you have ever lost within one month?

0–4	5–9	10–14	15–19	20+

3. What is your maximum weight gain within a week?

0–1	1.1–2	2.1–3	3.1–5	5.1+

4. In a typical week, how much does your weight fluctuate?

0–1	1.1–2	2.1–3	3.1–5	5.1+

5. Would a weight fluctuation of 5 lb affect the way you live your life?

Not at all	Slightly	Moderately	Very much

6. Do you eat sensibly in front of others and binge alone?

Never	Rarely	Often	Always

7. Do you give too much time and thought to food?

Never	Rarely	Often	Always

8. Do you have feelings of guilt after overeating?

Never	Rarely	Often	Always

9. How conscious are you of what you are eating?

Not at all	Slightly	Moderately	Extremely

10. How many pounds over your desired weight were you at your maximum weight?

0–1	1–5	6–10	11–20	21

1 *Never = 0, Rarely = 1, Sometimes = 2, Usually = 3, Always = 4*

2 *0–4 = 0, 5–9 = 1, 10–14 = 2, 15–19 = 3, 20+ = 4*

3 *0–1 = 0, 1.2–2 = 1, 2.1–3 = 2, 3.1–5 = 3, 5.1+ = 4*

4 *0–1 = 0, 1.1–2 = 1, 2.1–3 = 2, 3.1–5 = 3, 5.1+ = 4*

5 *Not at all = 0, Slightly = 1, Moderately = 2, Very much = 3*

6 *Never = 0, Rarely = 1, Often = 2, Always = 3*

7 *Never = 0, Rarely = 1, Often = 2, Always = 3*

8 *Never = 0, Rarely = 1, Often = 2, Always = 3*

9 *Not at all = 0, Slightly = 1, Moderately = 2, Extremely = 3*

10 *0–1 = 0, 1–5 = 1, 6–10 = 2, 11–20 = 3, 21 = 4*

Add up total score to find your index of restraint. Now refer to the analysis.

Questionnaire adapted from 'Internal and External Components of Emotionality in Restrained and Unrestrained Eaters' devised by J. Polivy, C.P. Herman and S. Walsh in the Journal of Abnormal Psychology, 1978, 87, page 497.

What the scores mean

High scorers on this scale *(mid-20s and above)* are chronic dieters – people who find it easier to count the days off diets rather than the days on them. They are extremely weight conscious and very preoccupied with what they eat. They are 'restrained'. Anorexics and bulimics, victims of the binge/vomit disease, are very restrained indeed. In fact, some bulimics have got the highest possible restraint score of 35.

A high score also indicates an 'ideal' weight some way below the set range and an increased susceptibility to stress-induced eating (maybe as a direct result of the stress of having to keep one's weight so low). Use the blank diary pages, further on, to help determine whether this is the case.

Moderate scorers *(low 20s and high teens)* may be conscious of what they eat as much for health as for weight reasons and may rarely diet or weigh themselves.

Low scorers *(15 and below)* are people who tend to eat what they like, regardless of how nutritious or fattening it is. They are not particularly concerned with what they weigh and rarely perceive it as a 'problem'. They are 'unrestrained'. Many score as low as 5; none is likely to be reading this book.

Which diet for which score?

(High scorers *(mid 20s and above)* are advised to follow the 24-week programme from week 1, even if weight initially increases slightly as food intake returns to more normal levels. Although quantities of food included in the earlier weeks of the diet may seem large, it will help weight to stabilize and will instil more appropriate eating patterns. Keep to the diet until you reach your goal – it may only take a few weeks – and then repeat Week 1, gradually increasing food intake until you establish an appropriate maintenance level.

Lower scorers *(early 20s and below)* should use the diet plan to lose as much weight as you need, starting at week 12 or even 20. The Blitz or 14-day Special diets might appeal as a quick means to moderate weight loss if objectives are more limited or weight needs to be lost quite quickly for a special occasion.

PAST IMPERFECT, FUTURE BETTER...

Diets, like history, have a habit of repeating themselves. Writing down why your diets usually fail in the space provided below may help make this one the exception. Your first safeguard is awareness; your second, the insight to pick an appropriate diet. See suggestions, *opposite.*

WHY DO DIETS FAIL (AND HOW CAN YOU SUCCEED)?

Reason	Suggested strategy	Diet
Boredom at prospect of so much further to go	Set limited objectives, shorter deadlines: e.g. a non-edible reward for every 1.8 kg/4 lb lost or a week off a month.	Start programme at week 20; earlier if you need to lose more weight, but take a week off every 4 weeks, or even every 3 (including 2 juice diet days), then continue with the diet.
Boredom with repetitive, unappetizing food	Choose an interesting diet with unusual food combinations fresh herbs and spices, exotic fruit, seafood and good cuts of meat. Spending more on less will make what you do eat seem special. Discover the wide choice of herb teas and tisanes available. Enjoy an occasional glass of champagne.	24-week programme, starting week 1, 12 or 20, depending on goal; the Vegetarian diet for a complete change.
Lack of will power	Write failure into the diet by allowing yourself to break it. (See notes on Indulgences page 54).	24-week programme.
Lack (or loss) of incentive	Go to health spa for a few days to get started or reinspired; make a contract with a friend; join a weightwatching group or exercise class.	Start with or switch to the Blitz diet for an encouraging initial loss, then return to the longer-term programme.
Loss of confidence in ability to lose weight at all	Pick your moment, such as when returning from holiday or any time when you have extra energy and a positive attitude.	Any, as long as it is a) balanced and b) different in every respect from the ones that have preceded it, i.e. the long-term programme if you usually crash diet or the High-Fibre/Low-Fat diet if you normally pick a low-carbohydrate one.
Weight sticking	Do you really *need* to continue with the diet? Re-read notes on 'set point' on the previous page. If you decide you do, continue with the diet and take more exercise. Vow not to look at the scales for a fortnight: use a tape measure instead.	
Erratic lifestyle	Choice of diet is crucial: it MUST be flexible and easy to follow.	24-week programme. Blitz or one of the 14-day special diets. Be well prepared by buying as much as possible beforehand.
Busy professional/social life	Most diets adapt easily to restaurant menus and most restaurants will adapt easily to your wishes, providing lemon juice in place of vinaigrette, unbuttered vegetables, etc. So ask...	Avoid diets that dictate exactly what you must and must not eat. Follow long-term programme, using dinner party menus for entertaining.
Snacking	Be prepared. Cut fine strips of carrot, celery, apple, cauliflower, etc, each morning and keep in refrigerator. Eat lunch and breakfast in stages.	One that subdivides easily: the 3 meals in the long-term programme can break down to 6 mini ones or even more...
Keeping the family company	Convert them to your healthier way of eating or make sure that you provide for yourself while they eat, so you do not have to sit, watch and be tempted...	24-week programme (starting week 1, 12 or 20). Most meals can be made more substantial and/or appealing to children by clever additions.
Surrounded by food	Out of sight is out of mind. Remove temptation where possible and where not possible pack in opaque containers. Buy as much as you need – no more. If necessary, shop more often.	
Arguments/emotional upheavals	Awareness is your best defence. Fill in the diary section over the page to see if there is a link between your mood and the amount or *type* of food you eat. Sometimes, a particular food becomes linked subconsciously with a particular state of mind, so that we not only reward or console ourselves by eating, which is itself inappropriate, but by eating the same sort of food – invariably the stodgy, unhealthy, highly-processed and fattening kind. Help yourself to break the pattern by being more aware of it and by resolving to eat only healthy foods.	A moderate diet, such as part or all of the 24-week programme, will actually help you to break the mood/food pattern by introducing healthier foods and making you more aware of how and when you choose to indulge (see page 54).

THE DIET DIARY

IMPORTANT DIARY PAGES MUST BE FILLED IN BEFORE DIET STARTS IN ORDER TO ASSESS HABITUAL EATING PATTERNS

We all eat for all sorts of reasons other than the need for food. Use this diary to help you determine what they are. If not actual sensations of hunger, such as stomach rumbles, what prompts you to have a meal? Convention (1 pm = 'lunchtime'), coercion, emotional stress, or have you never even thought about it?

It is important to continue with your diary for the full five days in order to get a reliable pattern. Individual days can be misleading. Remember that you are looking for factors that *consistently* determine the way you eat (or overeat) and the diary should highlight what these are. Once it does, the way forward will be clear. Combine diet with careful restructuring of lifestyle. Re-

lease nervous energy, comply with convention or mitigate boredom in more appropriate ways.

Write down everything you eat and drink in the columns provided on these pages. Don't worry if the lists seem very long. It is quite normal to be surprised, even alarmed, by the quantities you eat when everything is listed individually.

When you have completed your diary, look through it to see how well balanced and nutritious your diet is. As junk food can actually be a *cause* of overeating (see page 50), adjustments of quality as well as quantity may be in order. Bear in mind too that food, like drugs, can alter neurotransmitters in the brain and may affect mood and behaviour. Use the final column on your blank page to identify what these foods might be, noting in particular coffee, tea, alcohol and sugar-laden foods.

Day of the week: _____ Date: _____
Time: _____ Amount: _____ Food & drink: _____ Situation and mood before eating

---

Day of the week: _____ Date: _____
Time: _____ Amount: _____ Food & drink: _____ Situation and mood before eating

Day of the week: _____   Date: _____   Food & drink: _____   Situation and mood before eating
Time: _____   Amount: _____

_____   _____   _____   _____
_____   _____   _____   _____
_____   _____   _____   _____
_____   _____   _____   _____
_____   _____   _____   _____
_____   _____   _____   _____
_____   _____   _____   _____
_____   _____   _____   _____
_____   _____   _____   _____
_____   _____   _____   _____
_____   _____   _____   _____
_____   _____   _____   _____
_____   _____   _____   _____

Day of the week: _____   Date: _____   Food & drink: _____   Situation and mood before eating
Time: _____   Amount: _____

_____   _____   _____   _____
_____   _____   _____   _____
_____   _____   _____   _____
_____   _____   _____   _____
_____   _____   _____   _____
_____   _____   _____   _____
_____   _____   _____   _____
_____   _____   _____   _____
_____   _____   _____   _____
_____   _____   _____   _____
_____   _____   _____   _____
_____   _____   _____   _____
_____   _____   _____   _____
_____   _____   _____   _____
_____   _____   _____   _____

Day of the week: _____   Date: _____   Food & drink: _____   Situation and mood before eating
Time: _____   Amount: _____

_____   _____   _____   _____
_____   _____   _____   _____
_____   _____   _____   _____
_____   _____   _____   _____
_____   _____   _____   _____
_____   _____   _____   _____
_____   _____   _____   _____
_____   _____   _____   _____
_____   _____   _____   _____
_____   _____   _____   _____
_____   _____   _____   _____
_____   _____   _____   _____
_____   _____   _____   _____

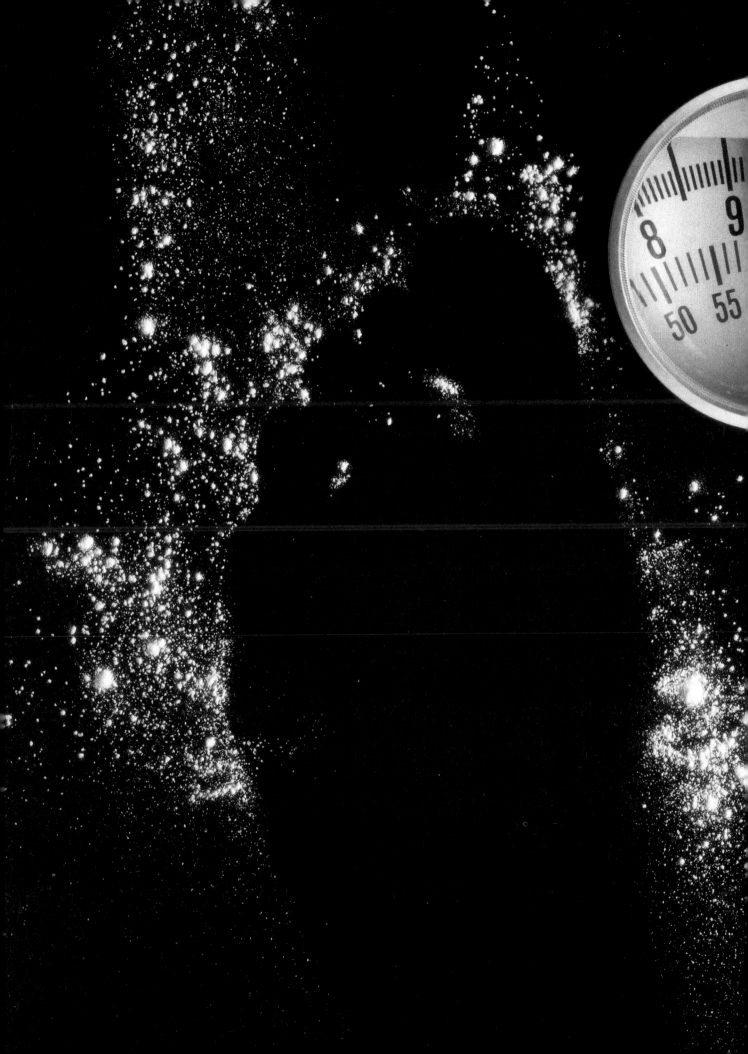

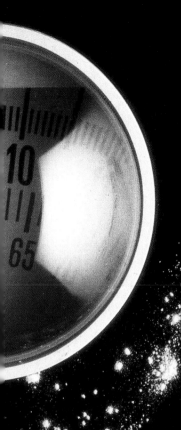

The 24-week diet programme

HOW TO USE THE PROGRAMME

This eating programme is graduated downwards, getting stricter as it continues... 1500 calories a day for the first eight weeks, 1200 calories for the next eleven weeks and 1000 calories, as low as nutritionists recommend for extended periods, for the last five. This will help keep weight loss steady, energy and spirits up, frustration down. Plateau phases are avoided by reducing food intake as the diet progresses. Where you start depends on how much you have to lose...

Start right at the beginning, week one, if you have more than 12.5 kg (28 lb) to lose; week eight if you have between 9 and 12.5 kg (20-28 lb); week 12 if you have between 6.5 and 9 kg (14-20 lb); week 16 if you have between 3.5 and 6.5 kg (8-14 lb) and week 20 if you have 3.5 kg (8 lb) or less. Starting earlier rather than later will make for more lasting differences in weight, shape, eating habits. So allow plenty of time. If you reach your goal before the end of the programme, gradually increase intake to keep weight stable by repeating two of the early (1500-calorie) weeks before stopping the diet altogether.

Resolve now to follow the diet as closely as you can. Buy fruit, vegetables, fish and meat as fresh as possible, find shops that sell wholewheat bread and wholewheat pasta (not difficult – most supermarkets now stock them as well as health food stores) and take the trouble to follow the recipes where given.

The programme has been devised in line with the most recent research findings and recommendations. It is healthy as well as slimming – rich in complex (starchy) carbohydrates, low in refined carbohydrates and fat, moderate in protein and high in fresh fruit and vegetables, often raw for maximum nutritional value. Sugar is kept to a minimum. Salt should be kept down, too (see page 46).

Once familiar with the diet, you will find it very flexible. Breakfasts and light meals are coded according to calorific value and listed on the following pages, so as to give as wide a choice as possible. Main meals are given each day and are specially planned, week by week, to include at least one vegetarian, one fish and one iron-rich meal, some poultry and red meat. Red meat, although rich in minerals such as zinc, is limited to just once or twice a week because the latest studies advise moderation of all animal fats. Dishes in dark type have recipes which can be found in the Recipe index at the back (pages 94-123).

Lists of vegetables are given beneath each of the main meals. Where the meal contains rice, pastry, pulses, potato or pasta (as in lasagne), or where these are listed separately (as in vegetable curry and rice), choose just one; otherwise, choose three (preferably one of them potato if listed). Green and mixed salads should be very lightly dressed with a dessertspoon of Lemon and Mustard, Lemon and Tarragon, Cucumber and Yoghurt or Cottage Cheese and Chive dressings (find recipes for these in the Recipe index).

If you do not like the main meal, replace that entire day for another within the appropriate section (i.e. weeks 1-8; 9-19; 20-24), but try to keep the balance right by exchanging like for like (fish for fish, for example), and remember to switch light meals too so that the total calorific value for the day remains the same.

Each week allows a certain number of 'indulgences'. These are coded 🧺🧺🧺, listed at the top of each week and reduced as the diet progresses. The Indulgences not only make the diet more enjoyable, but also help prevent strong cravings taking a hold and sabotaging all the good work done so far. Consult the lists on page 54.

While it is important to follow the diet closely, you may have to allow yourself some latitude if you have a busy social life. Concentrate on keeping intake moderate. Choose, or ask for, simply prepared meat and fish (no rich sauces), unbuttered vegetables, salads with a little dressing, fresh fruit instead of heavy desserts. Alcohol, which counts as an indulgence, can be drunk in moderation.

Drink at least six glasses of water a day (bottled or tap) and any amount of herb teas, tisanes and tea (with lemon). Try decaffeinated coffee, or coffee with chicory, for a change and discover the huge range of herbal teas and tisanes available. They not only keep you calmer, but taste delicious too...

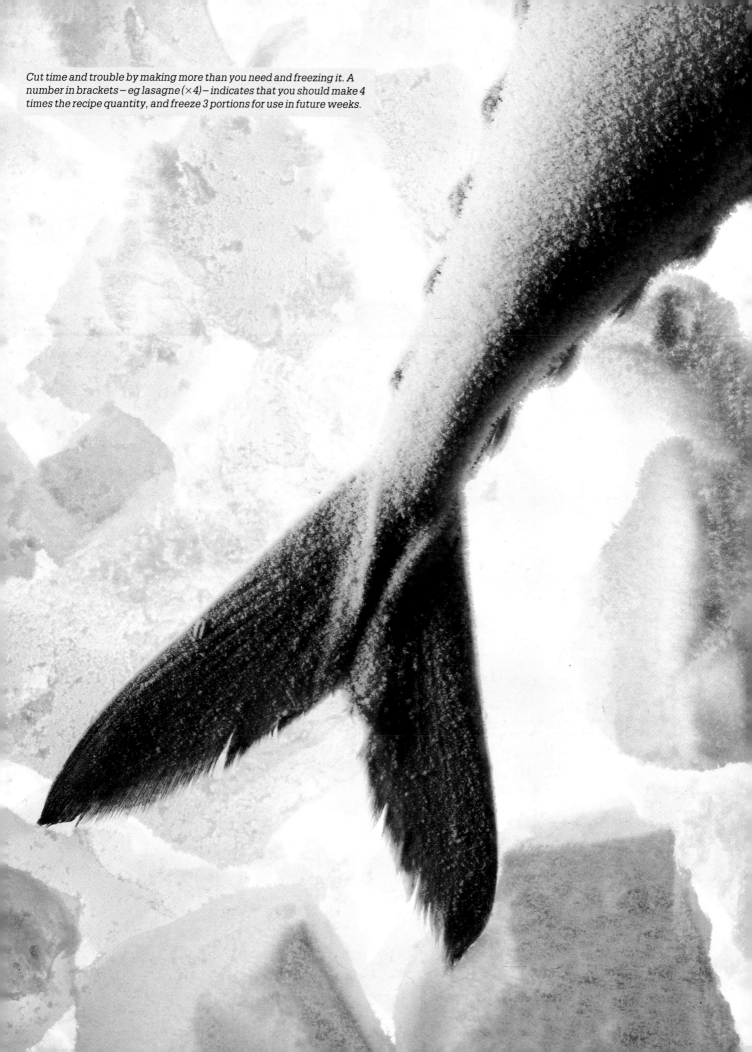

Cut time and trouble by making more than you need and freezing it. A number in brackets – eg lasagne (×4) – indicates that you should make 4 times the recipe quantity, and freeze 3 portions for use in future weeks.

BREAKFASTS

Different lists are given for different stages of the diet. Choose any menu and eat it at any time of day – not necessarily first thing or all at once. Try varying your breakfasts to see how well you feel and how much energy you have. From a metabolic point of view, protein is digested more efficiently in the early part of the day – so eggs, fish, even cheese and lean meat, European style, make an excellent breakfast.

WEEKS 1-12/300 CALORIES

MENU I

1 small peach/2 small fresh figs/
2 clementines/1 medium slice honeydew melon/125g (4 oz) raspberries/1 whole grapefruit
AND
1 bowl of muesli: 15g (½ oz) oatflakes, 15g (½ oz) chopped hazelnuts, 25g (1 oz) sultanas [golden raisins] and 15g (½ oz) wheatgerm, with 150 ml (¼ pint) (⅔ cup) skimmed milk

or

1 large scrambled egg with skimmed milk, 1 grilled rasher bacon [1 broiled bacon slice], 1 x 25g (1 oz) slice wholewheat toast and scraping of butter

or

125g (4 oz) smoked salmon with 2 x 25g (1 oz) slices wholwheat bread with scraping of butter, lemon juice and pepper

or

75g (3 oz) grilled [broiled] kipper fillet with 1 tomato and 1 slice wholewheat toast with scraping of butter

or

25g (1 oz) bran flakes/cornflakes/ grapenuts/raisin bran/wheatgerm with 1 tbsp plain yogurt and 150 ml (¼ pint) (⅔ cup) skimmed milk; 1 x 25g (1 oz) slice wholewheat toast with scraping of butter and 1 tsp honey, jam or marmalade

or

1 medium brown roll with 1 tsp butter and 2 tsp honey, jam or marmalade

or

1 small croissant with 1 tsp honey or jam
AND
cup of coffee (preferably decaffeinated), tea or herb tea – black with lemon or small dash of skimmed milk

MENU II

25g (1 oz) bran flakes/cornflakes/ grapenuts/raisin bran/1 Shredded Wheat/ 2 Weetabix/40g (1½ oz) bran cereal with 150 ml (¼ pint) (⅔ cup) skimmed milk

or

1 small carton plain yogurt with 2 tsp honey, 15g (½ oz) chopped hazelnuts and a sprinkling of wheatgerm

or

1 large mango

or

½ cantaloupe melon filled with 175g (6 oz) strawberries and 125g (4 oz) raspberries

or

1 large poached or coddled egg with 25g (1 oz) thinly sliced Parma ham/smoked ham
AND
2 x 25g (1 oz) wholewheat toast/1 bran muffin/3 pieces rye crispbread with 1 tsp butter, 1 tsp honey, jam or marmalade

or

1 x 25g (1 oz) slice light rye bread with ½ sliced hard-boiled egg layered with 15g (½ oz) thinly sliced Esrom, Gouda, Edam or Havarti cheese and some slices of tomato
AND
cup of coffee (preferably decaffeinated), tea or herb tea – black, with lemon or small dash of skimmed milk

MENU III

200 ml (⅓ pint) (⅞ cup) freshly squeezed orange or grapefruit juice

or

150 ml (¼ pint) (⅔ cup) apple or pineapple juice

or

2 medium oranges/2 small pears/175g (6 oz) cherries/2 small apples/1 medium banana/1 medium nectarine
AND
125g (4 oz) hot poached smoked haddock mixed with ½ chopped hard-boiled egg, chopped parsley on 1 x 25g (1 oz) slice wholewheat toast with scraping of butter

or

1 large scrambled egg made with skimmed milk, with 125g (4 oz) poached mushrooms and chopped parsley with 1 rye crispbread

or

2 grilled rashers streaky bacon [2 broiled bacon slices] with 1 grilled [broiled] tomato and 1 x 25g (1 oz) slice wholewheat toast and scraping of butter

or

1 x 25g (1 oz) slice light rye bread with 40g (1½ oz) very thinly sliced Esrom, Danbo, Jarlsberg, Edam or Gouda cheese with thin slice of orange

or

25g (1 oz) peanut butter on 1 rye crispbread
AND
cup of coffee (preferably decaffeinated), tea or herb tea – black, with lemon or small dash of skimmed milk

MENU I

150 ml (¼ pint) (⅔ cup) freshly squeezed orange or grapefruit juice/1 orange/1 pear/ 125g (4 oz) fresh pineapple/125g (4 oz) fresh guava/5 fresh apricots or plums/175g (6 oz) strawberries/½ fresh mango

or

1 satsuma, 125g (4 oz) raspberries or 2 fresh apricots with 2 tbsp plain yogurt
AND
1 x 40g (1½ oz) slice wholewheat toast with scraping of butter and honey, jam or marmalade

or

25g (1 oz) bran flakes/cornflakes/ grapenuts/raisin bran/2 Weetabix/1 large Shredded Wheat with 150 ml (¼ pint) (⅔ cup) skimmed milk and no sugar

or

1 medium poached, boiled or coddled egg with 2 rye crispbreads and scraping of butter

or

75g (3 oz) smoked salmon with squeeze of lemon juice and black pepper/50g (2 oz) smoked ham, both with 1 rye crispbread and scraping of butter

or

2 grilled rashers streaky bacon [2 broiled bacon slices] with 1 tomato
AND
cup of coffee (preferably decaffeinated), tea or herb tea – black, with lemon or small dash of skimmed milk

MENU II

25g (1 oz) bran flakes/cornflakes/ grapenuts/raisin bran/2 Weetabix/1 large Shredded Wheat with 150 ml (¼ pint) (⅔ cup) skimmed milk, no sugar

or

75g (3 oz) dried and soaked prunes with 2 tbsp plain yogurt

or

1 medium banana/125g (4 oz) paw-paw with 150g (5 oz) carton plain yogurt

or

2 fresh nectarines

or

2 grilled rashers streaky bacon [2 broiled bacon slices], 1 tomato and 125g (4 oz) poached mushrooms
AND
1 rye crispbread with scraping of butter and jam, honey or marmalade
AND
cup of coffee (preferably decaffeinated), tea or herb tea – black, with lemon or small dash of skimmed milk

MENU III

½ medium grapefruit/½ medium ogen melon/1 medium satsuma
AND
2 x 25g (1 oz) slices wholewheat toast, scraping of butter and jam, honey or marmalade

or

2 grilled rashers streaky bacon [2 broiled bacon slices], 1 tomato and 125g (4 oz) poached mushrooms

or

1 x 25g (1 oz) slice light rye bread/2 slices rye crispbread with 25g (1 oz) thinly sliced Esrom, Danbo, Jarlsberg, Edam or Gouda cheese

or

1 large boiled, poached or coddled egg with 1 x 25g (1 oz) slice wholewheat toast and scraping of butter
AND
cup of coffee (preferably decaffeinated), tea or herb tea – black, with lemon or small dash of skimmed milk

There is no good evidence to decree that you must start the day with something to eat, though most people feel better for doing so – but exactly what and how much they feel better for eating varies considerably. In one British study, a group of volunteers were all asked to change their breakfast habits for a few weeks – the large breakfast eaters having very little or nothing at all and the small breakfast eaters having a full meal. The result? Everyone felt *worse* for the change. Mental alertness, and concentration were particularly affected. It seems we naturally incline to what suits us best.

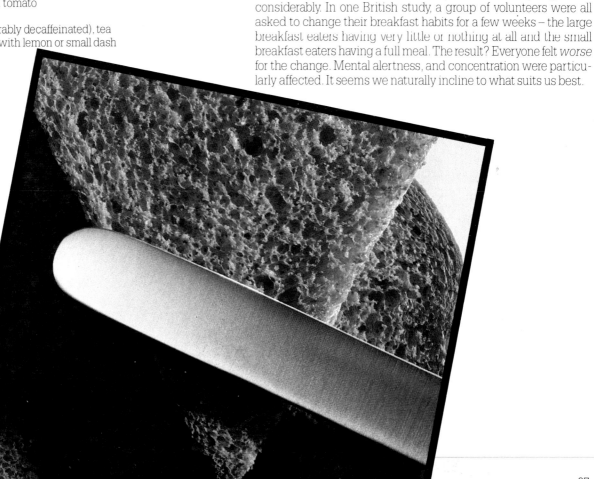

LIGHT MEALS

A 650 CALORIES

- Watercress soup/Carrot soup/Celery soup/Potato, carrot and onion soup WITH 2 slices wholewheat bread and butter, 50g (2 oz) any cheese AND green salad with **French dressing**
- Gazpacho/Cucumber and mint soup/Orange and tomato soup/Consommé WITH 125g (4 oz) French bread and 25g (1 oz) butter
- **Three bean salad** with **French** or **Blue cheese dressing** WITH 150g (5 oz) grapes/small carton plain yogurt and 2 tsp honey
- Salad Niçoise: 75g (3 oz) tuna (drained), 125g (4 oz) cold cooked new potato, 125g (4 oz) green beans, 1 tomato, 10 olives, 1 sliced hard-boiled egg, watercress, chopped lettuce, **French dressing** WITH 2 slices wholewheat/rye bread/wholewheat roll and butter
- Special salad: 1 sliced hard-boiled egg, 25g (1 oz) browned pine nuts, 1 slice bread made into croûtons, tomatoes, chicory [endive], lettuce, radicchio, watercress, 40g (1½ oz) any hard cheese (grated), **Thousand Island** or **Lemon and tarragon dressing**
- Club sandwich: 2 slices wholewheat toast, 50g (2 oz) any cheese, 2 grilled rashers streaky bacon [broiled bacon slice], 1 hard-boiled egg, 1 tsp mayonnaise salad/garnish WITH apple or banana
- Toasted cheese: 2 slices wholewheat bread toasted on one side, spread with 1 tsp mustard (optional) and 50g (2 oz) any hard cheese grilled [broiled] WITH large mixed salad with 1 tbsp **French dressing** AND 1 banana/small carton natural yogurt and 1 tsp honey
- Sandwiches: 3 slices wholewheat bread (fresh or toasted) WITH: 50g (2 oz) any cheese/150g (5 oz) chicken with 1 tsp mayonnaise/125g (4 oz) sardines with 1 tsp mayonnaise/100g (3½ oz) cooked ham/75g (3 oz) smoked salmon and little cream cheese/1 hard-boiled egg with 50g (2 oz) tuna and a little mayonnaise AND small carton plain yogurt and 2 tsp honey/150g (5 oz) grapes/apple and orange
- 2 large eggs scrambled with skimmed milk, 2 grilled rashers streaky bacon [broiled bacon slices], 1 tomato, 2 slices wholewheat toast and butter AND 1 apple/75g (3 oz) grapes/1 orange
- **Soufflé cheese omelette/Spinach soufflé** WITH wholewheat roll and butter, green salad with **French** or **Egg and caper dressing** AND 1 apple/75g (3 oz) grapes/1 orange
- **Quick pizza** WITH mixed salad with **French** or **Blue cheese dressing** AND banana/small carton plain yogurt with 1 tsp honey
- 2 poached eggs WITH 50g (2 oz) any hard cheese (grated) and 2 slices wholewheat toast and butter AND 1 orange/1 pear/1 apple/2 peaches
- Wholewheat fettuccine/macaroni/rigatoni/shells/spaghetti with **Cheese and ham** or **Tomato and basil sauce** WITH green salad and 50g (2 oz) any chopped browned nuts and **French dressing**
- 175g (6 oz) jacket potato WITH: 40g (1½ oz) sour cream, 75g (3 oz) smoked salmon, mixed salad and **Lemon and mustard** or **Herb dressing**/3 grilled [broiled] rashers streaky bacon, 40g (1½ oz) any hard cheese grated WITH large mixed salad with above dressings
- 1 sliced avocado pear WITH 1 pink grapefruit and a little **French dressing** AND 1 slice wholewheat bread with scraping of butter
- 150g (5 oz) grilled [broiled] beefburger with 25g (1 oz) any cheese, melted, WITH 1 wholewheat roll, lettuce, cucumber and tomato
- 1 medium smoked trout, 2 slices wholewheat bread and butter WITH green salad and **Herb dressing** AND 1 orange/2 tangerines/4 plums
- 150g (5 oz) smoked mackerel WITH green salad and **French Lemon and tarragon dressing** AND apple and orange/large banana

B 550 CALORIES

- French onion soup WITH large mixed salad and 25g (1 oz) any chopped nuts with 1 tbsp **French** or **Blue cheese dressing**
- Gazpacho/Cucumber and mint soup/Orange and tomato soup/Consommé WITH 75g (3 oz) French bread and butter
- Minestrone/Corn and fish chowder/Cream of onion soup WITH 2 slices wholewheat bread and butter, 25g (1 oz) any cheese AND apple and orange/1 banana and a few nuts/150g (5 oz) grapes/small carton plain yogurt and 1 tsp honey
- Melon, pear and cucumber salad/Mediterranean seafood salad/Curried mushroom salad/Fennel and orange salad/Chinese cabbage and chicken salad WITH 75g (3 oz) French bread and butter/wholewheat roll and butter AND apple and orange/150g (5 oz) grapes/small carton plain yogurt and 2 tsp honey
- **Three bean salad** WITH 1 tbsp **French, Blue cheese** or **Lemon and tarragon dressing** AND 1 slice wholewheat toast and butter
- Salad Niçoise: as A but with 50g (2 oz) tuna
- Avocado salad: ½ avocado pear, 25g (1 oz) Mozzarella cheese, 1 grilled rasher streaky bacon [broiled bacon slice], tomato, lettuce, cucumber, watercress, endive [chicory], 1 tbsp **French** or **Egg and caper dressing**
- Club sandwich: as A but without fruit
- Toasted cheese sandwich: as A but without fruit/yogurt
- Toasted peanut butter sandwich: 2 slices wholewheat toast and 50g (2 oz) peanut butter and small carton plain yogurt with 1 tsp honey
- Sandwiches: as A but without fruit or yogurt
- 2 large scrambled eggs WITH 2 grilled rashers streaky bacon [broiled bacon slices], 1 slice wholewheat toast and butter AND 1 apple/1 orange and a few grapes/6 plums/75g (3 oz) grapes
- **Quick pizza** WITH mixed salad and 1 tbsp **French** or **Egg and caper dressing**
- **Smoked salmon quiche/Tomato and courgette [zucchini] pie** WITH mixed salad and 1 tbsp **French** or **Blue cheese dressing** AND 1 banana/1 apple and a few grapes/small carton plain yogurt with 1 tsp honey and sprinkling of wheatgerm
- Wholewheat pasta as A but WITH 15g (½ oz) chopped nuts
- **Lasagne** WITH green salad and **French dressing** AND 1 orange/2 tangerines/4 plums
- **Jacket potatoes** with fillings 2 or 4 (page 107) WITH mixed salad, a sprinkling of nuts and 1 tbsp **Lemon and mustard** or **Herb dressing**
- Corn on the cob WITH 25g (1 oz) butter and 2 slices wholewheat bread or toast
- 1 large globe artichoke/150g (5 oz) asparagus WITH 40g (1½ oz) melted butter/3 tbsp **French dressing** AND 2 slices wholewheat/rye bread, 40g (1½ oz) any cheese/75g (3 oz) smoked salmon
- ½ avocado pear sliced WITH ½ pink grapefruit, sprinkled with parsley and a little **French dressing** AND 1 wholewheat roll and butter AND 40g (1½ oz) any cheese
- 1 large slice cantaloupe melon or 4 fresh figs WITH 75g (3 oz) Parma ham AND 2 slices wholewheat bread with butter, 25g (1 oz) any cheese
- 100g (4 oz) grilled [broiled] beefburger WITH 1 wholewheat roll/175g (6 oz) cottage cheese AND mixed salad with **French** or **Blue cheese dressing**

Light meals are coded A, B, C or D according to calorific value and listed below. Each list gives a wide variety of ideas and includes food which can either be prepared simply at home or well in advance and taken to the office with you…

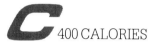 **400 CALORIES**

- French onion soup WITH 1 slice wholewheat bread and butter
- Watercress soup/Carrot soup/Celery soup/Potato, carrot and onion soup WITH 1 slice wholewheat/rye bread and butter, 25g (1 oz) any cheese
- Gazpacho/Cucumber and mint soup/Orange and tomato soup/Consommé WITH 1 slice wholewheat/rye bread and butter AND mixed salad with sprinkling chopped nuts and **Lemon and tarragon** or **Egg dressing**
- As first five salads from B WITH 1 slice wholewheat/rye bread and butter AND fruit/yogurt as listed
- Small serving **Three bean salad** without dressing
- Salad Niçoise: 50g (2 oz) tuna (drained), 125g (4 oz) green beans, 1 sliced hard-boiled egg, 1 tomato, lettuce, watercress, 10 olives, **French dressing** WITH 1 crispbread and scraping of butter
- Sandwiches: 2 slices wholewheat bread (fresh or toasted) with scraping of butter WITH: 50g (2 oz) any hard cheese/75g (3 oz) lean ham/40g (1½ oz) peanut butter/125g (4 oz) prosciutto/50g (2 oz) chicken liver, duck or game pâté/65g (2½ oz) tuna (drained)/3 grilled rashers streaky bacon [broiled bacon slices]/1 hard-boiled egg with 25g (1 oz) tuna and a little mayonnaise/100g (4 oz) smoked salmon/75g (3 oz) prawns [shrimps] with 1 tsp mayonnaise/75g (3 oz) sardines (drained) AND lettuce, tomato, cucumber, watercress garnish
- 65g (2½ oz) taramasalata with 1 piece warmed or toasted pitta bread
- 2 scrambled eggs WITH 25g (1 oz) smoked salmon and 1 slice wholewheat toast and butter
- **Soufflé cheese omelette/Spinach soufflé** WITH mixed salad and sprinkling chopped browned nuts and 1 tbsp **French** or **Thousand Island dressing**
- **French vegetable quiche** WITH large mixed salad and a little **French** or **Herb dressing**
- 2 poached eggs WITH 2 slices wholewheat toast and butter
- **Leek and thyme quiche** WITH mixed salad and **French, Egg and caper** or **Thousand Island dressing**
- Wholewheat pasta, as B but with no dressing on salad
- 175g (6 oz) jacket potato WITH 50g (2 oz) sour cream and 75g (3 oz) smoked salmon/2 rashers grilled streaky bacon [broiled bacon slices] and 20g (¾ oz) any hard cheese (grated), mixed salad and **Herb dressing/Fillings 1 or 3** (page 107) WITH small green salad 15g (½ oz) chopped nuts and **Lemon and tarragon dressing/ Fillings 2 or 4** WITH green or mixed salad and **Blue cheese** or **French dressing**
- ½ mango/½ cantaloupe melon/5 figs/large pear WITH 50g (2 oz) prosciutto or Parma ham AND 1 slice dark rye bread/2 crispbreads with scraping of butter
- ½ large avocado pear WITH ½ pink grapefruit sprinkled with chopped parsley and 1 tbsp **French dressing** AND 1 piece rye crispbread
- 150g (5 oz) artichoke hearts WITH 1 hard-boiled egg with lettuce, endive [chicory], cucumber sprinkled with chopped browned nuts and **French** or **Egg and caper dressing**
- 1 medium grilled [broiled] kipper WITH 1 piece wholewheat toast and butter
- 120g (4 oz) grilled [broiled] beefburger WITH 1 slice wholewheat bread/120g (4 oz) cottage cheese/mixed salad with **Cucumber and yogurt** or **Herb dressing**
- 1 small smoked trout WITH mixed salad and **French dressing** AND 1 slice wholewheat bread and butter

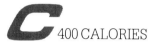 **300 CALORIES**

- French onion soup WITH 1 crispbread
- Watercress soup/Carrot soup/Celery soup/Potato, carrot and onion soup WITH 1 slice wholewheat rye bread and butter
- Gazpacho/Cucumber and mint soup/Orange and tomato soup/Consommé WITH 1 slice wholewheat/rye bread and butter and 50g (2 oz) any cheese
- Minestrone/Corn and fish chowder/Cream of onion soup WITH 1 slice wholewheat or rye bread
- Lentil soup WITH 2 slices wholewheat bread and scraping of butter. As first five salads from B WITH 1 slice wholewheat/rye bread and scraping of butter
- Crunchy salad
- Brown rice and nut salad AND 1 apple/1 orange/75g (3 oz) grapes/ small carton plain yogurt
- Sandwiches: 2 slices wholewheat bread (fresh or toasted) with a scraping of butter WITH: 25g (1 oz) hard cheese/40g (1½ oz) cooked ham/50g (2 oz) chicken/50g (2 oz) corned beef/1 hard-boiled egg/ 50g (2 oz) prawns [shrimps]/1½ grilled rashers streaky bacon [broiled bacon slices] AND lettuce, tomato, cucumber, watercress garnish
- Toasted bacon sandwich: 2 slices wholewheat toast with 2 grilled rashers streaky bacon [broiled bacon slices] and tomato (optional) AND 1 apple/orange/75g (3 oz) grapes
- Open sandwich: 1 slice pumpernickel and scraping of butter WITH 50g (2 oz) smoked cheese/50g (2 oz) prawns [shrimps] with lettuce and cucumber and 1 tbsp mayonnaise/50g (2 oz) chicken with ¼ avocado, watercress and tomato
- 2 scrambled eggs WITH 1 slice wholewheat toast/50g (2 oz) smoked salmon
- **Soufflé cheese omelette/Spinach soufflé** WITH lettuce, watercress and tomato salad
- 2 egg omelette WITH 75g (3 oz) poached mushrooms
- **Leek and thyme quiche**
- **Spinach and cottage cheese quiche** WITH mixed salad and 1 tbsp **French dressing**
- **Smoked salmon quiche/Tomato and courgette [zucchini] pie** WITH green salad and 1 tbsp **Lemon and tarragon** or **Herb dressing**
- **Piperade** WITH green salad and 1 tbsp **French dressing**
- 1 Baked egg WITH 2 slices wholewheat toast (no butter)
- 40g (1½ oz) wholewheat pasta WITH **Americana sauce**/7g (¼ oz) butter with garlic, parsley or basil/2 tsp pesto sauce AND mixed salad and 1 tbsp **French** or **Lemon and tarragon dressing**
- 175g (6 oz) jacket potato WITH: **Filling 1** (page 107) **Fillings 2 or 3** WITH small carton plain yogurt and 1 apple/**Filling 4** WITH mixed salad (no dressing)
- ½ avocado pear with 1 tbsp **French dressing**
- ½ mango/½ cantaloupe melon/5 figs/large pear WITH 75g (3 oz) prosciutto ham AND 1 rye crispbread
- 75g (3 oz) smoked salmon with lemon juice and black pepper WITH 2 slices wholewheat bread and scraping of butter
- 1 small smoked trout WITH mixed salad and 1 tbsp **French** or **Lemon and tarragon dressing**
- 1 large globe artichoke/150g (5 oz) asparagus WITH 40g (1½ oz) melted butter/3 tbsp **French dressing**

WEEK 1

MONDAY

Lamb noisette with garlic and rosemary
Vegetables: jacket baked potato, swede (rutabaga), Brussels sprouts, mangetout, green beans or cauliflower

150 g/5 oz carton plain yogurt with tsp honey

NB Soak fruit for tomorrow

TUESDAY
B

Courgette (zucchini) and tomato pie (×2)
Vegetables: spinach, boiled parsnip, green beans, broccoli or green salad

Winter fruit compote

WEDNESDAY

Mediterranean seafood sauce (×5)
75 g/3 oz boiled tagliatelle (25 g/1 oz/½ cup raw weight)
Vegetables: green or mixed salad, courgettes (zucchini) or green beans

Strawberry sorbet (×5)

THURSDAY

Liver provençal
75 g/3 oz boiled brown rice (25 g/1 oz/2 tbsp raw weight)
Vegetables: spinach, green beans or carrots

Banana, honey and nut fool (×6)

NB Soak prunes for tomorrow

FRIDAY

Pork fillet (tenderloin) with prunes
Vegetables: mashed potato (with skimmed milk), **red cabbage with apple**, green beans, braised celery, cauliflower or marrow (squash)

150 g/5 oz carton natural yogurt with 2 tsp honey and 25 g/1 oz wheatgerm

SATURDAY

1 cup consommé

Poached salmon steak
Vegetables: boiled new potato, courgettes (zucchini), peas, mangetout or green salad

100 g/4 oz grapes

SUNDAY

75 g/3 oz roast chicken (about 3 slices) with **Parsley and thyme stuffing** and 2 tbsp **Low fat gravy**
Vegetables: boiled potato, broccoli, carrots, cabbage, mangetout or 2 baked tomatoes

25 g/1 oz Camembert, Brie or smoked cheese with 1 rye crispbread

---

Fill in your weight, below. Charts are given every two weeks but you can make a weekly note, too, if you like…No more often than that though, because weight is not lost at a constant rate and daily fluctuations may reflect random variations rather than real changes.

In women, these random variations are largely caused by temporary shifts in body water that take place throughout the menstrual cycle as hormone levels rise and fall. A rise in oestrogen and progesterone just before menstruation, for example, causes the body to retain more water and become heavier. So be aware of this and know that a small gain in weight at this time reflects a gain in water, not fat.

Always use the same scales and weigh yourself on the same day each week, or fortnight, and at the same time. Keep scales on a solid flat surface, not carpet, and move them as little as possible. If you are serious about monitoring your weight, invest in proper quality scales. Although larger and heavier than the commercial type, they will fit in the corner of a bathroom or walk-in cupboard and have the advantage of a locking mechanism to keep everything stable while being moved.

Check scales for accuracy if they have been moved about or stored away: place a fixed known weight on the centre and take your reading directly in line with the indicator. If the reading is not exactly that of the fixed weight, your scales need adjusting. You may be able to do this yourself, but if the scales have been damaged, dropped or allowed to rust badly, they may need servicing or even replacing.

NB Weighing yourself has its limitations. Scales do not show whether you are losing lean or fat or just plain water and that's important, because it is what you lose that determines your shape at the end of the diet. So keep a subjective eye on your shape. Combine exercise with diet to firm up problem areas and use a measuring tape as an additional guide to progress.

Early weight losses on crash diets may be dramatic but they are deceptive, being losses not of fat but of glycogen, a granular carbohydrate stored in the liver and muscles, which binds with three times its weight in water.

Three pounds of water lost for every pound of glycogen! No wonder crash dieters feel their diet is working. But what they do not appreciate is that glycogen is always replaced, water retained again, and weight regained on a return to more normal eating.

There is, anyway, a limit to how much glycogen you can lose. Non-dieters probably have 2.7-3.6 kg (6-8 lb) of glycogen in their bodies, of which they might lose half. Habitual dieters have rather less because their systems have not had the chance to replenish themselves. Once glycogen stores are depleted, weight loss slows down and may even stop. The honeymoon period of rapid weight loss can never last indefinitely, even if you jump from one diet to another. Very restricted diets rarely require you to follow them for more than a fortnight because once the glycogen stores have been stripped they will appear to have stopped 'working'. Follow them for that amount of time and you will lose lots of weight but you will also regain it almost immediately.

The way to lasting weight loss is to keep glycogen levels stable and that means keeping intake moderate and the proportion of starchy carbohydrates reasonably high. This is why this diet starts off so gently and places such emphasis on wholemeal foods such as wholewheat bread and pasta. Although the amount of weight lost in the early stages may be disappointing in comparison with previous diets, at least you can be confident that every pound lost is a true pound lost and not just a fleeting phenomenon. You will appreciate the difference when the diet is over and you manage to keep off the weight you have lost.

*keeping glycogen levels up will also make you feel better, more energetic, see page 63.

some arithmetic . . .

1 kg (2.2 lb) of glycogen	= 4000 Calories
1 kg (2.2 lb) of water	= zero Calories
1 kg (2.2 lb) of fat	= 7000 Calories

If you lose 1kg (2.2lb) of glycogen, you will lose 4kg (9lb) overall because you will also lose 3kg (6.6lb) of water. This loss represents just 4000 calories. It can be regained in the space of one weekend.

If you lose 4kg (9lb) of fat, the loss will register identically on the scales, but this time represents 28,000 calories. This could only be regained after several *weeks* of overeating . . .

As the upper limit to the rate at which you can mobilize fat out of the fat cells, into the bloodstream and out of the body is about 1000 calories a day (that means burning 1000 calories more than you eat), and as it takes a deficit of 7000 calories to shift a kilogram of fat, the most you should aim to lose in a week is one kilogram (2.2lb). Any more will be glycogen/water or lean tissue . . . Neither is advisable.

	Weight	Bust	Waist	Hips	Thighs
Start					
Week 2					

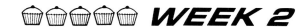

MONDAY

175 g/6 oz fillet (tenderloin) or rump steak grilled (broiled) with herbs, all fat removed
Vegetables: poached mushrooms, cabbage with caraway seeds, or green beans

½ medium ogen melon filled with 175 g/6 oz fresh strawberries or segments of 1 large orange

TUESDAY

Fish pie (×3)
Vegetables: green beans, 2 grilled (broiled) tomatoes, spinach, carrots or green salad

150 g/5 oz carton any fruit yogurt

WEDNESDAY

Braised kidneys (×3)
75 g/3 oz boiled brown rice (25 g/1 oz/2 tbsp raw weight)
Vegetables: carrots, cauliflower, marrow (squash), peas or mixed salad

1 mashed banana sprinkled with 25 g/1 oz hazelnuts

THURSDAY

Wholewheat pan pizza (×3)
Vegetables: green or mixed salad, braised fennel or spinach

1 stewed cooking apple, sweetened to taste, with 25 g/1 oz chopped dates and 150 g/5 oz carton natural yogurt

FRIDAY

Trout with almonds
Vegetables: boiled new potato, broccoli, mangetout, green beans or mixed salad

25 g/1 oz any hard cheese with 2 water biscuits

SATURDAY

Wholewheat macaroni with cheese and ham
Vegetables: 2 grilled (broiled) tomatoes, peas, broccoli, green or mixed salad

Fruit salad: 100 g/4 oz fresh pineapple, 100 g/4 oz grapes and 1 sliced banana

NB Soak fruit for tomorrow

SUNDAY

Chicken florentine
Vegetables: boiled new potato, swede (rutabaga), leeks, carrots, Brussels sprouts or poached mushrooms

150 g/5 oz any dried fruit (figs, apricots, prunes)

WEEK 3

MONDAY

A
Middle Eastern rice
Vegetables: green or mixed salad

150 g/5 oz carton plain yogurt with tsp honey

TUESDAY

C
Liver with orange (×2)
75 g/3 oz boiled brown rice (25 g/1 oz/2 tbsp raw weight)
Vegetables: broccoli, courgettes (zucchini), spinach or green salad

25 g/1 oz any hard cheese and 1 apple or pear

WEDNESDAY

B
Leek and thyme quiche
Vegetables: green beans, broccoli, green or mixed salad

Orange and pear fruit salad

THURSDAY

A
Sole with lemon and prawns (shrimp)
Vegetables: boiled new potato, 2 baked tomatoes, broccoli, leeks or green salad

100 g/4 oz stewed plums, sweetened to taste, with 150 g/5 oz carton plain yogurt

NB Marinate chicken for tomorrow

FRIDAY

B
Skewered chicken
Vegetables: jacket baked potato, carrots, broccoli, mangetout, 2 grilled (broiled) tomatoes, cauliflower or leeks

Peach and orange sorbet (×6)

SATURDAY

A
Spinach soufflé
Vegetables: boiled new potato, green or mixed salad, green beans, courgettes (zucchini) or poached mushrooms

1 nectarine or 100 g/4 oz grapes

SUNDAY

C
Lamb with apricot stuffing
Vegetables: green beans, cabbage, marrow (squash), cauliflower or carrots

Banana, honey and nut fool (×5)

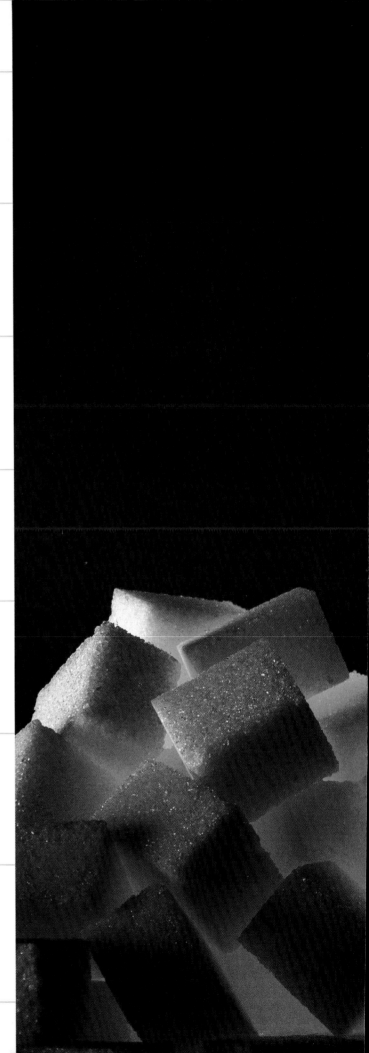

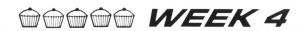

The metabolic flame burns energy in the form of accumulated sugar and fat reserves, and it burns brightest when you move fastest, eat most. When you diet, your metabolic rate drops sharply – by 6 per cent by the end of the first week and by 15-20 per cent at the end of the third. Raise it by keeping active...

MONDAY

Sole florentine
Vegetables: boiled new potato, braised celery, peas, carrots, broccoli or mixed salad

1 stewed cooking apple, sweetened to taste, with 150 g/5 oz carton plain yogurt

TUESDAY

Wholewheat spaghetti with chicken livers
Vegetables: green or mixed salad, peas, green beans or tomatoes

25 g/1 oz any blue cheese and 1 pear

WEDNESDAY

Veal escalope with tomatoes
Vegetables: boiled new potato, spinach, cauliflower, cabbage, courgettes (zucchini) or green beans

150 g/5 oz carton plain yogurt with 2 tsp honey and 25 g/1 oz wheatgerm

THURSDAY

Lasagne (×4)
Vegetables: green or mixed salad, spinach or poached mushrooms

25 g/1 oz dates, 25 g/1 oz walnuts and large apple

NB Soak fruit for tomorrow

FRIDAY

Vegetable curry (×4)
65 g/3 oz boiled brown rice (25 g/1 oz/2 tbsp raw weight)
Vegetables: green or mixed salad

Winter fruit compote

SATURDAY

Ham with cider sauce
Vegetables: jacket baked potato, broad (fava) beans, carrots, green beans or mangetout

Autumn baked apple

SUNDAY

1 cup consommé

Herb chicken
Vegetables: boiled potato, broccoli, cauliflower, peas, courgettes (zucchini) or spinach

100 g/4 oz fresh pineapple or 1 large orange

MONDAY

Pork curry (×2)
75 g/3 oz boiled brown rice (25 g/1 oz/2 tbsp raw weight)
Vegetables: sliced cucumber with 3 tbsp plain yogurt, green or mixed salad

1 banana and 25 g/1 oz raisins or 15 g/½ oz walnuts and 150 g/5 oz carton plain yogurt

TUESDAY

Liver provençal
75 g/3 oz boiled brown rice (25 g/1 oz/2 tbsp raw weight)
Vegetables: green or mixed salads, green beans

1 apple or large orange or pear

WEDNESDAY

Spinach roulade
Vegetables: poached mushrooms, green beans, 2 baked tomatoes, sweetcorn (kernel corn) or mixed salad

½ grapefruit with crunchy topping (25 g/1 oz wheatgerm, 1 tsp honey with cinnamon and spices to taste) placed under hot grill

THURSDAY

Bitkis (×4)
Vegetables: green beans, carrots, cauliflower, green or red cabbage, green or mixed salad

50 g/2 oz hard cheese with celery or cucumber

NB Soak fruit for tomorrow

FRIDAY

Baked fish with ginger
Vegetables: mashed potato, **red cabbage with apple**, carrots, leeks, broccoli, braised celery or mangetout

150 g/5 oz dried fruit (apricots, figs, prunes, etc)

SATURDAY

Fillet steak (tenderloin) with green peppercorns and herbs
Vegetables: jacket baked potato, green beans, cauliflower, carrots, green or mixed salad

Fruit salad: 100 g/4 oz fresh chopped pineapple, 50 g/2 oz grapes and ½ banana

SUNDAY

2 lamb cutlets, grilled (broiled), with 2 tsp redcurrant jelly, all fat removed
Vegetables: baked jacket potato, swede (rutabaga), sweetcorn (kernel corn), cauliflower, carrots or peas

25 g/1 oz any hard cheese with a water biscuit

	Weight	Bust	Waist	Hips	Thighs
Week 4					
Week 6					

Dieting slows down the metabolic rate and the more drastic the diet, the greater the slowdown. Anyone who has watched the scales sticking after just a few days' dieting will know this; and will know also that the only way to persuade the scales on down again is by scaling the diet down too. To lose more you have to eat less…and less…and less…until you end up subsisting on virtually nothing.

The dilemma is common, the reasons more complex, but the truth is that any diet that takes you, *or threatens to take you,* below your natural comfortable weight will become progressively harder as your body becomes more and more determined to defend its rightful healthy weight – that which psychologists call the 'set point'. Crash diets, which shock your body into the most spirited defence, are the least effective of all. Keep metabolism on an even keel by following a diet that reduces the quantities of food so gently that your body has a chance to adapt naturally to the new level without over-reacting.

'Metabolic rate' refers to the basal, or resting, rate. This is taken when the body is still. It is a measure of internal activity – the amount of energy used simply to keep the body going, to maintain essential biochemical processes such as oxygen exchange, protein synthesis and tissue repair.

The basal rate is the figure on which all other energy calculations depend, such as how much an hour's jogging or yoga is worth. Because basal rates can vary considerably from person to person, so can the amount of energy used by various activities. Charts stating that an hour's jogging uses so many calories, and an hour's running so many more, fail to take this into account. An hour's activity will never be worth exactly the same for everyone in terms of calories used or weight lost.

WHAT INFLUENCES YOUR METABOLIC RATE? As a rule, the larger and heavier you are and the more lean tissue you have, the higher your metabolic rate. Lean tissue (organs and muscle) is a key factor because there is much more going on there than in fat, which is relatively inert. Women, who have a higher ratio of fat to muscle than men and tend to be smaller and lighter, generally have lower metabolic rates.

IS THE SURVIVAL OF THE FITTEST ALSO THE SURVIVAL OF THE FATTEST? If those with the most adaptable metabolisms were best able to survive drought and famine and so to pass on their genes, as Darwin suggested, then yesterday's natural survivors are the overweight population of today…

Three things cause metabolism to drop when dieting:

1. You are getting lighter.

2. The body cannot distinguish between fashion and famine and reacts as though dieting were the latter, conserving its energy by functioning in a lower metabolic gear. This happens very quickly, probably after just four days.

3. As part of the emergency alert, metabolically-expensive lean tissue is jettisoned and inactive fat conserved, so lowering metabolic rate still further.

Metabolic rate not only drops when you diet, but also rises when you *overeat*. This was first noted in 1902 by a psychologist called Neumann who carried out an experiment on himself, eating about 2000 calories more than usual every day for several months. He found that although he put on weight to begin with, his weight soon stabilized at its new, higher level and ceased to rise thereafter.

Recent research suggests that the mechanism which allowed him to do this derives from a tissue known as brown fat, which has the function of burning off extra calories as heat rather than storing them as fat.

Brown fat may be a critical factor in determining who stays slim and who gets fat. People who tend to put on weight easily seem to have less brown fat, or less *active* brown fat, than people who eat all they like and still remain lean. In one experiment, where fat and lean people were exposed to cold, the lean group was found to be able to maintain their body temperature through the *internal* generation of heat, while that of the fat group dropped.

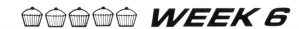

 MONDAY

Mediterranean seafood sauce (×4)
75 g/3 oz boiled brown rice (25 g/1 oz/2 tbsp raw weight)
Vegetables: peas, spinach or green salad

150 g/5 oz carton plain yogurt with 25 g/1 oz chopped dates and 25 g/1 oz raisins

 TUESDAY

Pork casserole
Vegetables: jacket baked potato, peas, red cabbage with apple, green beans, green or mixed salad

Apple or pear with 75 g/3 oz grapes

 WEDNESDAY

Smoked salmon quiche (×2)
Vegetables: green or mixed salad, green beans, courgettes (zucchini) or cucumber salad

1 fresh mango or 2 large oranges

 THURSDAY

Indian chicken
Vegetables: boiled new potato, braised fennel, green beans, marrow (squash), green or mixed salad

25 g/1 oz Stilton or 40 g/1½ oz Danish Blue and 1 apple or pear

 FRIDAY

Steak and kidney casserole (×3)
75 g/3 oz boiled tagliatelle (25 g/1 oz/½ cup raw weight)
Vegetables: green beans, braised fennel, spring greens, carrots or broccoli

Peach and orange sorbet (×5)

 SATURDAY

Lasagne (×3)
Vegetables: green or mixed salad

Fruit salad: 100 g/4 oz fresh pineapple, 100 g/4 oz grapes and 1 banana

NB Soak fruit for tomorrow

 SUNDAY

Chinese stuffed pepper (×2)
Vegetables: leeks, cauliflower, poached mushrooms, courgettes (zucchini), salsify or mixed salad

Winter fruit compote

WEEK 7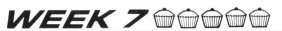

MONDAY

B

Lamb kebab
75 g/3 oz boiled brown rice (25 g/1 oz/2 tbsp raw weight)
Vegetables: poached mushrooms, green or mixed salad

25 g/1 oz Gouda or Edam and 2 water biscuits

TUESDAY

B

Liver stroganoff (×2)
75 g/3 oz boiled tagliatelle (25 g/1 oz/½ cup raw weight)
Vegetables: cauliflower, mangetout, Brussels sprouts, swede (rutabaga), green or mixed salad

Orange and pear fruit salad

WEDNESDAY

C

French vegetable quiche (×2)
Vegetables: green or mixed salad, spinach, green beans or celeriac

150 g/5 oz carton plain yogurt with 25 g/1 oz chopped dates, 25 g/1 oz hazelnuts and few raisins

THURSDAY

A

Skewered chicken
Vegetables: boiled new potato, sweetcorn (kernel corn), broccoli, green or mixed salad or poached mushrooms

1 apple, large orange or pear

FRIDAY

A

Poached salmon steak
Vegetables: boiled new potato, mangetout, cauliflower, green beans or green salad

Baked apple with blackcurrant sauce

SATURDAY

B

Chilli con carne (×2)
Vegetables: boiled new potato, carrots, cabbage, braised celery, green or mixed salad
Banana, honey and nut fool (×4)

SUNDAY

C

Barbecue lamb (×2)
Vegetables: jacket baked potato, courgettes (zucchini), cauliflower, spring greens, leeks or broccoli

25 g/1 oz Camembert, Brie or smoked cheese and 1 apple or pear

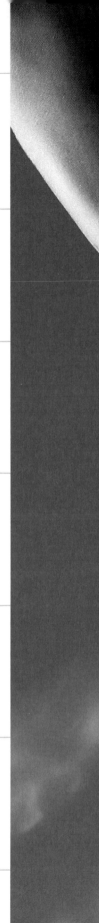

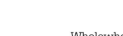

Activity is the key. Lose weight through a combination of diet and exercise and your shape will change dramatically...

MONDAY

Wholewheat pan pizza (×2)
Vegetables: green or mixed salad, spinach, mangetout or green beans

Fresh fruit salad: apple, orange, ½ medium ogen melon and 100 g/4 oz grapes

TUESDAY

Baked fish with ginger
Vegetables: boiled new potato, poached mushrooms, celeriac, cauliflower, mangetout, green or mixed salad

Peach and orange sorbet (×4)

WEDNESDAY

Cannelloni
Vegetables: **Pepperoni, ratatouille**, green or mixed salad

50 g/2 oz any hard cheese with 1 water biscuit

NB Soak prunes for tomorrow

THURSDAY

1 cup consommé

Pork fillet (tenderloin) with prunes
Vegetables: Brussels sprouts, **red cabbage with apple**, boiled parsnip, green beans, broccoli or cauliflower

1 banana

FRIDAY

Chicken florentine
Vegetables: boiled new potato, broad (fava) beans, spinach, cauliflower or broccoli

150 g/5 oz carton plain yogurt with 1 chopped apple and 25 g/1 oz chopped dates

SATURDAY

Steak au poivre: 175 g/6 oz fillet (tenderloin) or rump steak, grilled (broiled) with 12 black peppercorns pressed onto meat, fat removed
Vegetables: jacket baked potato, puréed swede (rutabaga), spinach, green or mixed salad

150 g/5 oz stewed rhubarb, sweetened to taste, and 150 g/5 oz carton plain yogurt

SUNDAY

Chicken véronique
Vegetables: boiled new potato, carrots, spring greens, courgettes (zucchini) or mangetout

50 g/2 oz any hard cheese and cucumber or celery

MONDAY

Skate with capers: 175 g/6 oz wing of skate, grilled (broiled) and served with 6 capers heated with 7 g/¼ oz butter

Vegetables: boiled new potato, green beans, poached mushrooms, salsify or braised celery

100 g/4 oz grapes or 1 banana

TUESDAY

Beef goulash (×4)

75 g/3 oz boiled tagliatelle (25 g/1 oz/½ cup raw weight)

Vegetables: 2 baked tomatoes, mangetout, spring greens, green or mixed salad

Baked apple with blackcurrant sauce

WEDNESDAY

Spinach soufflé

Vegetables: courgettes (zucchini), leeks, 2 baked tomatoes, green or mixed salad

Green fruit salad

THURSDAY

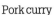

Pork curry

75 g/3 oz boiled brown rice (25 g/1 oz/2 tbsp raw weight)

Vegetables: green beans, green or mixed salad

25 g/1 oz Camembert with 2 rye crispbreads

FRIDAY

Stuffed aubergine (eggplant)

Vegetables: jacket baked potato, peas, carrots, mangetout, celeriac or green salad

1 peach, 1 small orange or 50 g/2 oz grapes

SATURDAY

Lasagne (×2)

Vegetables: spinach, green or mixed salad

½ grapefruit with crunchy topping (see Week 5 Day 3)

SUNDAY

Chicken with almonds

Vegetables: mashed potato, braised celery, spinach, peas, broccoli or green beans

1 large slice cantaloupe melon

Most diets concentrate on how much weight you can expect to lose in a given period and do not bother too much about where that weight is coming from, but new research is showing that the *type* of weight you lose is as important, from the point of view of your final shape, as the *amount*.

Studies at the University of Glasgow have shown that if you lose weight by dieting alone and take no exercise, up to one-third of the weight lost will be lean tissue (mainly muscle) not fat. This proportion rises with the severity of the diet. On an extended fast about half the weight lost is lean.

As muscle keeps you firm and fat makes you flabby, the most effective strategy is one which enables you to lose nearly 100 per cent fat while keeping, or even gaining, muscle. Do this by following a moderately restricted, nutritious eating plan and by keeping active both while losing weight and afterwards. Switching surplus fat for stronger muscles will result in a leaner, better-looking body and your metabolic rate will not drop as low ...

	Weight	Bust	Waist	Hips	Thighs
Week 8					
Week 10					

Fat is not just bulkier than muscle, but lighter too. If you habitually crash diet, you may gradually alter the composition of your body, upping the ratio of fat to lean, so although you may not weigh any more you will look different. Slimness is not just a matter of what the scales indicate, but of the shape you are in. You can be lean, or fat, but the more you crash diet, the more your chances of switching from the first to the second increase...

Q. Which exercise is the best to take up?

A. Any regular, fairly vigorous exercise, such as swimming, cycling, running or aerobic dancing, will help shed fat and conserve muscle. Choose an activity that you enjoy and which fits in with your way of life. Build up the time spent exercising and the level of intensity as you get fitter. This may also have a second, weight reducing effect by keeping your metabolic rate raised for some hours after the exercise has finished...

NB *'Passive exercise' is no substitute for active, on-your-feet exercising; nor is massage. Machines claiming to act by electrical stimulation of the muscle will not produce a visible slimming effect. 'The amount of energy dissipated by the muscle contractions is minimal,' states the Royal College of Physicians' 1983 report 'Obesity', 'and it is clear that the public should be advised against the use of these devices, which are often expensive as well as being ineffective techniques for slimming...'*

 WEEK 10

MONDAY

Liver with orange
Vegetables: boiled new potato, green beans, carrots, peas or green salad

25 g/1 oz grapes

TUESDAY

175 g/6 oz fillet (tenderloin) or rump steak, grilled (broiled) with herbs, all fat removed
Vegetables: watercress salad, green beans, swede (rutabaga), salsify, asparagus, 2 baked tomatoes or cauliflower

50 g/2 oz fresh pineapple

WEDNESDAY

100 g/4 oz **stuffed roast shoulder of lamb** (about 3 thin slices), all fat removed, with 2 tbsp **low fat gravy**
Vegetables: braised celery, **red cabbage with apple**, Brussels sprouts, carrots, broccoli, or boiled parsnip

1 apple, large orange or pear

THURSDAY

Wholewheat spaghetti with tomato and basil
Vegetables: peas, courgettes (zucchini), celeriac, green or mixed salad

1 banana

FRIDAY

Cottage pie (×2)
Vegetables: carrots, cabbage, leeks, marrow (squash), swede (rutabaga) or green beans

1 peach, 3 plums or 50 g/2 oz grapes

SATURDAY

Sole with herbs and wine
Vegetables: boiled new potato, mangetout, salsify, green beans, broccoli or green salad

25 g/1 oz smoked cheese and 1 water biscuit

SUNDAY

Pork chop with cider
Vegetables: boiled parsnip mashed with pepper and 1 tsp butter, **red cabbage with apple**, carrots, green beans, leeks or peas

Red fruit salad

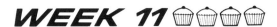

MONDAY

Bitkis (×3)
Vegetables: green salad, poached mushrooms, courgettes (zucchini), green beans or butter beans

Green fruit salad

TUESDAY

2 lamb cutlets, grilled (broiled), with 2 tsp redcurrant jelly, all fat removed
Vegetables: jacket baked potato, ratatouille, spinach, courgettes (zucchini), 2 grilled (broiled) tomatoes, broccoli or cauliflower

WEDNESDAY

Aubergine (eggplant) pie
Vegetables: green beans, poached mushrooms, sweetcorn (kernel corn) or green salad

½ grapefruit

THURSDAY

Herring with mustard sauce
Vegetables: boiled new potato, mangetout, salsify, broad (fava) beans, green beans or green salad

1 apple, large orange or pear

FRIDAY

Chilli con carne
Vegetables: boiled new potato, carrots, green beans, green or mixed salad

25 g/1 oz any hard cheese with celery

SATURDAY

Sole with lemon and prawns (shrimp)
Vegetables: boiled new potato, mangetout, broccoli, watercress, peas or mixed salad

1 fresh mango or 2 oranges

SUNDAY

Chicken florentine
Vegetables: green beans, broccoli, baked onion, cauliflower, 2 baked tomatoes or braised fennel

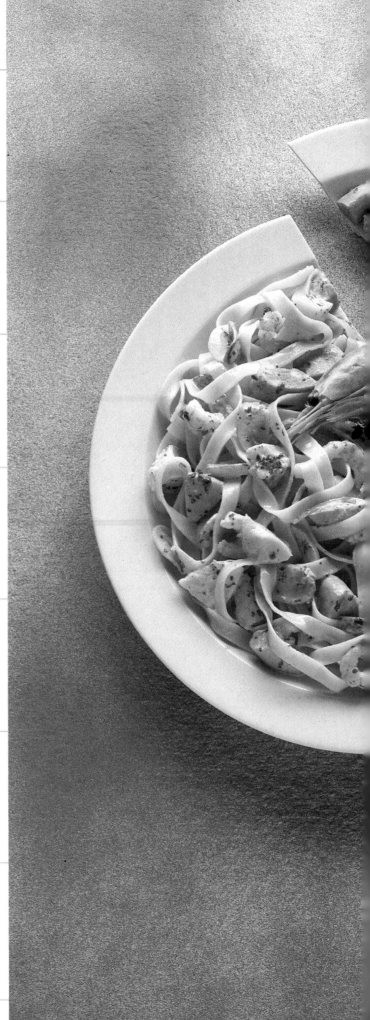

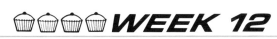
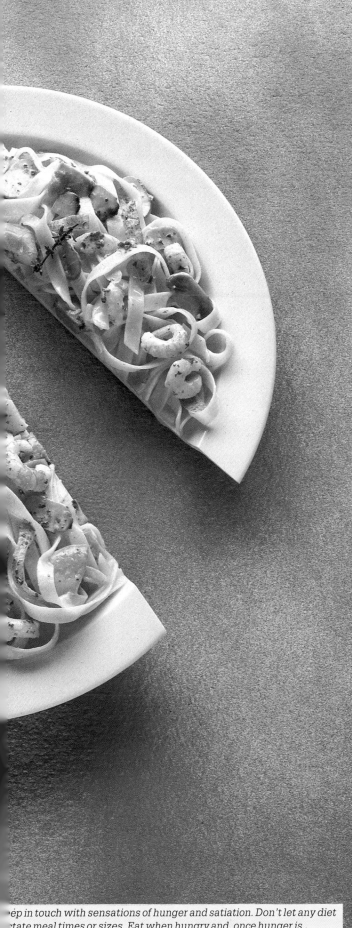

MONDAY

Liver provençal
75 g/3 oz boiled tagliatelle (25 g/1 oz/½ cup raw weight)
Vegetable: green or mixed salad or spinach

150 g/5 oz carton plain yogurt with 2 tsp honey and sprinkling of wheatgerm

TUESDAY

Smoked haddock roulade (×2)
Vegetables: courgettes (zucchini), mangetout, broccoli, green or mixed salad

100 g/4 oz passion fruit, 175 g/6 oz fresh strawberries or 50 g/2 oz grapes

WEDNESDAY

French vegetable quiche
Vegetables: spinach, green beans, sweetcorn (kernel corn), green or mixed salad

½ grapefruit or 1 clementine

THURSDAY

Chicken véronique
Vegetables: boiled new potato, green salad, broccoli, spring greens, cauliflower or green beans

25 g/1 oz Camembert or Brie and 1 rye crispbread

FRIDAY

Cannelloni
Vegetables: 2 grilled (broiled) tomatoes, **ratatouille**, green or mixed salad

50 g/2 oz fresh pineapple or 50 g/2 oz grapes

SATURDAY

Trout with almonds
Vegetables: boiled new potato, green beans, salsify, peas, broccoli, asparagus or green salad

150 g/5 oz carton plain yogurt with 2 tsp honey

SUNDAY

Beef goulash (×3)
75 g/3 oz boiled brown rice (25 g/1 oz/2 tbsp raw weight)
Vegetables: 2 baked tomatoes, carrots, Brussels sprouts, spring greens or marrow (squash)

1 peach or medium slice honeydew melon

...ep in touch with sensations of hunger and satiation. Don't let any diet ...tate meal times or sizes. Eat when hungry and, once hunger is ...tisfied, STOP.

	Weight	Bust	Waist	Hips	Thighs
Week 12					
Week 14					

MONDAY

Wholewheat macaroni with cheese and ham
Vegetables: spinach, mangetout, peas,
poached mushrooms or green salad

Strawberry sorbet (×4)

TUESDAY

Vegetable curry (×2)
75 g/3 oz boiled brown rice (25 g/1 oz/2 tbsp
raw weight)

1 tangerine/satsuma or peach

WEDNESDAY

Bitkis (×3)
Vegetables: carrots, green beans, braised
fennel, green or mixed salad

100 g/4 oz grapes

THURSDAY

Fish pie (×2)
Vegetables: broccoli, mangetout, carrots, green
or mixed salad

½ grapefruit

FRIDAY

Beef carbonnade
Vegetables: jacket baked potato, **red cabbage
with apple**, broccoli, peas or spring greens

150 g/5 oz carton plain yogurt with 1 peach,
100 g/4 oz raspberries or 50 g/2 oz grapes

NB Marinate the chicken for tomorrow

SATURDAY

Skewered chicken
Vegetables: jacket baked potato, 2 grilled
(broiled) tomatoes, courgettes (zucchini), green
or mixed salad

25 g/1 oz any hard cheese with celery or
cucumber

SUNDAY

2 lamb cutlets, grilled (broiled), with 2 tsp
redcurrant jelly, all fat removed
Vegetables: new potato, baked onion, peas,
sweetcorn (kernel corn), cauliflower, carrots or
mixed salad

½ ogen melon

Although 'hunger' and 'appetite' are often interchangeably, there are some important distinctions. While hunger is a physiological sensation, caused by lack of food and allied to specific processes such as stomach contractions, appetite is less well defined and appears to be governed as much by external cues as internal ones.
For example: the food itself – how appealing it looks, how good it smells and how much you like it; your mood (how excited/tense/depressed/distracted/bored you are); a multitude of other external factors, largely influenced by conditioning, such as 'If it's 1 pm, it must be lunchtime...'

There is now good evidence that people who are overweight tend to be more susceptible to these factors. Hunger seems to be less important in determining the way they eat, appetite more.

EXPERIMENT with hunger when you eat... stopping every so often, waiting a few moments, then sitting back and asking, 'Am I still hungry?' Is the hunger still there or has it gone? Look for an absence of the sensation, not a feeling of fullness or physical discomfort. If you are still hungry, eat a little more; then repeat the test.

A third of the adult British population attempts to slim each year and spends over £200 *million* on slimming products designed to help them do so – more often to the profit of the manufacturers than to themselves.

Most slimming products aim to suppress appetite. Few work in the long term. They can be divided, as follows, into three groups:

1. FIBRE-BASED BULKING AGENTS containing bran, guar gum or methyl cellulose, which swell in the stomach when swallowed with water, supposedly producing a sensation of fullness. In practice, a substantial amount of fibre would have to be taken in this way – much more than the maximum doses in these products – and the stomach soon adapts to the sensation of distension anyway.

2. SWEETS designed to raise blood/sugar levels so rapidly and substantially that they will signal to the brain that hunger is satisfied. In reality, the body reacts quickly to

return these levels to normal by secreting insulin which facilitates the removal of glucose from the blood into the cells, so any effect on appetite is very brief.

3. ANAESTHETIC CHEWING GUM which numbs the mouth so that pleasure derived from food, such as taste and texture, is minimized and the food, theoretically, loses its appeal. The sheer number of different factors influencing the appetite are stacked against this one too, as is the fact that the anaesthetic effect wears off quite quickly.

The most rigid diets are often the most appealing because their iron rules provide the discipline that dieters usually lack, but they do have their dangers. One of the less obvious is that they alienate you from feelings of hunger and satiation by stipulating exactly when and what and how much you must eat. You cannot afford to acknowledge hunger if hungry most of the time...

Years spent crash dieting may cause you to abandon hunger as a cue for eating and to depend upon less reliable cues, such as availability, mood or time of day. This may not be apparent while the current diet is going well and weight is being lost, but once you have finished the diet or your willpower falters, disordered eating habits can wreak havoc. The compulsive eating trap is a common one. One-third of all patients attending US obesity clinics describe episodes of binge eating after crash dieting and the true proportion is probably a lot higher than that.

AVOID regular use of laxatives. They won't speed weight loss, can become addictive and may be dangerous as they deplete the body of essential minerals, particularly potassium. Loss of potassium is especially hazardous because it can affect the heart by inducing spontaneous contraction of the cardiac muscle. Other side-effects include dehydration, impaired kidney function, epilepsy and even death.

MONDAY

Steak and kidney casserole (×2)
75 g/3 oz boiled brown rice (25 g/1 oz/2 tbsp raw weight)
Vegetables: green beans, braised celery or peas

100 g/4 oz passion fruit, 175 g/6 oz fresh strawberries or 50 g/2 oz grapes

TUESDAY

Mediterranean seafood sauce (×3)
75 g/3 oz boiled tagliatelle (25 g/1 oz/½ cup raw weight)
1 vegetable: green or mixed salad

Green fruit salad

WEDNESDAY

Piperade
Vegetables: jacket baked potato, spinach, broccoli, green beans, green or mixed salad

Autumn baked apple

THURSDAY

Sole florentine
Vegetables: boiled new potato, 2 grilled (broiled) tomatoes, poached mushrooms or green salad

Banana, honey and nut fool (×3)

FRIDAY

Stuffed pepper with tomato sauce (×2)
75 g/3 oz boiled pasta shells (25 g/1 oz/½ cup raw weight)
Vegetable: green salad

25 g/1 oz Stilton or 40 g/1½ oz Danish Blue and 1 apple or pear

SATURDAY

Chicken with peach and ginger
Vegetables: boiled new potato, spinach, mangetout, broccoli, cauliflower or green salad

150 g/5 oz carton plain yogurt with 2 tsp honey and sprinkling wheatgerm

SUNDAY

175 g/6 oz fillet (tenderloin) or rump steak, grilled (broiled) with herbs, all fat removed
Vegetables: 2 grilled (broiled) tomatoes, cauliflower, green beans, **red cabbage with apple**, green or mixed salad

½ ogen melon or 1 tangerine/satsuma

WEEK 15 🧁🧁🧁🧁

MONDAY

B

Lamb kebab
75 g/3 oz boiled brown rice (25 g/1 oz/2 tbsp raw weight)
Vegetables: peas, poached mushrooms, spinach or green salad

Red fruit salad

TUESDAY

C

Liver stroganoff
75 g/3 oz boiled tagliatelle (25 g/1 oz/½ cup raw weight)
Vegetables: broccoli, green beans, leeks or green salad

Strawberry sorbet (×3)

WEDNESDAY

C

Spinach roulade
Vegetables: poached mushrooms, 2 grilled (broiled) tomatoes, sweetcorn (kernel corn), green beans, broccoli or salsify

150 g/5 oz carton any fruit yogurt

THURSDAY

B

Sole with lemon and prawns (shrimp)
Vegetables: boiled new potato, green beans, mangetout, peas, cauliflower or green salad

1 apple, large orange or pear

NB Soak fruit for tomorrow

FRIDAY

C

Sweet and sour chicken
Vegetables: beansprouts, poached mushrooms, mangetout, green beans, cauliflower or peas

Winter fruit compote

SATURDAY

A

Chinese stuffed pepper
Vegetables: green or mixed salad

Green fruit salad

SUNDAY

D

100 g/4 oz **stuffed roast shoulder of lamb** (about 3 slices) with 2 tbsp **low fat gravy**
Vegetables: jacket baked potato, baked onion, green beans, cauliflower or **red cabbage with apple**

25 g/1 oz Camembert, Brie or smoked cheese with celery or a few grapes

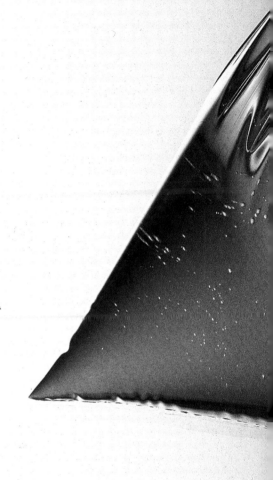
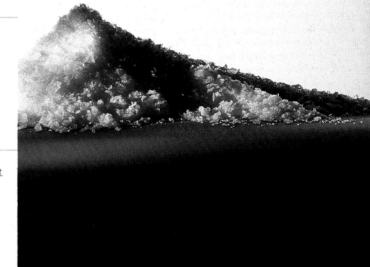

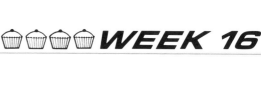

A — MONDAY

Wholewheat pan pizza
Vegetables: green or mixed salad

150 g/5 oz stewed rhubarb or 100 g/4 oz stewed plums, sweetened to taste, with 150 g/5 oz carton plain yogurt

B — TUESDAY

Baked fish with ginger
Vegetables: boiled new potato, mangetout, poached mushrooms, green beans or green salad

100 g/4 oz grapes or 1 banana

C — WEDNESDAY

Cannelloni
Vegetables: **pepperoni**, spinach, green or mixed salad

1 apple, large orange or pear

B — THURSDAY

Herb chicken
Vegetables: boiled new potato, mangetout, spring greens, peas, broccoli or carrots

1 peach, 100 g/4 oz raspberries, 3 plums or 50 g/2 oz grapes

D — FRIDAY

Herring with mustard sauce
Vegetables: boiled new potato, mangetout, sweetcorn (kernel corn), green or mixed salad

Banana, honey and nut fool (×2)

D — SATURDAY

Braised kidneys (×2)
75 g/3 oz boiled brown rice (25 g/1 oz/2 tbsp raw weight)
Vegetables: carrots, mangetout or green salad

25 g/1 oz Camembert, Brie or smoked cheese and 1 rye crispbread

C — SUNDAY

175 g/6 oz fillet (tenderloin or rump steak), grilled (broiled) with 6 crushed black peppercorns pressed onto both sides, all fat removed
Vegetables: spinach, green beans, broccoli, marrow (squash), 2 baked tomatoes or green salad

1 apple or pear with 75 g/3 oz grapes

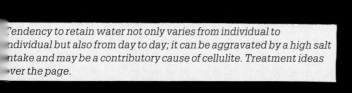
Tendency to retain water not only varies from individual to individual but also from day to day; it can be aggravated by a high salt intake and may be a contributory cause of cellulite. Treatment ideas over the page.

MONDAY

2 lamb cutlets, grilled (broiled), all fat removed
Vegetables: 2 grilled (broiled) tomatoes, green beans, courgettes (zucchini), spinach or poached mushrooms

Green fruit salad

TUESDAY

Oriental red mullet
Vegetables: boiled new potato, broad (fava) beans, braised celery, **ratatouille** or mixed salad

Strawberry sorbet (×2)

WEDNESDAY

Chicken with peach and ginger
Vegetables: mashed potato, mangetout, courgettes (zucchini), braised fennel, peas or green salad

½ grapefruit

THURSDAY

Vegetable lasagne
Vegetables: spinach, green beans, peas or green salad

½ ogen melon or 1 tangerine/satsuma

FRIDAY

Liver provençal
Vegetables: baked jacket potato, cauliflower, peas, braised celery, swede (rutabaga) or carrots

150 g/5 oz carton plain yogurt

SATURDAY

Fish pie
Vegetables: spinach, mangetout, green beans, carrots or green salad

Autumn baked apple

SUNDAY

175 g/6 oz fillet (tenderloin) or rump steak, grilled (broiled) with herbs, all fat removed
Vegetables: mashed potato, broccoli, **ratatouille, red cabbage with apple** or green salad

Peach and orange sorbet (×3)

CUTTING DOWN YOUR SALT INTAKE

	Eat freely
Meat	beef, rump and sirloin steak, lamb, pork, veal, chicken, duck, grouse, partridge, pheasant, turkey, venison
Fish	cod (raw or grilled), halibut, eel, trout, herring roe
Dairy foods	unsalted butter, cod liver oil, vegetable oils
Cereals	barley, flour, rice, rye, soya flour, spaghetti, puffed or shredded wheat
Fruit	all fruit except those listed, *right*
Vegetables	artichokes, asparagus, aubergines (eggplant), French (green) and runner (string) beans, Brussels sprouts, cauliflower, chicory, endive, leeks, lettuce, marrow (squash), onions, parsnips, peas, green peppers, potatoes, salsify, spring greens, tomatoes
Nuts	almonds, Brazil nuts, hazelnuts, peanuts, walnuts
Drinks	herbal teas, fruit juices, lager, cider, red wine, rosé wi. sparkling wine
Seasonings	mustard, pepper

Cellulite may be a cosmetic problem, and not a medical one, but it is a problem all the same – especially to the women who have it.

A lamentable lack of scientific research has led beauticians to concentrate more on cures than on causes for these infuriatingly intractable pockets of fat, though whether there is a proven cure is doubtful. In fact, there is no good evidence that *any* of the remedies on offer at exclusive salons have a significant effect. Self-help, however, might, *see opposite.*

Cellulite is sometimes described as 'fat gone wrong' because, unlike ordinary fat which disappears with dieting, cellulite tends to become *more* marked and visible as weight is lost. If this is your problem now, a combination approach – directed at reducing excess water, restoring circulation, purifying the system and firming contours – is in order. But don't expect to see results for at least 3 months: it is a long, slow process.

1. **EXERCISE** can help by firming muscles, boosting circulation. Particularly recommended: running, skipping, cycling (indoor cycles especially), jumping and trampolining.
2. **DIET** can have very positive effects. Cut right down on salt (see listings *above*), using a seasoning substitute to make food palatable. Eat plenty of raw vegetables, fresh fruits and (particularly) foods high in vitamin B6 (known to be helpful for counteracting puffiness and bloating): lamb's

	moderation	Avoid
	pigeon, offal (ox, lamb, pig or calf sweetbreads	canned meat, kidney, chicken liver, pork pie, bacon, ham, salami, sausages
	k, lemon sole, plaice, whiting, g, mackerel, salmon, whitebait, s	kipper, canned salmon, sardines, crab and tuna, lobster, scampi, oysters, scallops, smoked fish, prawns (shrimps)
	gg yolk, yogurt, cheese	salted butter, dried milk and margarine
	nacaroni, oatmeal, muesli, rye eads, bread	most brand cereals, oatcakes, biscuits (crackers) and pastry
	urrants, melons, passion fruit, pricots and figs, raisins and s (golden raisins)	olives in brine
	eans, kidney beans, broccoli, le, cucumber, lentils, mushrooms, tatoes, canned tomatoes, routs, beetroot (beet), carrots, radishes, watercress, spinach	canned carrots, peas, potatoes, sweetcorn (kernel corn); 'instant' potato
	uts, desiccated coconut	salted peanuts
	beers, white wine, sherry, th	brand hot chocolate and milk-based drinks
	vinegar, chutneys	baking powder, yeast and beef extract, bottled sauces, tomato purée, salt

liver, mackerel, nuts, wholegrains and wheatgerm.

3. MASSAGE helps stimulate the tissues directly under the skin, so *possibly* freeing trapped waste deposits and eliminating pockets of water, but you do not need the expensive variety from beauty salons. Rub the area briskly with a rough flannel or, European-style, with a natural-fibre brush, in long, firm strokes towards the heart for 5 minutes every day; then wash or shower.

NB Reducing salt intake will have health benefits, too. A high intake may lead to high blood pressure, a major contributory factor to coronary heart disease. As much as 30 per cent of the population may be at risk.

Professor Arnold Bender of the University of London's Queen Elizabeth College, and a leading authority on salt in the diet, says that we all get more than enough salt in our diet because about one-third of the salt we consume is *already* present in the food we eat and that is enough to satisfy our physiological needs. Another third is added during cooking to make food more palatable, the final third to 'season' it once on the plate...

	Weight	Bust	Waist	Hips	Thighs
Week 16					
Week 18					

MONDAY

Bitkis
75 g/3 oz boiled brown rice (25 g/1 oz/2 tbsp raw weight)
Vegetables: green or mixed salad, green beans or courgettes (zucchini)

100 g/4 oz grapes

TUESDAY

Lamb with garlic and rosemary
Vegetables: boiled new potato, courgettes (zucchini), 2 baked tomatoes, green beans, **red cabbage with apple** or asparagus

½ grapefruit with crunchy topping (see Week 5 Day 3)

WEDNESDAY

Mediterranean seafood sauce (×2)
75 g/3 oz boiled tagliatelle (25 g/1 oz/½ cup raw weight)
Vegetables: spinach, peas, mangetout, mixed or green salad

Banana, honey and nut fool

THURSDAY

175 g/6 oz fillet (tenderloin) or rump steak, grilled (broiled) with herbs, all fat removed
Vegetables: jacket baked potato, **ratatouille**, green beans, cauliflower or green salad

25 g/1 oz Camembert, Brie and 1 rye crispbread

FRIDAY

Aubergine (eggplant) pie
75 g/3 oz pasta shells (25 g/1 oz/½ cup raw weight)
Vegetables: green or mixed salad

150 g/5 oz carton plain yogurt with 1 tsp honey

SATURDAY

Lasagne
Vegetables: spinach, green or mixed salad

Peach and orange sorbet (×2)

SUNDAY

Barbecue lamb
Vegetables: poached mushrooms, **red cabbage with apple**, broccoli, cauliflower, sweetcorn (kernel corn), spinach or green salad

Autumn baked apple

WEEK 19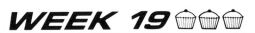

MONDAY

A

Skate with capers: 150 g/5 oz wing of skate, grilled (broiled) and served with 6 capers heated with 7 g/¼ oz butter
Vegetables: boiled new potato, broccoli, salsify, mangetout, or green salad

½ ogen melon filled with 100 g/4 oz fresh chopped pineapple or segments of large orange

TUESDAY

Beef goulash (×2)
Vegetables: jacket baked potato, 2 baked tomatoes, carrots, peas, green beans, marrow (squash) or cabbage

150 g/5 oz carton plain yogurt with 2 tsp honey and sprinkling wheatgerm

WEDNESDAY

Courgette (zucchini) and tomato pie
Vegetables: broccoli, carrots, spinach, spring greens, mangetout or green salad

1 apple, large orange or pear

THURSDAY

Kidneys in red wine
75 g/3 oz boiled brown rice (25 g/1 oz/2 tbsp raw weight)
Vegetables: cauliflower, swede (rutabaga), spring greens, leeks, peas or green salad

1 banana

FRIDAY

B

Stuffed pepper with tomato sauce
Vegetables: poached mushrooms, carrots, green or mixed salad

1 peach, 100 g/4 oz fresh raspberries or 2 tangerines/satsumas

SATURDAY

C

Smoked salmon quiche
Vegetables: mangetout, green beans, green or mixed salad

Peach and orange sorbet

SUNDAY

Chicken with almonds
Vegetables: braised celery, courgettes (zucchini), mangetout, broccoli or green beans

25 g/1 oz Danish Blue or Roquefort and 1 water biscuit

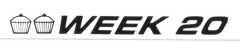

 A

Vegetable curry (×2)
75 g/3 oz boiled brown rice (25 g/1 oz/2 tbsp raw weight)
Vegetables: green or mixed salad or sweetcorn (kernel corn)

100 g/4 oz fresh pineapple

MONDAY

 D

175 g/6 oz fillet (tenderloin) or rump steak, grilled (broiled) with herbs, all fat removed
Vegetables: jacket baked potato, 2 grilled (broiled) tomatoes, watercress, braised fennel, swede (rutabaga), salsify or mixed salad

1 apple, large orange or pear

TUESDAY

 D

Lamb with garlic and rosemary
Vegetables: jacket baked potato, Brussels sprouts, cauliflower, broccoli, baked onion or braised celery

½ ogen melon or 1 tangerine/satsuma

WEDNESDAY

 D

Smoked haddock roulade
Vegetables: courgettes (zucchini), spinach, 2 grilled (broiled) tomatoes, poached mushrooms or cauliflower

Green fruit salad

THURSDAY

 D

Cottage pie
Vegetables: cabbage, carrots, swede (rutabaga), mangetout, leeks or green salad

1 small banana

FRIDAY

 D

Wholewheat macaroni with cheese and ham
Vegetables: peas, broccoli, 2 grilled (broiled) tomatoes, green or mixed salad

1 peach, 3 plums or 50 g/2 oz grapes

SATURDAY

 D

Chicken florentine
Vegetables: mashed potato, broad (fava) beans, braised leeks, braised fennel, **red cabbage with apple**, green beans or green salad

100 g/4 oz grapes

SUNDAY

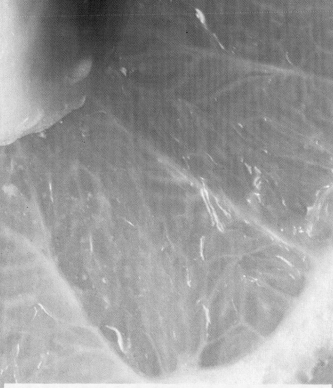

One of the most enduring dietary myths . . . eating half a grapefruit before a meal helps burn off fat. More myths over the page . . .

MONDAY

Liver provençal
75 g/3 oz boiled tagliatelle (25 g/1 oz/½ cup raw weight)
Vegetables: spinach, carrots, peas, marrow (squash), spring greens or mangetout

½ grapefruit

TUESDAY

Skewered chicken
Vegetables: 2 grilled (broiled) tomatoes, mangetout, poached mushrooms, green or mixed salad

50 g/2 oz fresh pineapple

WEDNESDAY

Baked fish with ginger
Vegetables: boiled new potato, broccoli, braised fennel, leeks or green beans

1 banana

THURSDAY

Piperade
Vegetables: braised celery, fennel, cauliflower, green beans, green or mixed salad

50 g/2 oz grapes

FRIDAY

Lamb kebab
Vegetables: jacket baked potato, braised celery, courgettes (zucchini), poached mushrooms or green salad

150 g/5 oz carton natural yogurt with 2 tsp honey and sprinkling wheatgerm

SATURDAY

Sole florentine
Vegetables: boiled new potato, carrots, cauliflower, 2 grilled (broiled) tomatoes or mangetout

1 apple, large orange or pear

SUNDAY

Beef goulash
75 g/3 oz boiled tagliatelle (25 g/1 oz/½ cup raw weight)
Vegetables: green beans, carrots, marrow (squash), baked onion, peas or green salad

½ ogen melon or 1 tangerine/satsuma

---

8 more myths...

A calorie is a calorie is a calorie. All calories may be equally fattening but they are not equally nourishing, see opposite.

Margarine is less fattening than butter. Both contain exactly the same number of calories (80 per 10 g).

Yogurt is not fattening. Natural fat-free or low-fat yogurts are relatively low in calories (about 70 in a small carton) but whole milk or fruit-flavoured yogurts are almost twice that. Despite their health-giving image, fruit yogurts are also extremely high in sugar (about 17 per cent).

Fruit is not fattening. Bananas have twice the calories of apples and cherries and 4 times the calories of grapefruit. Although most fruits have little or no fat, avocados contain large amounts.

Slimming breads are less fattening than other breads. Unless the information on the wrapper states how low the bread is in calories (and it's lower per slice than the average), it may not be any less fattening. Some granary breads are less fattening than 'slimming' breads and much better for you.

There's no difference between honey and sugar. Both are fattening, but honey contains fructose, which is sweeter than sugar (sucrose), so you use less of it, and water, which makes it lower in calories anyway.

Eating foods in certain combinations activates enzymes which prevents them being absorbed by the gut... (Judy Mazel, 'Beverly Hills Diet', 1981). 'Blatantly wrong-headed and potentially dangerous' ('British Journal of Hospital Medicine', February, 1982).

Eating carrots is the healthiest way to keep slim. Eating excessive quantities of carrots can be bad for you. Complications include amenorrhoea (absent or irregular periods), temporary infertility and discoloration of the skin, which actually turns orange.

The US Department of Agriculture has cautioned that it is difficult to get all the nutrients we need on less than 1600 calories a day. This means that slimmers, whose diets are always some way below this, must make extra sure that what they eat is nutritious and well-balanced.

Even people subsisting on diets containing much more than 1600 calories may not be getting all the nutrients necessary to good health – the correct balance of amino acids in protein, for example, or the right fatty acids or enough of the fibre, vitamins, minerals and trace elements that their bodies require to function at their best. Today's typical highly-refined diet overfeeds and undernourishes, putting on weight while taking away vitality and wellbeing. In addition to providing next-to-nothing nutritionally, it also draws heavily upon valuable stores of certain key nutrients – most notably magnesium and the B vitamins, especially B1 (thiamin). In one Japanese study, early signs of the thiamin-deficiency disease, beriberi, were found among affluent and apparently 'well-fed' teenagers living on junk food diets.

NB Under-nutrition can lead to overeating. If your diet is composed largely of refined foods and 'empty' calories, such as those contained in sugar and alcohol, you may have to eat 1000 calories or more *over* the basic 1600 or so that you need just to get the vital nutrients that your body requires. It is much more difficult to become slim and to remain slim on an unbalanced diet because hunger is influenced by quality of food as well as quantity. If the quality of what you eat is inadequate, messages of hunger will continue to be sent until the shortfall is made up.

IMPORTANT. Now that you are on the last phase of the diet, with calories cut to just 1000, each calorie must count for as much as possible. There is no room in your diet for junk foods of limited nutritional value. Increase nutrient density by taking a daily multivitamin and mineral tablet, eating organically grown fruit and vegetables raw or very briefly cooked and buying all foods as fresh as possible.

	Weight	Bust	Waist	Hips	Thighs
Week 20					
Week 22					
Week 24					

MONDAY

Soufflé cheese omelette
Vegetables: **ratatouille**, broccoli, poached mushrooms, green or mixed salad

25 g/1 oz grapes

TUESDAY

Trout with almonds
Vegetables: boiled new potato, braised fennel, mangetout, green beans, green or mixed salad

100 g/4 oz fresh pineapple

WEDNESDAY

100 g/4 oz fillet (tenderloin) or rump steak, grilled (broiled) with herbs, all fat removed
Vegetables: boiled new potato, **ratatouille**, spring greens, green or mixed salad

½ grapefruit with crunchy topping (See Week 5 Day 3)

THURSDAY

Cannelloni
Vegetables: 2 grilled (broiled) tomatoes, **pepperoni**, green or mixed salad

1 tangerine/satsuma or 1 oz fresh pineapple

FRIDAY

Braised kidneys
75 g/3 oz boiled brown rice (25 g/1 oz/2 tbsp raw weight)
Vegetables: carrots, broccoli, marrow (squash), peas or mixed salad

1 small peach or 25 g/1 oz grapes

SATURDAY

Chicken with peach and ginger
Vegetables: green salad, mangetout, green beans, salsify, peas or courgettes (zucchini)

Green fruit salad

SUNDAY

Lamb with garlic and rosemary
Vegetables: jacket baked potato, 2 baked tomatoes, **red cabbage with apple**, cauliflower or spring greens

1 small slice melon

WEEK 23

MONDAY

 C

Mediterranean seafood sauce
75 g/3 oz boiled tagliatelle (25 g/1 oz/½ cup raw weight)
Vegetables: green or mixed salad, courgettes (zucchini) or green beans

75 g/3 oz fresh pineapple or 50 g/2 oz grapes

TUESDAY

D

Tarragon chicken: 225 g/8 oz chicken portion, cooked in foil with skin removed and a slice of onion, a sprig of fresh tarragon, seasoning and lemon juice.
Vegetables: boiled new potato, braised celery, broccoli or leeks

1 banana

WEDNESDAY

D

Steak and kidney casserole
Vegetables: green beans, mangetout, 2 baked tomatoes, spinach, Brussels sprouts or spring greens

Red fruit salad

THURSDAY

 B

Vegetable curry
75 g/3 oz boiled brown rice (25 g/1 oz/2 tbsp raw weight)
Vegetables: green or mixed salad

½ grapefruit

FRIDAY

 D

Smoked salmon roulade
Vegetables: boiled new potato, braised fennel, green beans, peas, spinach or green salad

1 apple, orange or pear

SATURDAY

 C

Wholewheat spaghetti with chicken livers
Vegetables: peas, 2 grilled (broiled) tomatoes, spinach, green or mixed salad

1 small peach, 2 plums or 25 g/1 oz grapes

SUNDAY

  D

Lamb kebab
Vegetables: jacket baked potato, swede (rutabaga), parsnip, **red cabbage with apple,** cauliflower, carrots or green salad

Strawberry sorbet

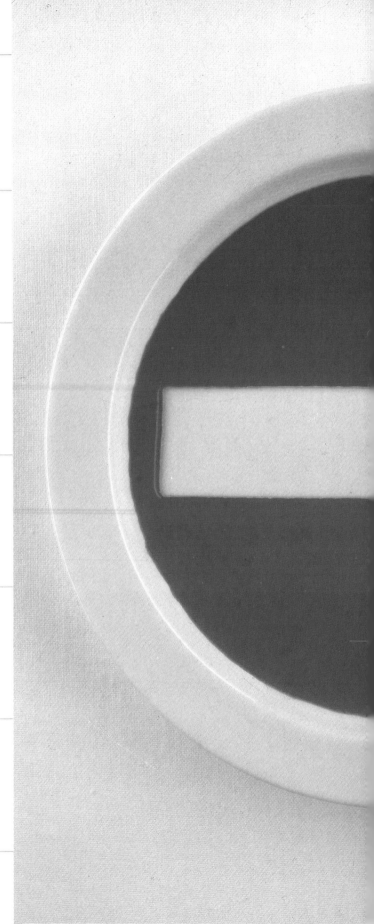

Knowing when to stop dieting is as important as being able to keep to your diet. The key is comfort: stop at a weight you can comfortably maintain. You will know you have gone too far if you find it a constant struggle to keep to your new weight.

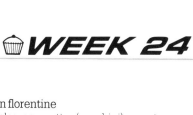

Chicken florentine
Vegetables: courgettes (zucchini), carrots, leeks, broccoli, cauliflower or beetroot (beet)

½ ogen melon or 1 tangerine/satsuma

MONDAY

Spinach soufflé
Vegetables: green beans, 2 grilled (broiled) tomatoes, poached mushrooms, green or mixed salad

150 g/5 oz carton plain yogurt

NB Soak prunes for tomorrow

TUESDAY

Pork fillet with prunes
Vegetables: cabbage, spinach, braised celery, marrow (squash), spring greens, baked onion or carrots

1 apple, large orange or pear

WEDNESDAY

200 g/7 oz plaice (flounder) fillet, grilled (broiled) with herbs
Vegetables: boiled new potato, mangetout, green beans, peas, 2 grilled (broiled) tomatoes, poached mushrooms or green salad

75 g/3 oz fresh pineapple

THURSDAY

Wholewheat spaghetti with tomato and basil
Vegetables: spinach, peas, green beans, green or mixed salad

1 peach, 3 plums, 100 g/4 oz raspberries or 50 g/2 oz grapes

FRIDAY

Indian chicken
Vegetables: boiled new potato, courgettes (zucchini), asparagus, green or mixed salad

½ grapefruit

SATURDAY

150 g/5 oz fillet (tenderloin) or rump steak, grilled (broiled) with herbs, all fat removed
Vegetables: **red cabbage with apple**, Brussels sprouts, green beans, green or mixed salad

1 banana or 100 g/4 oz grapes

SUNDAY

INDULGENCES

As temptation is a part of any diet, there are no forbidden fruits on this one. Some high-calorie foods are allowed every week, even in the final stages when overall calorie count is cut right down.

These Indulgences are meant to encourage a more flexible attitude to food. Being allowed to 'break' your diet from time to time and indulge in a favourite food, or drink, should help avoid the all-or-nothing starve/stuff mentality that sabotages many diets almost as soon as they have started. If all foods are allowed there can be no excuse for defaulting.

Each week of the diet gives a code of indulgences allowed. Check particular favourites against these lists and, if your heart's desire is not on them, work out exactly how much you can allow yourself within the stated limit.

100 CALORIES

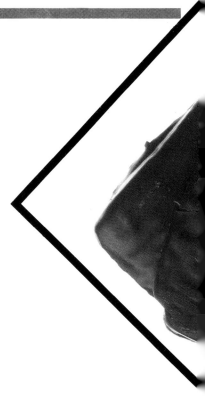

50g (2 oz) dried apricots
1 mashed banana with 1 tsp sugar
50g (2 oz) chestnuts
½ medium ogen melon with 50g (2 oz) port OR 25g (1 oz) port and 75g (3 oz) strawberries OR 175g (6 oz) strawberries
1 large nectarine
125g (4 oz) fresh pineapple with 2 tsp single (light) cream
250g (8 oz) fresh cherries
1 passion fruit with 125g (4 oz) paw-paw OR 2 medium peaches
3 small dried figs
2 fresh figs with 125g (4 oz) grapes
100g (3½ oz) palm hearts with lemon juice and chopped parsley
25g (1 oz) Austrian smoked cheese with 1 rye crispbread
25g (1 oz) Lancashire/Double Gloucester/Roquefort cheese
40g (1½ oz) sausage roll (made with shortcrust pastry)

2 grilled (broiled) fish fingers
25g (1 oz) Parma ham with 1 large fresh peach
125g (4 oz) prawns (shrimps) in shells with lemon juice and 25g (1 oz) wholewheat bread
25g (1 oz) smoked cod's roe with lemon juice, on 25g (1 oz) wholewheat toast
2 tsp mayonnaise
2 Bourbon biscuits (cookies)
1 shortbread biscuit (cookie)
1 plain cup cake
1 small jam tart
50g (2 oz) chocolate ice cream
100g (3½ oz) chocolate frozen mousse
75g (3 oz) fruit yogurt
1 thin pancake (crêpe) with lemon juice and ¾ tsp sugar
75g (3 oz) egg custard
1 large meringue with 1 tbsp whipping cream
25g (1 oz) fruit pastilles
150 ml (¼ pint) (⅔ cup) grape juice
1 cup of Ovaltine: 1 tsp Ovaltine with 200 ml (⅓ pint) (⅞ cup) skimmed milk

1 cup hot chocolate: 2 tsp drinking chocolate and 200 ml (⅓ pint) (⅞ cup) skimmed milk
300 ml (½ pint) (1¼ cups) Coca Cola
4 tbsp (2 fl oz) (¼ cup) spirit (any) mixed with slimline tonic/bitter lemon/soda
300 ml (½ pint) (1¼ cups) dry or sweer cider
1 large glass of champagne
300 ml (½ pint) (1¼ cups) lager
generous glass dry or medium sherry
25g (1 oz) any liqueur, except Chartreuse

200 CALORIES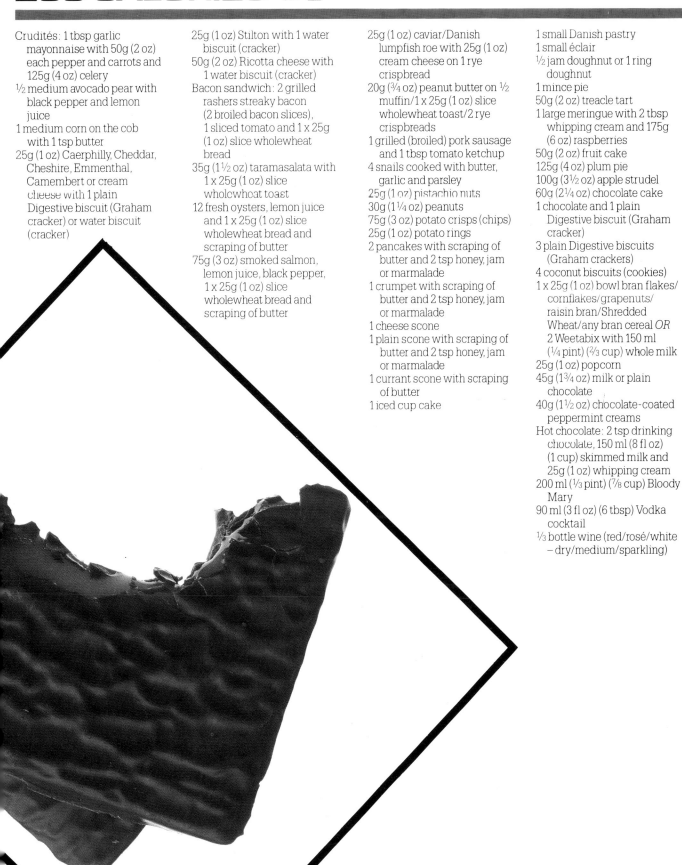

Crudités: 1 tbsp garlic mayonnaise with 50g (2 oz) each pepper and carrots and 125g (4 oz) celery

½ medium avocado pear with black pepper and lemon juice

1 medium corn on the cob with 1 tsp butter

25g (1 oz) Caerphilly, Cheddar, Cheshire, Emmenthal, Camembert or cream cheese with 1 plain Digestive biscuit (Graham cracker) or water biscuit (cracker)

25g (1 oz) Stilton with 1 water biscuit (cracker)

50g (2 oz) Ricotta cheese with 1 water biscuit (cracker)

Bacon sandwich: 2 grilled rashers streaky bacon (2 broiled bacon slices), 1 sliced tomato and 1 x 25g (1 oz) slice wholewheat bread

35g (1½ oz) taramasalata with 1 x 25g (1 oz) slice wholewheat toast

12 fresh oysters, lemon juice and 1 x 25g (1 oz) slice wholewheat bread and scraping of butter

75g (3 oz) smoked salmon, lemon juice, black pepper, 1 x 25g (1 oz) slice wholewheat bread and scraping of butter

25g (1 oz) caviar/Danish lumpfish roe with 25g (1 oz) cream cheese on 1 rye crispbread

20g (¾ oz) peanut butter on ½ muffin/1 x 25g (1 oz) slice wholewheat toast/2 rye crispbreads

1 grilled (broiled) pork sausage and 1 tbsp tomato ketchup

4 snails cooked with butter, garlic and parsley

25g (1 oz) pistachio nuts

30g (1¼ oz) peanuts

75g (3 oz) potato crisps (chips)

25g (1 oz) potato rings

2 pancakes with scraping of butter and 2 tsp honey, jam or marmalade

1 crumpet with scraping of butter and 2 tsp honey, jam or marmalade

1 cheese scone

1 plain scone with scraping of butter and 2 tsp honey, jam or marmalade

1 currant scone with scraping of butter

1 iced cup cake

1 small Danish pastry

1 small éclair

½ jam doughnut or 1 ring doughnut

1 mince pie

50g (2 oz) treacle tart

1 large meringue with 2 tbsp whipping cream and 175g (6 oz) raspberries

50g (2 oz) fruit cake

125g (4 oz) plum pie

100g (3½ oz) apple strudel

60g (2¼ oz) chocolate cake

1 chocolate and 1 plain Digestive biscuit (Graham cracker)

3 plain Digestive biscuits (Graham crackers)

4 coconut biscuits (cookies)

1 x 25g (1 oz) bowl bran flakes/ cornflakes/grapenuts/ raisin bran/Shredded Wheat/any bran cereal OR 2 Weetabix with 150 ml (¼ pint) (⅔ cup) whole milk

25g (1 oz) popcorn

45g (1¾ oz) milk or plain chocolate

40g (1½ oz) chocolate-coated peppermint creams

Hot chocolate: 2 tsp drinking chocolate, 150 ml (8 fl oz) (1 cup) skimmed milk and 25g (1 oz) whipping cream

200 ml (⅓ pint) (⅞ cup) Bloody Mary

90 ml (3 fl oz) (6 tbsp) Vodka cocktail

⅓ bottle wine (red/rosé/white – dry/medium/sparkling)

Special diets

Diets are not just about eating less but about eating well. Good nutrition, always important, is especially vital when breastfeeding or pregnant or when following a restricted diet for health or ethical reasons. In this chapter you will find healthy eating plans for prospective and nursing mothers, a high-fibre, very low-fat diet (highly recommended for men) and a vegetarian diet, designed both for those already committed to this healthy way of eating and for those anxious to try something new. A healthy diet that keeps interest up, boredom down, has the best possible chance of success.

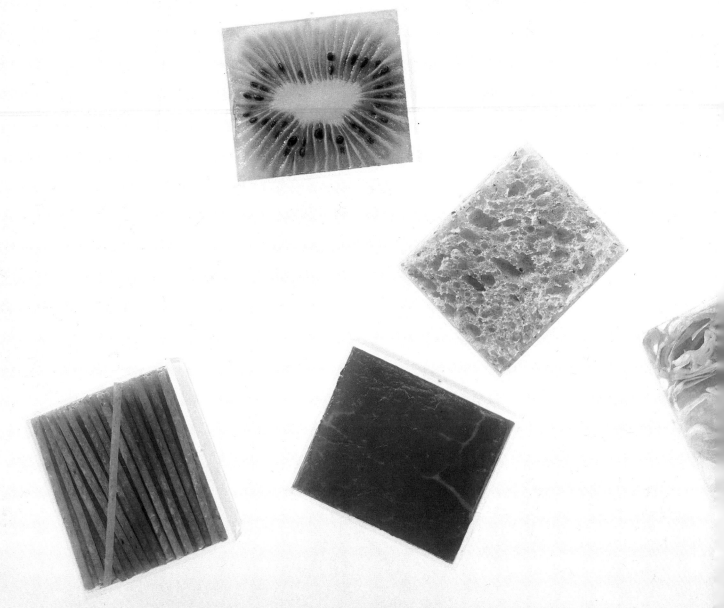

There are diets for other special circumstances too. If you want to lose a little weight quickly for a holiday or special occasion, for example, you can follow one of the short sharp Blitz diets, safe in the knowledge that you are not undernourishing yourself – though you should be aware that this is not the best way of losing weight in the long term. Re-read the introduction to find out why. The 24-hour juice fasts will refresh and revitalize, whether or not you want to lose weight, and make an excellent break from too much rich, heavy food and alcohol. Try one for a day and see how much better you feel... An analysis of essential nutrients – calories, carbo-hydrates, protein, fibre, relevant vitamins and minerals – is given for each diet. Figures in brackets after each nutrient indicate the recommended daily allowance (U.K. only).

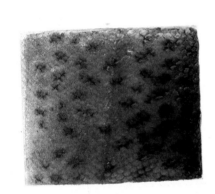

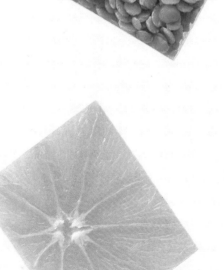

JUICE DIETS

These fruit and vegetable juices will provide a refreshing rest from the excesses of rich food, unbalanced eating patterns and an unhealthy lifestyle. Set aside one day when demands are not too great. Allow yourself 3 cocktails, all the same or different, and alternate with plentiful glasses of water.

Providing it is undertaken for a period of no more than two days, fasting can be a great relief to the system – particularly if it is habitually overloaded with alcohol and rich or refined foods. In general, you can expect to feel bad on the first day, better on the second. These feelings of general malaise (headaches, irritability, weakness) are thought to be due both to lack of food and to withdrawal symptoms of foods to which one is 'allergically addicted'. These masked allergies are very difficult to track down and should only be investigated under the direction of an environmentally and nutritionally orientated doctor. Yet another possible explanation for these symptoms is that after a period without food the metabolism switches to a state called ketosis, in which it starts burning fats rather than sugars. This can release fat-soluble toxins which may have some transient bad effects as they are swept out of the system.

Prolonged fasting can have some serious side-effects: protein, mineral and vitamin deficiencies, fainting, dizziness, possible liver disorder and even death. Most doctors now consider that prolonged fasts should only be taken as a means of weight control under the strictest medical supervision.

	Vegetable I	Vegetable II	Fruit I	Fruit II
Calories	81	56	133	187
Protein	38%	29%	5%	6%
Fat	5%	7%	NONE	NONE
Carbohydrate	57%	64%	95%	94%
Fibre (g)	14.3	5.1	5.6	6.9
Vitamin C (mg)	48.3	163.6	23.8	84.3
Potassium (mg)	1443	993	463	879
Magnesium (mg)	95	47	24	35
Sodium (mg)	587	41	8	10

Fasting may help clear the mind and cleanse the system but it is not an effective long-term strategy for losing weight. When you fast, as much as 65 per cent of the weight lost is due to a breakdown of lean tissue – not fat. The result is a far from ideal body shape and a steep drop in metabolic rate – as much as 40 per cent on extended fasts – making some weight regain inevitable once the fast is broken.

VEGETABLE JUICES
Weigh vegetables after trimming. Wash them well, especially the ones that grow above the ground, which may have been sprayed with harmful chemicals. Shake dry.

FRUIT JUICES
Wash all fruit carefully, remembering that even if it looks clean, it has probably been sprayed with chemicals. Remove stones (pits), but leave apple cores, skin, etc.

Vegetable Juice I

Metric/Imperial	American
75 g/3 oz spinach, leaves and tender stalks only	3 oz spinach, leaves and tender stalks only
150 g/5 oz carrots	5 oz carrots
150 g/5 oz fennel	5 oz fennel
75 g/3 oz celery	3 oz celery

Put all ingredients through a juicer.

Fruit Juice I

Metric/Imperial	American
2 dessert apples (preferably Cox's or Granny Smith's)	2 Granny Smith apples
2 apricots or 2-3 plums	2 apricots or 2-3 plums
½ mango or paw-paw, or 2 passion fruit, or 1 lime	½ mango or paw-paw, or 2 passion fruit, or 1 lime

Put all ingredients through a juicer.

Vegetable Juice II

Metric/Imperial	American
175 g/6 oz tomatoes	6 oz tomatoes
125 g/4 oz cucumber	4 oz cucumber
75-125 g/3-4 oz green pepper or chicory	3-4 oz green pepper or endive
25 g/1 oz watercress or parsley	1 oz watercress or parsley

Put all ingredients through a juicer.

Fruit Juice II

Metric/Imperial	American
1 large ripe pear	1 large ripe pear
1 large orange	1 large orange
125 g/4 oz black grapes	4 oz black grapes

Put all ingredients through a juicer.

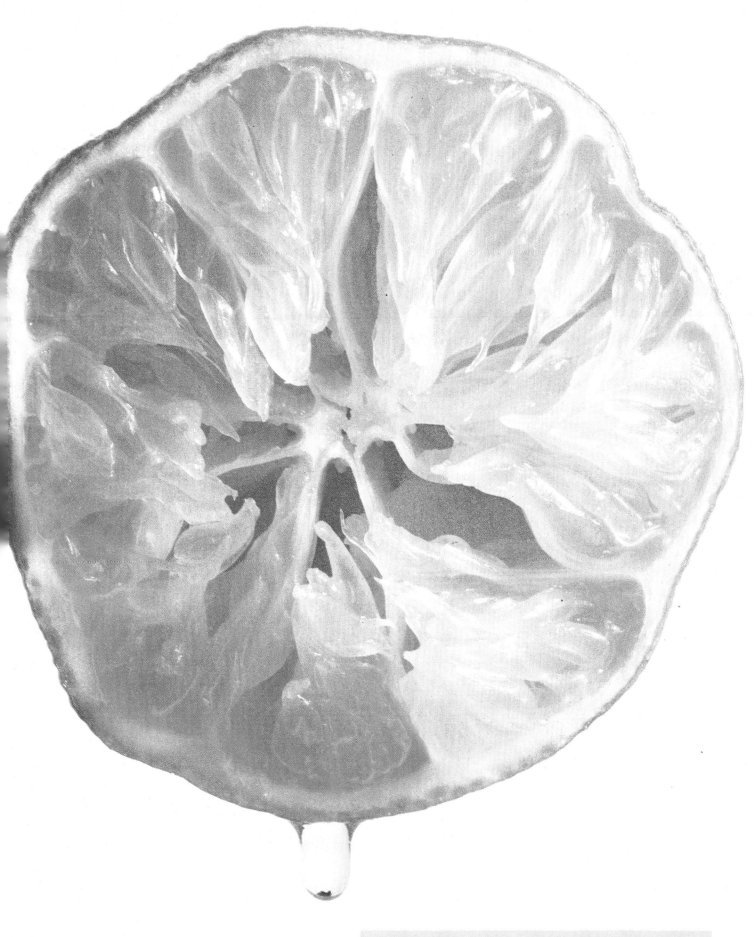

On fasts and juice diets you tend to lose a great deal of retained fluid and, with it, the important minerals potassium, magnesium and sodium. These fruit and vegetable juices have been specially formulated to compensate for this and so keep levels up...

Calories 750 • Protein 31% (10%) • Fat 18% (30-35%) • Carbohydrate 51% (60-55%) • Fibre 20 g

5-DAY BLITZ

Low- or no-carbohydrate diets should be 'strongly discouraged' says the Royal College of Physicians in its 1983 report, *Obesity*, even if you only want to follow them for a short period of time. To lose weight rapidly, choose a diet high in starchy carbohydrates (wholewheat bread, wholegrain cereals and pasta, lentils and pulses) and low in fats instead, like the diets given here.

	BREAKFASTS	LIGHT MEALS	MAIN MEALS
DAY 1	None	Milk: 600 ml/1 pint (2½ cups) whole milk Fruit: 3 oranges (100 g/3½ oz each) and 2 apples (125 g/4 oz each)	None
DAY 2	BREAKFAST ALLOWANCE FROM DAY 2: 25 g/1 oz Shredded Wheat, Weetabix, Weetaflakes *or* Puffed Wheat, with 10 g/⅓ oz bran	Tomato sandwich: 100 g/3½ oz tomatoes, 1 tsp low calorie mayonnaise and 50 g/2 oz wholewheat bread Fruit: 120 g/4 oz apple	Fillet steak: 125 g/4 oz fillet (tenderloin), grilled (broiled), using no oil. Season well and remove all fat. Vegetable: 100 g/3½ oz broccoli Strawberry ice: blend together 150 g/5 oz fresh or frozen strawberries, 6 tbsp water, and 10 g/⅓ oz dried skimmed milk until smooth. Freeze for about 3 to 4 hours until firm.
DAY 3	As day 2	Cheese and pepper sandwich: 50 g/2 oz chopped green pepper, 100 g/3½ oz cottage cheese and 50 g/2 oz wholewheat bread Fruit: 100 g/3½ oz orange	Fillet of plaice (flounder): 150 g/5 oz fillet, grilled (broiled) with a sprinkling of freshly chopped herbs. Serve with slices of lemon. Vegetable: 100 g/3½ oz carrots Stewed apples: 150 g/5 oz apples cooked with 15 g/½ oz raisins (no sugar)
DAY 4	As day 2	Cucumber and egg sandwich: 50 g/2 oz chopped cucumber, 50 g/2 oz hard-boiled egg, 1 tsp low calorie mayonnaise and 50 g/2 oz wholewheat bread Fruit: 150 g/5 oz pear	Paprika chicken: remove the skin from 100 g/3½ oz chicken breast and coat with French (Dijon-style) mustard and paprika to taste. Grill (broil) under a gentle heat until thoroughly cooked. Vegetable: 100 g/3½ oz cabbage Fruit: 100 g/3½ oz cherries or grapes
DAY 5	As day 2	Smoked salmon and watercress sandwich: 60 g/2½ oz smoked salmon, 50 g/2 oz chopped watercress, 1 tsp low calorie mayonnaise, lemon juice and 50 g/2 oz wholewheat bread Fruit: 125 g/4 oz apple	Eggs and spinach: 2 medium eggs poached and served with 100 g/3½ oz boiled and chopped spinach. Season well. Vegetable: 50 g/2 oz grilled (broiled) tomato Fruit: 1 banana

DAILY ALLOWANCE FROM DAY 2: 600 ml/1 pint (2½ cups) skimmed milk; unlimited water and herb teas. 1 daily multivitamin plus iron.

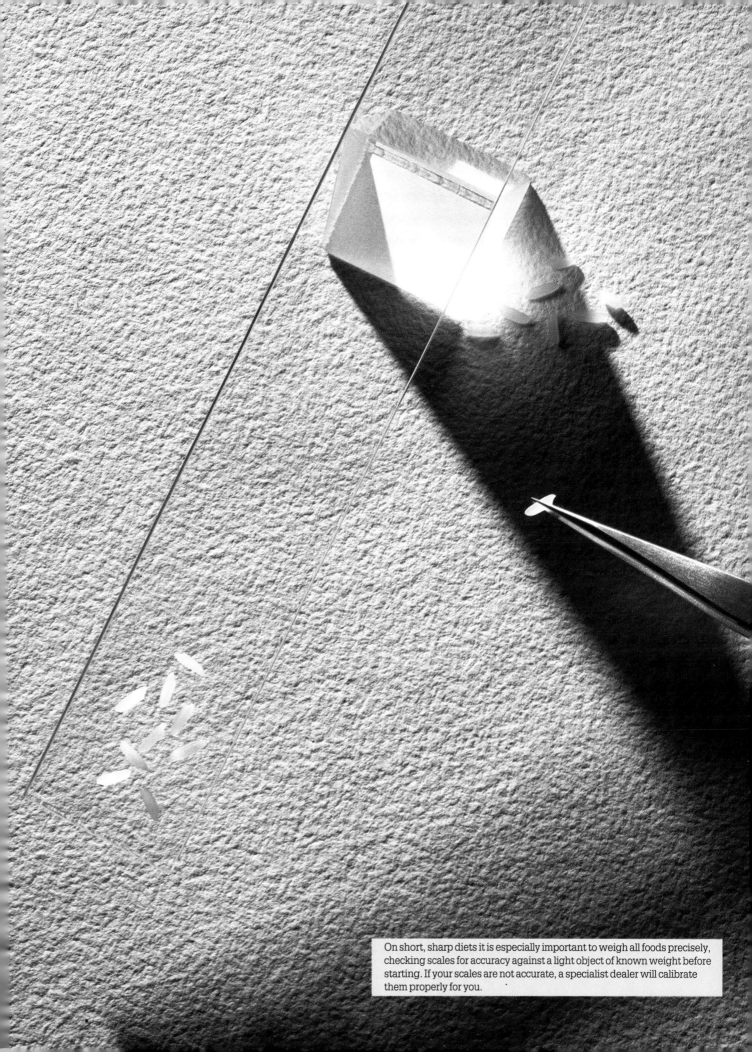

On short, sharp diets it is especially important to weigh all foods precisely, checking scales for accuracy against a light object of known weight before starting. If your scales are not accurate, a specialist dealer will calibrate them properly for you.

Calories 900 ● Protein 32% ● Fat 15% ● Carbohydrate 53% ● Fibre 28 g

10-DAY BLITZ

Short sharp diets can be great for getting into shape for a holiday or special occasion, but they must be followed by several weeks of moderate eating if you want to keep the weight off for any length of time.

Weight that is lost very quickly tends to be regained very quickly too, partly because the loss is largely glycogen instead of fat (see page 31) and partly because of a long-term drop in basal metabolic rate.

LIGHT MEALS

DAY 1

BREAKFAST ALLOWANCE: 25 g/1 oz Shredded Wheat, Weetabix, Weetaflakes *or* Puffed Wheat, with 7 g/¼ oz bran.

Cheese and caper sandwich: 50 g/2 oz cottage cheese, 15 g/½ oz capers and 50 g/2 oz wholewheat bread
Fruit: 1 apple

Pork casserole: follow recipe on page 113 but leave out the soy sauce and sugar and add 50 g/2 oz mushrooms 5 minutes before the end of cooking.
Vegetables: 100 g/3½ oz carrots
Oranges and figs: simmer 50 g/2 oz dried figs in 4 tbsp orange juice for 20 minutes or until soft. Allow to cool and mix with 100 g/3½ oz fresh orange slices.

DAY 2

As day 1

Liver pâté and tomato sandwich: 50 g/2 oz **liver pâté** (see Breastfeeding Diet, page 78) and 100 g/3½ oz sliced tomatoes with 50 g/2 oz wholewheat bread
Fruit: 100 g/3½ oz cherries or grapes

Baked jacket potato: 150 g/5 oz potato with 100 g/3½ oz seasoned cottage cheese.
Ratatouille (page 114)
Baked apple: 100 g/3½ oz apple filled with 15 g/½ oz raisins

DAY 3

As day 1

Baked beans on toast: 100 g/3½ oz baked beans and 50 g/2 oz tomato on 50 g/2 oz wholewheat toast
Fruit: 1 pear

Indian chicken (page 106)
Salad: 100 g/3½ oz lettuce, watercress, cucumber and green pepper
Banana and prunes: 100 g/3½ oz chopped banana mixed with 50 g/2 oz stewed prunes

DAY 4

As day 1

Corn and cheese sandwich: 50 g/2 oz cottage cheese, 40 g/1½ oz sweetcorn (kernel corn) flavoured with Tabasco (hot pepper sauce) with 50 g/2 oz wholewheat bread
Fruit: 1 orange

Plaice (flounder) in orange sauce: (see High fibre, Low fat Diet, Day 9, page 67)
Vegetables: 100 g/3½ oz broccoli or green beans
Banana and melon: 50 g/2 oz chopped banana mixed with 100 g/3½ oz chopped melon

DAY 5

As day 1

Cucumber sandwich: 50 g/2 oz sliced cucumber, 1 tsp low calorie mayonnaise with 50 g/2 oz wholewheat bread
Fruit: 1 orange

Lamb with garlic and rosemary (page 108)
Vegetable: 100 g/3½ oz shredded white cabbage cooked in just enough boiling water to cover. Serve well seasoned with freshly ground black pepper.
Fruit: 1 grapefruit

DAILY ALLOWANCE: 600 ml/1 pint (2½ cups) skimmed milk; unlimited water and herb teas; 1 daily multivitamin plus iron

It is a well known and accepted fact that dieting depresses the metabolism. Not so well known or accepted is the fact that it may remain depressed once the diet is over – *even if all the weight that was lost has been regained*. If metabolic rate does not recover to 100 per cent each time, it is not surprising that it gets more and more difficult to lose weight with each successive diet.

In one Scottish experiment, set up to assess the effects of yo-yoing weight levels on metabolic rate, volunteers were over-fed one month and under-fed the next so that their weight gains and losses would reflect the typical pattern of on/off dieters. After 18 months, when the results were analysed, every one of the volunteers showed a measurable drop in metabolic rate – one by as much as 15 per cent – even though they were back at the weight at which they had started.

Diets of less than 750 calories a day are nearly always self-defeating because glycogen levels become so depleted that most of the lost weight is regained almost immediately. People who fast or go on very stringent diets may, on breaking them, step up their intake to as little as 1,000 calories and still find themselves regaining weight over the next day or days.

A rapid loss of glycogen is not a good idea. It interferes with concentration and makes you feel listless, lethargic, depressed, headachy and hungry. Keep some carbohydrate in your diet and you will feel much better.

BREAKFASTS	LIGHT MEALS	MAIN MEALS	
As day 1	Soup julienne: mix 2 tsp beef extract with 200 ml/⅓ pint (⅞ cup) boiling water. Add 25 g/1 oz diced carrot and simmer for 10 minutes. Add 25 g/1 oz sliced leek and seasoning, and continue cooking until the vegetables are just tender. 75 g/3 oz wholewheat bread with 15 g/½ oz low fat spread Fruit: 1 pear	Fillet steak: 150 g/5 oz fillet (tenderloin), grilled (broiled), using no oil. Season well and remove all fat. Vegetables: 100 g/3½ oz grilled (broiled) mushrooms, 50 g/2 oz grilled (broiled) tomatoes and 100 g/3½ oz peas. Stewed apple: 100 g/3½ oz apple stewed without sugar	DAY 6
As day 1	Tomato sandwich: 100 g/3½ oz sliced tomatoes, 1 tsp low calorie mayonnaise and 50 g/2 oz wholewheat bread Fruit: 1 peach	**Kidneys in red wine** (page 108) Brown rice: 40 g/1½ oz boiled Salad: 100 g/3½ oz lettuce, watercress, cucumber and green pepper Orange jelly: dissolve 7 g/¼ oz (1 envelope) gelatine in 7 tbsp fresh orange juice. Leave in the refrigerator for 2 hours until set.	DAY 7
As day 1	Ham sandwich: 50 g/2 oz lean ham, 50 g/2 oz shredded lettuce, 1 tsp low calorie mayonnaise and 50 g/2 oz wholewheat bread Fruit: 1 apple	Baked fish: wrap 200 g/7 oz cod steak in foil with 50 g/2 oz sweetcorn (kernel corn), 2 sliced tomatoes, a little celery salt and freshly ground black pepper. Bake in a moderately hot oven, 200°C (400°F) or Gas Mark 6, for 15 minutes. Vegetable: 100 g/3½ oz broccoli Raspberry yogurt: 100 g/5 oz plain yogurt mixed with 100 g/3½ oz fresh or frozen raspberries NB Soak apricots for tomorrow	DAY 8
As day 1	Liver pâté and tomato sandwich: 50 g/2 oz **liver pâté** (see Breastfeeding Diet, page 78), 100 g/3½ oz sliced tomatoes and 50 g/2 oz wholewheat bread Fruit: 1 apple	Poached egg and potato: 1 poached egg with 150 g/5 oz mashed potato made with skimmed milk. Coleslaw: 50 g/2 oz cabbage, 25 g/1 oz grated carrot, 15 g/½ oz grated onion and 7 g/¼ oz shredded red pepper mixed with 7 g/¼ oz sultanas (golden raisins), 2 tsp low fat dressing (page 110) and seasoning. Fruit compote: 25 g/1 oz dried apricots stewed and mixed with 50 g/2 oz chopped banana	DAY 9
As day 1	Crab and tomato sandwich: 50 g/2 oz fresh or canned crabmeat, 50 g/2 oz sliced tomatoes, 1 tsp low calorie mayonnaise and 50 g/2 oz wholewheat bread Fruit: 1 pear	Lemon chicken escalope: remove the skin from 125 g/4 oz chicken breast and beat well. Coat with 7 g/¼ oz wholemeal flour and fry for 5 minutes each side in 2 tsp oil. Remove and keep warm. Add the juice of 1 lemon and seasoning to the pan. Bring to the boil, pour over chicken. Vegetable: 100 g/3½ oz runner (string) beans Blackberry and port mousse: stew 75 g/3 oz fresh or frozen blackberries with 1 tsp sugar until tender. Blend with 1 tbsp plain yogurt, 1 tsp lemon juice and 1 tsp port. Sprinkle over 7 g/¼ oz (1 envelope) gelatine and stir until dissolved. Leave in a cool place to set.	DAY 10

Calories 1200 • Protein 27% • Fat 16% (maximum recommended intake 35%) • Carbohydrate 57% • Fibre 33 g • Vitamin A 1069 mg (RDA) • Calcium 1187 mg

HIGH FIBRE, LOW FAT

The average westerner eats some 20 g/³⁄₄oz of fibre per 2000 calories. Although this diet contains nearly half that in terms of calories, its fibre content is more than half as much again.

In this diet, half your fibre comes from cereals and wholewheat bread and half from fruit, vegetables, beans and pulses. Once you have lost weight, keep to the principles and increase the quantities for an excellent weight-maintenance eating plan.

In its report on Dietary Fibre, the Royal College of Physicians has suggested that substantial health benefits may be gained by increasing the amount of fibre which we eat, particularly in the form of cereals.

Lack of fibre in the diet has been implicated in at least 12 diseases, from cancer of the colon and diverticulitis to gallstones and varicose veins. These diseases are known as the 'diseases of civilisation' because they are much commoner in industrialized countries than in less-developed ones, such as those in rural Africa, where fibre intake is 3 or 4 times higher.

Hand in hand with lack of fibre and a highly refined diet goes a surfeit of fat. It is no coincidence that many diseases which are linked with excessive fat intake, such as coronary heart disease, have also been linked with a low fibre intake.

Fibre regulates the rate at which food is broken down, digested and released into the bloodstream, so helping to ensure a smooth running digestive system and (good news for slimmers) providing a continuous supply of energy which keeps you feeling fuller longer...

Food in its natural state is high in fibre. If you take away the fibre, you are left with the pure 'refined' sugar. This 'refined' sugar rushes into the bloodstream and loads the body with far more sugar than it is capable of dealing with at any one time because it cannot produce enough insulin to keep the blood/sugar ratio at a sensible level. If you continually do this, the cells that produce the insulin may eventually give up the struggle and the result will be maturity-onset diabetes – a disease which is more common in developed countries, such as Britain and the USA, than in less-developed countries where food is still largely eaten in its natural state.

In the past, doctors were reluctant to accept that fibre might have some subtle beneficial effects because they considered that it was merely 'roughage' – indigestible food that passed unaltered through the gut and out the other end. Its laxative effects were attributed to the fact that it increased bulk and helped push everything along.

Although there is some truth in this, we now know that fibre is much more than an inert bulking agent and that it is actually broken down and, indeed, digested in the colon. Some of the by-products of this process have a chemical effect on the muscles of the colon wall, inducing them to be more active and helping to guard against constipation.

Fibre has another vital protective function, by giving the bacteria that colonize the lower reaches of the intestine something to work on. Highly refined food, which is digested well before it reaches the colon, does not keep the bacteria fully occupied with the result that they may start to produce toxic substances and carcinogens (cancer-producing agents).

As fibre is metabolized in the colon it produces breakdown products known as volatile fatty acids (VFAs). Cows and sheep are known to be able to re-absorb them and to use them as their chief source of energy, explaining why they can subsist quite happily on vast amounts of fibre in the form of grass or even straw. There is now some evidence that human beings produce VFAs too and that people on extremely high-fibre diets may derive a proportion of their energy from fibre, just as cows do. It is intriguing to think that, with just a little change in physiology, we might have been as well able to live on grass as we do now on bread.

As Vitamin A is found mainly in fats, such as butter and fish oils, you should be aware of alternative sources when you limit your fat intake. Eat more yellow or orange fruits and vegetables (carrots, apricots, etc) and dark green vegetables, such as watercress, spring greens and spinach.

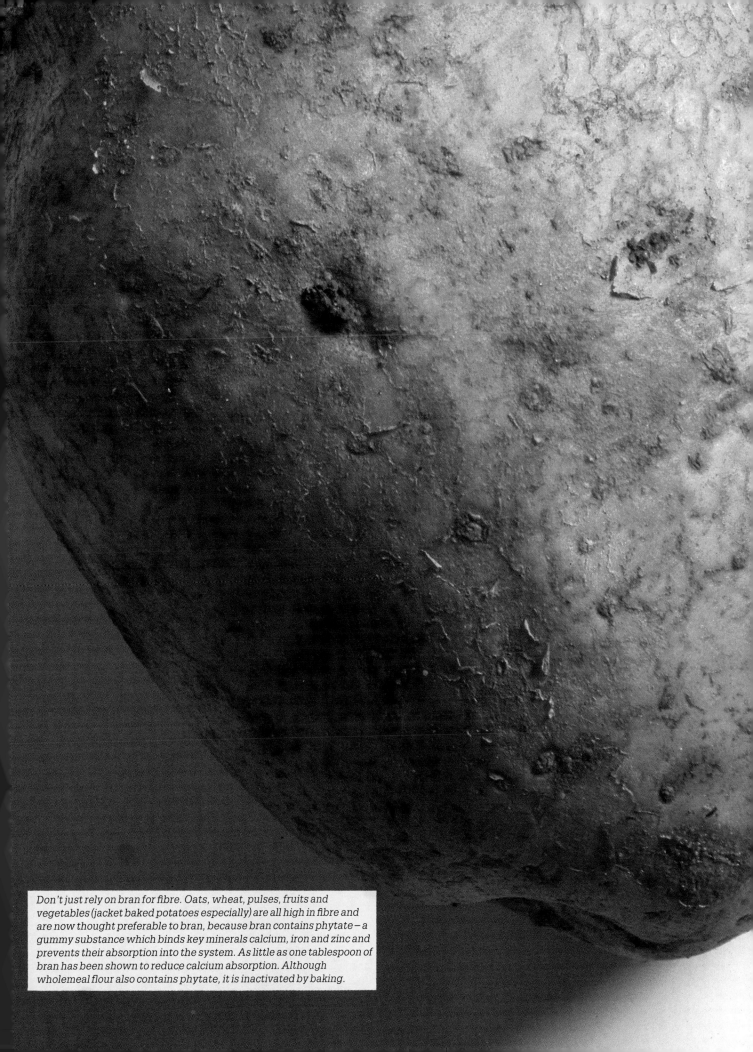

Don't just rely on bran for fibre. Oats, wheat, pulses, fruits and vegetables (jacket baked potatoes especially) are all high in fibre and are now thought preferable to bran, because bran contains phytate – a gummy substance which binds key minerals calcium, iron and zinc and prevents their absorption into the system. As little as one tablespoon of bran has been shown to reduce calcium absorption. Although wholemeal flour also contains phytate, it is inactivated by baking.

	BREAKFASTS	LIGHT MEALS	MAIN MEALS
DAY 1	BREAKFAST ALLOWANCE: 25 g/1 oz Shredded Wheat, Weetabix, Weetaflakes *or* Puffed Wheat	Tomato and peanut sandwich: 20 g/¾ oz peanut butter, 50 g/2 oz sliced tomato and 75 g/3 oz wholewheat bread Fruit: 2 pears	**Sweet and sour pork** Brown rice: 40 g/1½ oz boiled Vegetables: 100 g/3½ oz raw beansprouts Figs and oranges: soak 25 g/1 oz dried figs in 6 tbsp fresh orange juice for about 4 hours or until soft. If wished, simmer gently for 20 minutes, then cool and mix with 100 g/3½ oz fresh orange segments. NB Soak beans for tomorrow.
DAY 2	As day 1	Poached egg: 1 poached egg and 1 grilled (broiled) tomato on 75 g/3 oz wholewheat toast with 15 g/½ oz low fat spread 150 g/5 oz plain yogurt NB Soak lentils and make stock for tomorrow.	**Beef and bean casserole** Vegetable: 150 g/5 oz jacket baked potato Orange jelly: 150 ml/¼ pint (⅔ cup) fresh orange juice set with 1 tsp gelatine
DAY 3	As day 1	Lentil soup (page 109) 75 g/3 oz wholewheat bread Fruit: 2 pears	**Wholewheat pan pizza** (page 123) Coleslaw: 100 g/3½ oz grated white cabbage and 100 g/3½ oz grated carrot mixed with 20 g/¾ oz **low fat dressing**(page 110) and seasoning Fruit: 100 g/3½ oz grapes NB Soak prunes for tomorrow.
DAY 4	As day 1	Ham and lettuce sandwich: 50 g/2 oz cooked ham, 50 g/2 oz lettuce and 75 g/3 oz wholewheat bread with 15 g/½ oz low calorie mayonnaise Fruit: 2 apples	**Fish pie** (page 104) Use sweetcorn (kernel corn) in place of peas Vegetables: 100 g/3½ oz runner (string) beans Stewed prunes: 100 g/3½ oz prunes stewed without sugar
DAY 5	As day 1	Baked beans on toast: 200 g/7 oz baked beans and 50 g/2 oz grilled (broiled) tomato on 75 g/3 oz wholewheat toast Fruit: 1 banana	Lamb kebabs: 100 g/3½ oz cubed lean lamb, 25 g/1 oz quartered onion, 50 g/2 oz small whole tomatoes, 50 g/2 oz whole mushrooms and bay leaves, arranged alternately on a skewer, seasoned and grilled (broiled) or barbecued Brown rice: 40 g/1½ oz boiled Salad: 100 g/3½ oz watercress, 100 g/3½ oz chicory (endive) and 50 g/2 oz orange segments with 2 tsp **low fat dressing** (page 110) Raspberry yogurt: 150 g/5 oz fresh raspberries
DAY 6	As day 1	Cheese and pickle sandwich: 40 g/1½ oz Edam cheese, 2 tsp pickle and 75 g/3 oz wholewheat bread Fruit: 2 apples	**Lemon chicken escalope** (see 10-day Blitz Diet, page 63). Use 150 g/5 oz chicken. Vegetables: 100 g/3½ oz boiled potato and 100 g/3½ oz broccoli Apple compote: 150 g/5 oz apple stewed with 25 g/1 oz raisins
DAY 7	As day 1	Prawn and lettuce sandwich: 100 g/3½ oz prawns (shrimp), 50 g/2 oz lettuce and 20 g/¾ oz low calorie mayonnaise with 75 g/3 oz wholewheat bread	Roast meat: 100 g/3½ oz lean roast meat with 2 tbsp **low fat gravy** (page 110) Vegetables: 150 g/5 oz jacket baked potato, 100 g/3½ oz carrots and 100 g/3½ oz peas Peaches with plum sauce: 100 g/3½ oz stewed plums, stoned (pitted) and puréed, and served with 100 g/3½ oz poached, sliced fresh peaches NB Soak haricot beans for tomorrow.

DAILY ALLOWANCE: 600 ml/1 pint (2½ cups) skimmed milk

BREAKFASTS	LIGHT MEALS	MAIN MEALS	
WEEK 2 As day 1	Tomato sandwich: 100 g/3½ oz tomatoes, 20 g/¾ oz low calorie mayonnaise and 75 g/3 oz wholewheat bread Fruit: 2 apples	Bean and tuna fish salad: mix 50 g/2 oz cooked and cooled haricot beans with 50 g/2 oz drained tuna, 25 g/1 oz finely chopped onion, lemon juice, crushed garlic, freshly chopped parsley and seasoning. Vegetables: 150 g/5 oz boiled new potato and 100 g/3½ oz green pepper *Note:* to prepare the pepper, cut it in half, remove pith and seeds, and flatten. Place under a preheated grill (broiler) until the skin is blackened. Remove skin and serve at once. Banana yogurt: 150 g/5 oz plain yogurt with 100 g/3½ oz banana.	DAY 8
As day 1	**Lentil soup** (page 109) 75 g/3 oz wholewheat bread Fruit: 1 pear	Plaice in orange sauce: poach 200 g/7 oz plaice (flounder) fillet in 120 ml/4 fl oz (½ cup) fresh orange juice. Remove fish and keep warm. Thicken sauce with 1 tsp cornflour (cornstarch) mixed with 1 tsp water and season well. Serve with orange slices. Vegetables: 150 g/5 oz boiled new potato and 100 g/3½ oz runner (string) beans Fruit: 100 g/3½ oz grapes or cherries NB Soak beans for tomorrow.	DAY 9
As day 1	Beetroot open sandwich: 75 g/3 oz curd cheese, 2 tsp horseradish sauce and 100 g/3½ oz pickled or fresh sliced beetroot (beet) on 75 g/3 oz wholewheat bread Fruit: 2 oranges	**Chilli con carne** (page 101) Vegetable: 150 g/5 oz jacket baked potato Baked apple: 100 g/3½ oz apple, filled with 25 g/1 oz raisins and served with 65 g/2½ oz plain yogurt NB Soak apricots for tomorrow.	DAY 10
As day 1	Crab and beansprout sandwich: 50 g/2 oz fresh or canned crabmeat, 50 g/2 oz beansprouts and 75 g/3 oz wholewheat bread with 20 g/¾ oz low calorie mayonnaise Fruit: 200 g/7 oz grapes	**Poached chicken** Vegetables: 100 g/3½ oz carrots and 150 g/5 oz boiled potato Stewed apricots: 50 g/2 oz dried apricots soaked overnight and stewed in a little water until soft. Serve with 15 g/½ oz chopped walnuts	DAY 11
As day 1	Cucumber salad: slice ½ cucumber lengthways, scoop out the centre and chop. Mix with 50 g/2 oz curd cheese, 40 g/1½ oz chopped red pepper, 6 stoned (pitted) black olives and seasoning. Fill cucumber halves. 75 g/3 oz wholewheat bread Fruit: 2 pears	**Beef goulash** (page 98) Vegetables: 150 g/5 oz jacket baked potato and 100 g/3½ oz cauliflower Blackcurrant yogurt: 100 g/3½ oz fresh or frozen blackcurrants stewed until soft and cooled. Mix with 150 g/5 oz plain yogurt and add a little saccharine, if wished. NB Soak lentils for tomorrow.	DAY 12
As day 1	Tuna and tomato sandwich: 75 g/3 oz tuna, 100 g/3½ oz sliced tomato and 75 g/3 oz wholewheat bread Fruit: 1 banana	**Vegetable curry** (page 121) 40 g/1½ oz green mango chutney Brown rice: 40 g/1½ oz boiled Yogurt and cucumber: 50 g/2 oz chopped cucumber mixed with 50 g/2 oz plain yogurt. Chill before serving. Fruit: 200 g/7 oz melon	DAY 13
As day 1	Cheese and sweetcorn sandwich: 75 g/3 oz cottage cheese, 50 g/2 oz sweetcorn (kernel corn), 25 g/1 oz shredded lettuce and 75 g/3 oz wholewheat bread Fruit: 100 g/3½ oz grapes or cherries	**Roast beef:** 100 g/3½ oz lean roast beef served with 2 tbsp **low fat gravy** (page 110). Vegetables: 150 g/5 oz jacket baked potato, 150 g/5 oz peas and 100 g/3½ oz cauliflower Fruit salad: 150 g/5 oz sliced fresh peaches with 100 g/3½ oz fresh strawberries *OR* Cheese and biscuits: 25 g/1 oz Edam cheese with 1 Digestive biscuit (Graham cracker)	DAY 14

VEGETARIAN

Variety is the keynote of the vegetarian diet. Eat from as wide a range of foods as possible – mixing fruit with vegetables, nuts, seeds, cereals, eggs and dairy products – and you will have a diet that is lower in fat, higher in fibre and as adequate in protein as any other diet. And remember, vegetarians tend not only to be healthier and longer-living, but slimmer too...

Protein, often seized upon as a major problem for vegetarians, is the one component of the diet most of us get more than enough of. In recognition of this, official bodies, such as the Food and Agriculture Organisation, are now *reducing* their recommended intake of protein.

A second misconception is that because meat contains most protein it also contains the best. Eggs, milk, fish, cheese and whole rice (in that order) *all* provide better quality protein than red meat and poultry; while vegetable sources, such as nuts, seeds, grains and pulses, also provide some.

Vegans, who do not eat dairy foods, eggs or fish, should take care to mix their plant proteins. Of the 22 amino acids in protein, there are 8 that the body cannot make and that must therefore be found in the diet. The egg is a uniquely valuable protein source because it contains all 8, and in the right concentrations, while grains and pulses contain different and complementary amino acids. Combine them, as with beans on toast or lentil curry with rice, to get the protein you need.

MAKE SURE YOU GET ENOUGH of vitamins B12, B1, B2 and D and iron... especially if you are a vegan. B12 is particularly important for people choosing to make their diet completely free of animal products (dairy foods, eggs, even honey) because these are the major nutritional sources of the vitamin. Although supplementation is usually necessary, there are recorded cases of British vegans living 14 to 17 years without any form of B12 supplement, and still maintaining apparently normal levels of the vitamin. This has led nutritionists to theorize that some people are able to manufacture and absorb B12 in their own gut. But this emphatically does not apply to everyone.

B1 (thiamin) and B2 (riboflavin) can be found in pulses, yeast, wheatgerm (an excellent source of most of the B vitamins) and cereals and should not be a problem if the diet is varied. You should also be getting sufficient vitamin D if you get enough sunshine, as the primary source of the vitamin is sunlight; secondary sources are fatty fish, margarine and fish oil. The best, easily absorbed source of iron is meat and fatty fish like sardines. Secondary sources are eggs, soya and dark green vegetables. Taking a Vitamin C-rich fruit or vegetable with your meal will help increase iron uptake from your food by as much as 4 times.

Vegetarian diets can protect against high blood pressure. One study in Israel revealed that only 2 per cent of a group of vegetarians had high blood pressure compared with 26 per cent in a meat-eating group of similar age and social circumstance. In Australia a group of men actually *lowered* their abnormal blood pressures by switching to a vegetarian diet for 6 weeks. When they returned to eating meat, their blood pressures rose to their previous levels.

It is now generally agreed that excessive meat consumption and over-indulgence in animal fats can contribute to a damaging effect on the arteries, to coronary heart disease and to a whole number of cancers, including those of the bowel, colon, ovary, breast, pancreas and prostate. Eliminating meat from the diet automatically cuts out a major source of fat. We have become accustomed to thinking of meat as protein, but in fact even lean meat, with a little visible fat removed, still contains large amounts of fat up to 60 per cent or more of the total weight once water is discounted. Even if not intending to eliminate meat from the diet entirely, we should all cut down. Once a day is more than adequate, twice excessive.

NB *VERY RESTRICTIVE VEGETARIAN DIETS, SUCH AS MACROBIOTIC DIETS, NEED CAREFUL PLANNING AND SUPPLEMENTATION. GET PROFESSIONAL NUTRITIONAL ADVICE BEFORE EMBARKING ON THEM.*

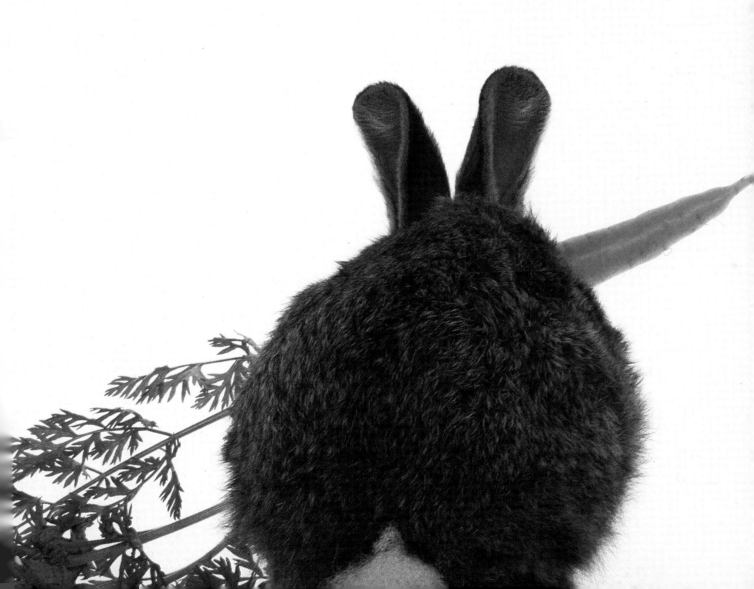

The ultimate vegetarian . . . Luckily, human herbivores don't have to rely on rabbit food to enjoy the health benefits that can be derived from a vegetarian diet, see left. Find protein in nuts, beans, pulses, wholegrains, lentils and dairy foods too.

	BREAKFASTS	LIGHT MEALS	MAIN MEALS
DAY 1	BREAKFAST ALLOWANCE: 25 g/1 oz Shredded Wheat, Weetabix, Weetaflakes *or* Puffed Wheat	Tomato sandwich: 100 g/3½ oz sliced tomatoes, 50 g/2 oz shredded lettuce, 2 tsp low calorie mayonnaise and 75 g/3 oz wholewheat bread Fruit: 2 apples	Eggs on vegetable purée Vegetable: 200 g/7 oz jacket baked potato Fruit: 1 pear Cheese: 50 g/2 oz Camembert
DAY 2	As day 1	Cottage cheese and fennel sandwich: 50 g/2 oz chopped fennel, 100 g/3½ oz cottage cheese and 75 g/3 oz wholewheat bread Fruit: 2 oranges	**Vegetable curry** (page 121) served with 40 g/1½ oz mango chutney. Brown rice: 50 g/2 oz boiled Fruit: 100 g/3½ oz fresh or frozen raspberries
DAY 3	As day 1	Beetroot open sandwich: 75 g/3 oz curd cheese mixed with 2 tsp horseradish sauce, 100 g/3½ oz sliced beetroot (beet) or tomato and 75 g/3 oz wholewheat bread Fruit: 1 apple	**Wholewheat pan pizza** (page 123) Salad: 150 g/5 oz lettuce, watercress, green pepper and cucumber Fruit: 1 pear NB Soak beans for tomorrow.
DAY 4	As day 1	Poached egg: 1 poached egg with 1 grilled (broiled) tomato on 75 g/3 oz wholewheat toast Fruit: 1 peach or pear	**Mixed bean salad** Salad: 150 g/5 oz watercress, grated carrot and chicory (endive) Ginger yogurt: 150 g/5 oz plain yogurt mixed with 50 g/2 oz chopped, crystallized stem (preserved) ginger
DAY 5	As day 1	Cheese and peanut sandwich: 15 g/½ oz sugar-free peanut butter mixed with 20 g/¾ oz curd cheese and 50 g/2 oz chopped apple with 75 g/3 oz wholewheat bread Fruit: 1 orange	Broccoli with cheese sauce: cook 150 g/5 oz broccoli tips until just tender. Prepare 150 ml/¼ pint (⅔ cup) **white sauce** (page 123) and add 50 g/2 oz grated Cheddar cheese. Pour the cheese sauce over the freshly cooked broccoli. Vegetable: 150 g/5 oz jacket baked potato Fruit: 200 g/7 oz melon
DAY 6	As day 1	Grapes and blue cheese sandwich: 25 g/1 oz seeded and halved grapes, 75 g/3 oz blue cheese, 25 g/1 oz curd cheese and 75 g/3 oz wholewheat bread Fruit: 100 g/3½ oz banana	**Gnocchi with tomato sauce** (page 105) Fruit: 1 pear
DAY 7	As day 1	100 g/3½ oz cooked, canned or fresh salsify Tomato salad: 100 g/3½ oz sliced tomatoes, freshly chopped basil, seasoning and **low fat dressing** (page 110) with 50 g/2 oz olives Fruit: 100 g/3½ oz grapes	Vegetable omelette: prepare an omelette using 2 eggs, a little skimmed milk, 2 tsp freshly chopped chives and seasoning. Cook in a non-stick frying pan (skillet) and fill with 100 g/3½ oz cooked broad (fava) beans or peas. Orange yogurt: 150 g/5 oz plain yogurt mixed with 100 g/3½ oz fresh orange segments

DAILY ALLOWANCE: 600 ml/1 pint (2½ cups) skimmed milk

BREAKFASTS	LIGHT MEALS	MAIN MEALS	
As day 1	Pickle and cheese sandwich: 50 g/2 oz Edam cheese, 25 g/1 oz sweet pickle and 75 g/3 oz wholewheat bread Fruit: 2 apples NB Soak lentils for tomorrow.	Stuffed tomatoes: slice the tops and scoop out the seeds from 2 large tomatoes. Fill with curd cheese flavoured with Tabasco (hot pepper sauce) and paprika, and sprinkle with freshly chopped herbs. Vegetable: 150 g/5 oz jacket baked potato Blackcurrant and banana dessert: stew 100 g/3½ oz fresh or frozen blackcurrants, cool, and purée in a blender. Stir in 50 g/2 oz chopped banana and serve chilled.	DAY 8
As day 1	Lentil soup (page 109) 75 g/3 oz wholewheat bread Fruit: 1 pear	Vegetable lasagne (page 121) Wholewheat pasta: 50 g/2 oz boiled Spiced grapefruit: 100 g/3½ oz fresh grapefruit, sprinkled with cinnamon and browned under a hot grill (broiler)	DAY 9
As day 1	Baked beans on toast: 150 g/5 oz baked beans and 50 g/2 oz tomato on 75 g/3 oz wholewheat toast Fruit: 1 orange	Cheese pie Red cabbage with apples (page 115) Fruit: 1 pear	DAY 10
As day 1	Avocado cheese sandwich: 40 g/1½ oz sliced avocado, 50 g/2 oz cottage cheese and 75 g/3 oz wholewheat bread Fruit: 2 apples NB Soak lentils for tomorrow.	Middle Eastern rice (page 111) Chicory and orange salad: 100 g/3½ oz chicory (endive) and 100 g/3½ oz fresh orange segments tossed in low fat dressing (page 110) Fruit: 200 g/7 oz melon	DAY 11
As day 1	Lentil soup (page 109) 75 g/3 oz wholewheat bread Fruit: 2 pears	Courgettes au gratin Hot beetroot: 100 g/3½ oz thinly sliced cooked beetroot (beet) heated through with the juice of 1 lemon or small orange Fruit and cheese: 200 g/7 oz sliced fresh plums with 50 g/2 oz curd cheese NB Soak lentils for tomorrow.	DAY 12
As day 1	Cheese and pineapple sandwich: 50 g/2 oz cottage cheese, 25 g/1 oz chopped pineapple and 75 g/3 oz wholewheat bread Fruit: 2 apples	Wholewheat spaghetti with tomato and basil sauce (page 123). Add 25 g/1 oz cooked lentils to the sauce. Oranges and figs: soak 50 g/2 oz dried figs in 6 tbsp orange juice for 4 hours or until soft. If wished, simmer gently for 20 minutes, then cool and mix with 100 g/3½ oz fresh orange slices.	DAY 13
As day 1	Cheese and tomato sandwich: 50 g/2 oz curd cheese, 50 g/2 oz finely chopped green pepper, 50 g/2 oz sliced tomato and 75 g/3 oz wholewheat bread Fruit: 100 g/3½ oz grapes	Mushroom omelette: prepare an omelette using 2 eggs and skimmed milk. Fill with 100 g/3½ oz poached mushrooms. 50 g/2 oz wholewheat bread with 15 g/½ oz low fat spread Salad: 150 g/5 oz mixed green vegetables Yogurt with raisins: 150 g/5 oz plain yogurt mixed with 15 g/½ oz raisins	DAY 14

PREGNANCY

Because eating well is essential when pregnant or breastfeeding, these diets are healthy eating programmes rather than stringent slimming regimens. They are designed to be as easy and flexible as possible. There is no need to weigh out quantities exactly; just follow the broad outlines of the diet using standard recipes where none are given and cutting down on fat and sugar where possible. If you want to use fat in your recipes and/or on bread or potatoes, substitute skimmed milk for half or even all the whole milk allowance.

There is increasing evidence that the nutritional status of *both* partners, but the woman especially, is important to the future health of the unborn child – particularly around the time of conception – when sperm and eggs are developing and cells are fusing and dividing. These processes draw on the body's *immediate* nutritional reserves, which must be adequate for the biochemical changes involved in the development of the fetus to go ahead normally.

Diet before conception as well as afterwards must therefore be a priority to give your baby the best possible start in life. Stop smoking, cut alcohol consumption right down and preferably out altogether, and revise your diet – making sure it is high in protein, iron and zinc (red meat is an outstandingly good source of all these), wholegrains and folic acid – well before stopping contraception. Folic acid, extremely important to the very early development of the fetus, can be found in most vegetables, liver, oranges, melons, avocados, nuts, broccoli and Brussels sprouts – the last two are particularly good sources. Eat them briefly cooked or raw in salads.

Feelings of nausea, with or without actual vomiting, often occur during early pregnancy. Help yourself by eating little and often. A dry biscuit (cracker) or piece of toast taken with a little tea or fruit juice can sometimes help reduce the sickness, particularly if taken on waking. As prolonged and frequent episodes of vomiting can deplete important nutrients, you should consult your doctor if vomiting persists.

As long as women are fairly active and well-fed before they conceive*, they need to eat very little more once they do become pregnant, according to on-going studies in Scotland, Holland, Thailand and the Gambia. These reveal that when women eat according to instinct, and not according to what they are told by their doctors, they raise their intake very little – by 100 calories a day or even less – with the exception of a brief period around the middle of their pregnancy when intake may rise more steeply.

These findings, which conflict very strongly with the old advice to 'eat for two', suggest that there is a biological control operating during pregnancy which conserves energy by slowing down the general level of activity, lowering metabolic rate and instituting other biochemical changes – rather in the same way that starvation/crash dieting is now understood to do (see page 34). Previous estimates of food requirements during pregnancy,

which have ignored this biological control factor, have therefore tended to be unrealistically high.

Many women date their weight problems from pregnancy and it is possible that if they feel they must eat much more than they want to when they become pregnant, they could be setting themselves up for weight problems later on. The key, it now appears, is to have the confidence to be guided by your body and listen to its needs. Your doctor will let you know if he considers you need to put on more weight at any stage. In the meantime, think more in terms of the quality of what you eat than the quantity. The diet here will give a guide.

Women who have a very sedentary lifestyle and are already subsisting on low-calorie intakes, say around 1,600, are an exception and will need to raise intake more substantially.

Obstetricians routinely advise a weight increase of around 12.5 kg (28 lb) over a pregnancy – though even here there are wide variations in the amount of weight gained with no apparent effects on the birthweight of the baby. If overweight at the start of pregnancy, however, it is possible that your obstetrician will advise restricting weight gain to about 7 kg (15½ lb) so that your weight after delivery will actually be less than at the start of your pregnancy. Let yourself be guided by your doctor.

BREAKFAST ALLOWANCES FOR DIET OVER THE PAGE:

A

1 egg (boiled, poached or scrambled);
2 slices wholewheat toast with 15 g/½ oz low fat spread and 25 g/1 oz marmalade;
150 ml/¼ pint (⅔ cup) unsweetened orange or grapefruit juice

B

40 g/1½ oz Shredded Wheat, Weetaflakes, Allbran or Weetabix and 1 tsp sugar (if necessary);
150 ml/¼ pint (⅔ cup) unsweetened orange or grapefruit juice

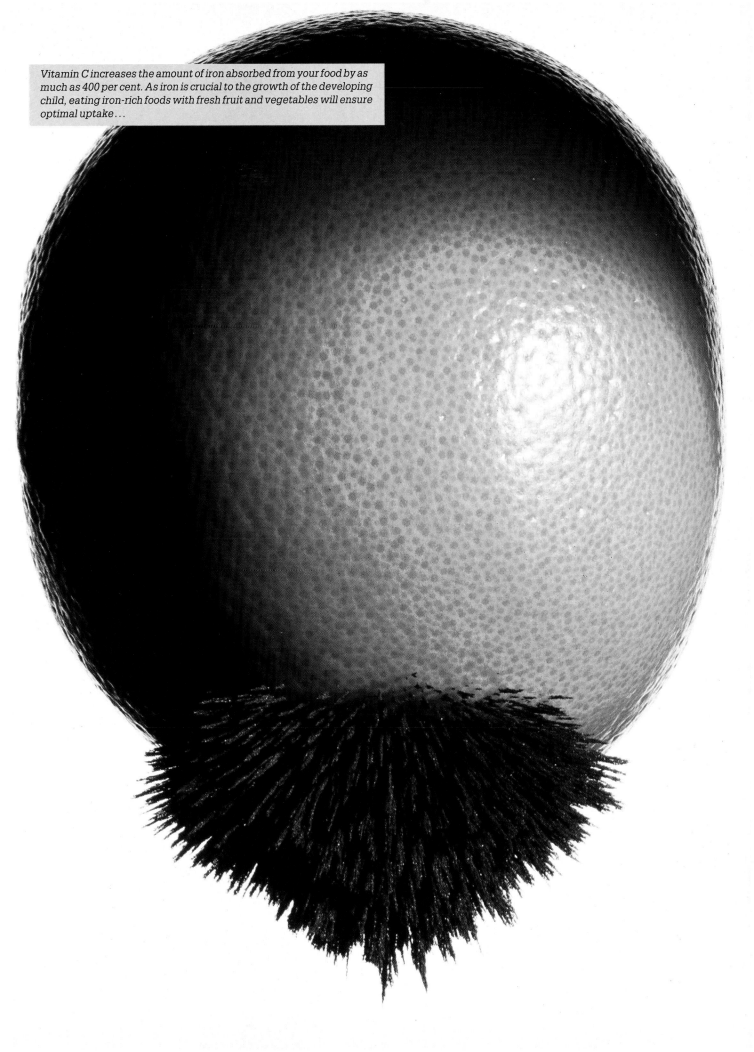

Vitamin C increases the amount of iron absorbed from your food by as much as 400 per cent. As iron is crucial to the growth of the developing child, eating iron-rich foods with fresh fruit and vegetables will ensure optimal uptake...

	BREAKFASTS	LIGHT MEALS	MAIN MEALS

DAY 1

LIGHT MEALS: Tongue and tomato sandwich: 60 g/2½ oz tongue, 100 g/3½ oz sliced tomato and 75 g/3 oz wholewheat bread with 15 g/½ oz low fat spread
Fruit: 1 orange

MAIN MEALS: **Lasagne** (page 108)
Salad: watercress and **low fat dressing** (page 110)
Fruit: 150 g/5 oz pear
Cheese: 60 g/2½ oz Camembert

DAY 2

LIGHT MEALS: Cheese and Indian pineapple salad: 50 g/2 oz pineapple, 60 g/2½ oz apple and 50 g/2 oz celery, diced and mixed together with 20 g/¾ oz low calorie mayonnaise, seasoning, pinch of curry powder and freshly chopped mixed herbs. Serve with 100 g/3½ oz cottage cheese, 75 g/3 oz wholewheat bread and 15 g/½ oz low fat spread.

MAIN MEALS: Lamb's liver: coat 150 g/5 oz lamb's liver in seasoned flour. Soften 50 g/2 oz sliced onion in 10 g/⅓ oz oil and add the liver. Take care not to overcook. Season and serve at once.
Vegetables: 150 g/5 oz boiled potato and boiled cabbage
Stewed apple and custard: 150 g/5 oz stewed apple with 150 g/5 oz custard

DAY 3

LIGHT MEALS: Poached egg: 1 poached egg on 75 g/3 oz wholewheat toast with 15 g/½ oz low fat spread
Vegetable: 1 tomato
Fruit: 1 banana
Tea: 60 g/2½ oz fruit cake

MAIN MEALS: **Watercress soup** (page 122)
Lamb with apricot stuffing
Vegetables: 150 g/5 oz boiled potato and 100 g/3½ oz green beans
Green fruit salad (page 106)

DAY 4

LIGHT MEALS: Kipper pâté: blend together 100 g/3½ oz cooked kipper fillet, 25 g/1 oz cottage cheese, crushed garlic, nutmeg, pepper and juice of ¼ lemon. Chill and serve with slices of lemon, 75 g/3 oz wholewheat bread with 20 g/¾ oz low fat spread
Salad: 50 g/2 oz watercress
Fruit: 100 g/3½ oz grapes or cherries
Tea: 60 g/2½ oz scone with 15 g/½ oz low fat spread and 30 g/1¼ oz jam (jelly)

MAIN MEALS: Beef kebab: 150 g/5 oz cubed lean beef and as many small whole tomatoes, mushrooms and onion quarters as desired. Season and grill (broil) to taste.
Brown rice: 60 g/2½ oz boiled
Salad: 100 g/3½ oz mixed green vegetables
Strawberry sorbet (page 118)

NB Soak apricots for tomorrow.

DAY 5

LIGHT MEALS: Cheese and lettuce sandwich: 60 g/2½ oz Cheddar cheese, 60 g/2½ oz shredded lettuce, 1 tbsp low calorie mayonnaise and 75 g/3 oz wholewheat bread
Fruit: 2 apples

MAIN MEALS: **Wholewheat spaghetti with chicken livers** (page 123)
(but leave out the sherry)
Apricot dessert: 150 g/5 oz stewed apricots mixed with 10 g/⅓ oz walnuts and 150 g/5 oz plain yogurt. Serve chilled.

DAY 6

LIGHT MEALS: Tuna and tomato sandwich: 60 g/2½ oz tuna, 100 g/3½ oz sliced tomatoes and 75 g/3 oz wholewheat bread with 15 g/½ oz low fat spread
Fruit: 1 banana
Tea: 2 Digestive biscuits (Graham crackers)

MAIN MEALS: **Beef goulash** (page 98)
Vegetables: 200 g/7 oz jacket baked potato and 150 g/5 oz broccoli
Winter fruit compote (page 123)

DAY 7

LIGHT MEALS: Ham and lettuce sandwich: 60 g/2½ oz lean ham, 60 g/2½ oz shredded lettuce, 1 tbsp low calorie mayonnaise and 75 g/3 oz wholewheat bread
Fruit: 100 g/3½ oz grapes or cherries
Tea: 1 slice wholewheat toast with butter and jam or honey

NB Soak lentils for tomorrow.

MAIN MEALS: Roast lamb: 150 g/5 oz lean roast lamb served with 2 tbsp **low fat gravy** (page 110)
Vegetables: 100 g/3½ oz jacket baked potato, 100 g/3½ oz peas and 100 g/3½ oz carrots
Apple crumble: 100 g/3½ oz serving with 2 tbsp single (light) cream

DAILY ALLOWANCE: 1.2 litres/1 pint (5 cups) whole milk

BREAKFASTS	LIGHT MEALS	MAIN MEALS	
	Lentil soup (page 109) 75 g/3 oz wholewheat toast with 15 g/½ oz low fat spread Yogurt: 150 g/5 oz plain yogurt Fruit: 100 g/3½ oz fresh orange segments	Cauliflower cheese: 300 g/10 oz serving Vegetable: 150 g/5 oz boiled potato Salad: 100 g/3½ oz sliced tomatoes with **low fat dressing** (page 110) Fruit salad: 150 g/5 oz fresh fruit salad	DAY 8
	Sardine and tomato sandwich: 100 g/3½ oz sardines, 100 g/3½ oz sliced tomatoes and 75 g/3 oz wholewheat bread with 15 g/½ oz low fat spread Fruit: 1 pear	**Kidneys in red wine** (page 108). Use 200 g/7 oz kidney. Brown rice: 60 g/2½ oz boiled Salad: watercress and chicory (endive) with **low fat dressing** (page 110) Rice pudding: 200 g/7 oz homemade or canned rice pudding with 30 g/1¼ oz rosehip syrup or 200 g/7 oz fresh fruit salad	DAY 9
	Smoked mackerel: 100 g/3½ oz smoked mackerel served with 50 g/2 oz watercress, slices of lemon and 75 g/3 oz wholewheat bread with 15 g/½ oz low fat spread Fruit: 200 g/7 oz grapes or cherries	Baked chicken: spread 1 chicken quarter with enough mustard and paprika to cover. Grill (broil), bake or barbecue for about 20-30 minutes until thoroughly cooked. Vegetables: 150 g/5 oz jacket baked potato and 150 g/5 oz carrots Rhubarb or prune fool: stew 150 g/5 oz rhubarb or stoned (pitted) prunes and blend with 100 g/3½ oz custard. Just before serving, add a swirl of single (light) cream.	DAY 10
	Pickle and beef sandwich: 50 g/2 oz corned beef, 100 g/3½ oz sliced tomato, 40 g/1½ oz sweet pickle and 75 g/3 oz wholewheat bread Fruit and nut yogurt: 150 g/5 oz plain yogurt mixed with 20 g/¾ oz raisins and 10 g/⅓ oz chopped mixed nuts	**Fish pie** (page 104) Vegetables: 150 g/5 oz runner (string) beans Fruit: 2 pears	DAY 11
	Cheese and lettuce sandwich: 60 g/2½ oz Cheddar cheese, 60 g/2½ oz shredded lettuce, 1 tbsp low calorie mayonnaise and 75 g/3 oz wholewheat bread Fruit: 2 apples	**Chicken Véronique** (page 100) Vegetables: 150 g/5 oz boiled potato and 150 g/5 oz broccoli Banana and ginger dessert: 50 g/2 oz chopped stem (preserved) ginger mixed with 100 g/3½ oz chopped banana and 150 g/5 oz plain yogurt. Serve chilled. NB Soak apricots for tomorrow.	DAY 12
	Baked beans on toast: 150 g/5 oz baked beans on 75 g/3 oz wholewheat toast with 15 g/½ oz low fat spread Fruit: 2 apples	**Veal escalope with ham** (page 121) Vegetables: 150 g/5 oz boiled potato and 150 g/5 oz peas Apple and apricot dessert: 100 g/3½ oz apples stewed with 50 g/2 oz dried apricots	DAY 13
	Salmon sandwich: 60 g/2½ oz canned or fresh salmon, 60 g/2½ oz shredded lettuce, 1 tbsp low calorie mayonnaise and 75 g/3 oz wholewheat bread Fruit: 200 g/7 oz melon	Roast beef: 150 g/5 oz lean roast beef with 2 tbsp **low fat gravy** (page 110) Vegetables: 100 g/3½ oz cauliflower with 150 g/5 oz carrots and 150 g/5 oz jacket baked potato Fruit and honey yogurt: 150 g/5 oz plain yogurt mixed with 120 g/4 oz fresh fruit, 1 tsp honey and 1 tsp wheatgerm	DAY 14

Protein 21% ● Fat 39% ● Carbohydrate 50% ● Fibre 34 g ● Calcium 2149 mg (1200 mg) ● B1 1.97 mg (1.1 mg) ● B2 4.30 mg (1.8 mg) ●
C 175 mg (60 mg) ● A (1,200 μg) ● Iron 16.45 mg (15 mg)

BREASTFEEDING

Breast milk is perfect for babies. It requires no preparation or sterilization and is always just the right temperature. Although its composition is largely controlled by the body in response to the baby's needs, it is also influenced by the mother's diet, which must therefore be extra nutritious.

This plan does not have to be followed exactly, but it does provide a good guide – incorporating plenty of dairy foods, including an extra pint of milk, for protein and calcium; fibre to offset constipation (a very common problem post-natally); and lots of fruit and vegetables, particularly carrots for vitamin A and dark green vegetables for folic acid.

Let yourself be guided by your hunger and keep meal times flexible, but try to eat and drink something when breastfeeding to help replace what you lose.

GETTING BACK INTO SHAPE... Attempting to slim in the first 6 weeks after the birth can reduce chances of producing milk and will certainly lower energy. Exercise is the more effective strategy. Start gently and build up gradually, giving yourself a full 9 months to get slim and fit again. It is important to start exercising as soon as you feel strong enough because the muscles are most responsive when they are healing.

Weight put on during pregnancy will tend to be lost quite slowly, but it will go as the baby's appetite increases. By the seventh week, when the baby starts taking more than you are putting in, weight should drop.

BE JUST AS CAREFUL about smoking, drinking and taking drugs as you were when pregnant. Harmful chemicals can still pass to the baby in the breast milk.

The new-born baby grows well on a low-salt, low-sugar diet. Breast milk, in particular, is low in salt. Yet intake is often raised dramatically after weaning – added either by the mother to suit her own taste or by food manufacturers to formulas and baby foods. The average salt intake of the weaned child may be more than 5 times its physiological requirement.

In some parts of the world, breastfeeding is reliably used as a method of family planning. The Kung! hunter/gatherer tribe in the Kalahari Desert, for example, manage to achieve an average space of four years between children in their families, not through any formal method of contraception but because the mother breastfeeds for three out of the four years.

In order to see whether the same protective effect might also apply to western-style breastfeeding, a research project was set up in Edinburgh with 12 nursing mothers. All of them, fortunately, wished to become pregnant again, and seven of them did – two before the return of their periods, indicating that menstruation cannot be relied upon as a mark of returned fertility.

These results do not rule out the contraceptive effectiveness of breastfeeding for western mothers, but they do show that the protective effects diminish with the western pattern of infrequent suckling, often supplemented with bottle or other type of infant food. In the study, there was a close correlation between conception and frequency and duration of breastfeeding. None of the women became pregnant until they were only feeding their child three times a day, or less, although two did actually ovulate (and so were potentially fertile) when breast feeding four times a day. This suggests that breastfeeding only becomes an effective contraceptive when taking place at least five times a day – preferably on demand – for periods of at least ten minutes a time.

BREAKFAST ALLOWANCE FOR DIET OVER THE PAGE:
A
1 egg (boiled, poached or scrambled); 50 g/2 oz wholewheat toast with 15 g/½ oz low fat spread and 25 g/1 oz marmalade; 150 ml/¼ pint (⅔ cup) unsweetened fruit juice
B
40 g/1½ oz Shredded Wheat, Weetaflakes, Weetabix *or* Allbran with 1 tsp sugar (if necessary); 150 ml/¼ pint (⅔ cup) unsweetened fruit juice

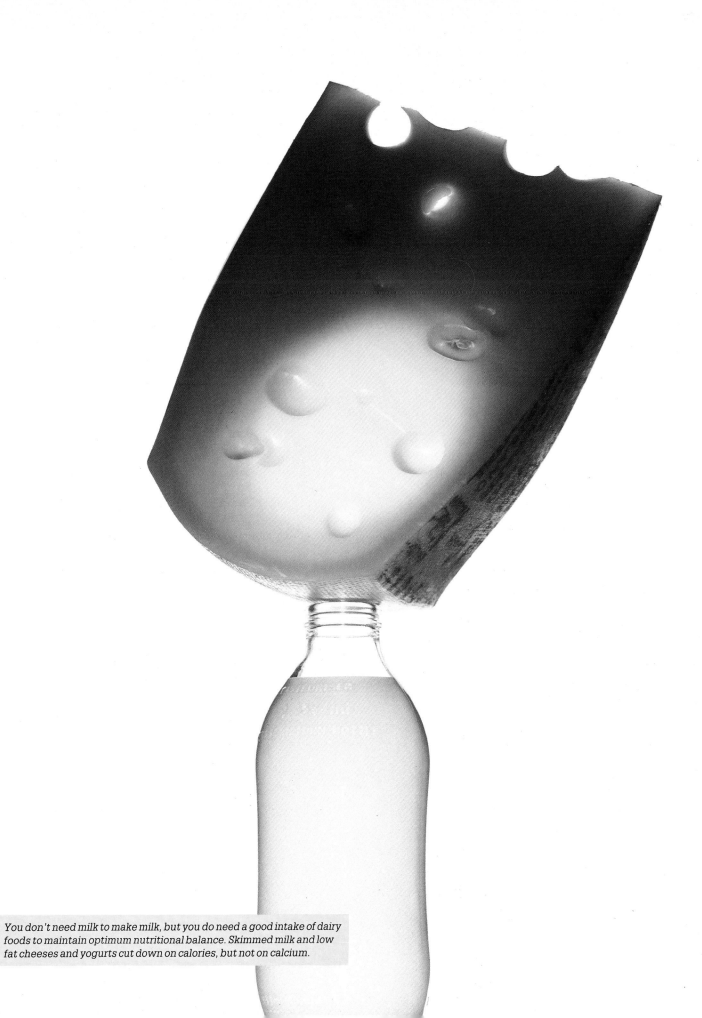

You don't need milk to make milk, but you do need a good intake of dairy foods to maintain optimum nutritional balance. Skimmed milk and low fat cheeses and yogurts cut down on calories, but not on calcium.

BREAKFASTS	LIGHT MEALS	MAIN MEALS

DAY 1

Lentil soup (page 109)
75 g/3 oz wholewheat toast with 15 g/½ oz low fat spread
Fruit: 1 banana

NB Soak lentils and make stock for tomorrow.

Lemon chicken escalope (see 10-day Blitz Diet, Day 10, page 63)
Vegetables: 150 g/5 oz boiled new potato and 150 g/5 oz broccoli served with 120 ml/4 fl oz (½ cup) **white sauce** (page 123)
Ice cream and apricots: 50 g/2 oz vanilla ice cream with 100 g/3½ oz fresh, canned or dried and soaked apricots

DAY 2

Meat and pickle sandwich: 60 g/2½ oz corned beef or cold lean meat, 40 g/1½ oz pickle, 50 g/2 oz watercress and 75 g/3 oz wholewheat bread with 15 g/½ oz low fat spread
Fruit: 1 pear

Cottage pie (page 102)
Vegetables: 100 g/3½ oz peas and 100 g/3½ oz carrots
Cheese and fruit: 25 g/1 oz crackers, 25 g/1 oz Edam cheese, 15 g/½ oz low fat spread and 100 g/3½ oz grapes

DAY 3

Cheese and tomato sandwich: 60 g/2½ oz Cheddar cheese, 100 g/3½ oz sliced tomatoes, 20 g/¾ oz low calorie mayonnaise and 75 g/3 oz wholewheat bread
Fruit: 1 orange

Lamb's liver (see Pregnancy Diet, Day 2, page 74)
Vegetables: 150 g/5 oz boiled new potatoes and 150 g/5 oz cabbage
Ginger dessert: 40 g/1½ oz stem (preserved) ginger with 3 tbsp single (light) cream

NB Soak prunes for tomorrow.

DAY 4

Herb omelette: prepare an omelette using 2 eggs, freshly chopped herbs and seasoning. Cook in a non-stick frying pan (skillet).
Salad: lettuce, watercress, cucumber and green pepper with **low fat dressing** (page 110).
75 g/3 oz wholewheat bread with 20 g/¾ oz low fat spread
Fruit: 100 g/3½ oz grapes

Pork fillet with prunes (page 114)
Vegetables: 150 g/5 oz boiled new potato and 100 g/3½ oz runner (string) beans
Apple meringue: peel; core and slice a large cooking apple and cook gently until soft. Transfer to an ovenproof dish and top with meringue. Place in a hot oven to brown the top and serve at once.

DAY 5

Sardines on toast: 60 g/2½ oz sardines and 100 g/3½ oz sliced tomatoes on 75 g/3 oz wholewheat toast with 15 g/½ oz low fat spread
Nut yogurt: 150 g/5 oz plain yogurt mixed with 25 g/1 oz chopped walnuts

Baked chicken with mushroom sauce: wrap 200 g/7 oz chicken breast in foil with 100 g/3½ oz mushrooms, 25 g/1 oz onion and seasoning. Bake in a moderately hot oven, 200°C (400°F) or Gas mark 6, for about 30 minutes. Prepare some **white sauce** (page 123), stir in the mushrooms and serve with the chicken.
Vegetables: 150 g/5 oz jacket baked potato and 150 g/5 oz spinach
Red fruit salad (page 115)

DAY 6

Pâté and tomato sandwich: 50 g/2 oz **liver pâté**, 100 g/3½ oz sliced tomatoes, 75 g/3 oz wholewheat bread and 15 g/½ oz low fat spread
Fruit: 1 apple
Tea: 2 Digestive biscuits (Graham crackers)

Whiting in lemon sauce
Vegetables: 150 g/5 oz boiled new potato and 150 g/5 oz peas
Fruit and cheese: 1 pear and 50 g/2 oz Camembert

DAY 7

Prawn sandwich: 50 g/2 oz prawns (shrimp), 25 g/1 oz shredded lettuce, 50 g/2 oz sliced tomatoes, 75 g/3 oz wholewheat bread and 20 g/¾ oz low calorie mayonnaise
Fruit: 2 Pears
Tea: 40 g/1½ oz scone with 10 g/⅓ oz low fat spread

Roast chicken: 150 g/5 oz roast chicken served with 50 g/2 oz bread sauce and 2 tbsp **low fat gravy** (page 110)
Vegetables: 150 g/5 oz boiled new potato, 100 g/3½ oz carrots and 100 g/3½ oz peas
Fruit yogurt: 150 g/5 oz plain yogurt mixed with fresh fruit

DAILY ALLOWANCE: 1.2 litres/2 pints (5 cups) whole milk

BREAKFASTS	LIGHT MEALS	MAIN MEALS	
	Lentil soup (page 109) 75 g/3 oz wholewheat toast with 15 g/½ oz low fat spread Cheese: 50 g/2 oz Edam Fruit: 1 apple	Beefburger: combine 200 g/7 oz minced (ground) lean chuck steak with a little minced onion, freshly chopped herbs and seasoning. Shape into patties and grill (broil) or barbecue. Serve with 50 g/2 oz sweet pickle. Vegetables: 150 g/5 oz boiled new potato and 100 g/3½ oz carrots Junket and fruit: 200 g/7 oz junket or 2 tbsp single (light) cream served with 100 g/3½ oz fresh or frozen blackberries or blueberries	DAY 8
	Poached egg and baked beans: 1 poached egg and 150 g/5 oz baked beans on 75 g/3 oz wholewheat toast with 15 g/½ oz low fat spread Fruit: 200 g/7 oz melon	Mixed grill: 200 g/7 oz lamb's kidneys grilled (broiled) with 15 g/½ oz lean bacon and 100 g/3½ oz tomatoes Brown rice: 50 g/2 oz boiled Vegetables: 150 g/5 oz cabbage and 100 g/3½ oz poached mushrooms Baked apple with plums and red wine (page 96)	DAY 9
	Ham sandwich: 60 g/2½ oz lean ham, 50 g/2 oz shredded lettuce, 15 g/½ oz low calorie mayonnaise and 75 g/3 oz wholewheat bread Fruit: 2 apples Tea: 40 g/1½ oz scone with 10 g/⅓ oz low fat spread	Baked fish: place 200 g/7 oz white fish in foil with 100 g/3½ oz sliced tomatoes, 100 g/3½ oz sweetcorn (kernel corn) and seasoning. Seal the foil and bake in a moderately hot oven, 200°C (400°F) or Gas Mark 6, for 15 minutes. Vegetables: 150 g/5 oz boiled new potato and 100 g/3½ oz peas Cheese and fruit: 50 g/2 oz Cheddar cheese and 100 g/3½ oz grapes	DAY 10
	Egg sandwich: 2 chopped hard-boiled eggs mixed with 15 g/½ oz low calorie mayonnaise, seasoning and 50 g/2 oz cress with 75 g/3 oz wholewheat bread Banana yogurt: 150 g/5 oz plain yogurt mixed with 100 g/3½ oz chopped banana	Avocado vinaigrette: 100 g/3½ oz sliced avocado served with low fat dressing (page 110) Lamb chops: 100 g/3½ oz lamb chop grilled (broiled) with fresh rosemary and garlic Vegetables: 150 g/5 oz jacket baked potato and 100 g/3½ oz carrots Rice pudding: 150 g/5 oz homemade or canned rice pudding with 2 tsp jam (jelly)	DAY 11
	Smoked mackerel pâté: blend together 100 g/3½ oz smoked mackerel, 50 g/2 oz cottage cheese, lemon juice and black pepper. Chill well and serve with 50 g/2 oz watercress and 75 g/3 oz wholewheat toast. Fruit: 2 pears	Cheese pie Ratatouille (page 114) Fruit yogurt: 150 g/5 oz plain yogurt mixed with 100 g/3½ oz orange slices and 100 g/3½ oz canned or fresh lychees	DAY 12
	Carrot, cheese and nut sandwich: 50 g/2 oz grated carrot, 25 g/1 oz Cheddar cheese, 15 g/½ oz chopped walnuts, seasoning and 75 g/3 oz wholewheat bread Fruit: 1 apple	Poached chicken: 150 g/5 oz poached chicken with 2 tbsp low fat gravy (page 110) Vegetables: 100 g/3½ oz broccoli and 50 g/2 oz poached mushrooms Fruit: 1 peach or banana	DAY 13
A	Tongue and tomato sandwich: 60 g/2½ oz tongue or lean meat, 25 g/1 oz chopped celery, 50 g/2 oz sliced tomato, 15 g/½ oz low calorie mayonnaise and 75 g/3 oz wholewheat bread Fruit: 200 g/7 oz melon Tea: 50 g/2 oz fruit cake	Roast meat: 125 g/4 oz lean roast meat with 2 tbsp low fat gravy (page 110) Vegetables: 150 g/5 oz jacket baked potato, 100 g/3½ oz carrots and 100 g/3½ oz cauliflower Rhubarb or prune fool: (See Pregnancy Diet, Day 10, page 75).	DAY 14

Entertaining

Eating less does not have to mean eating alone. Share a deliciously light meal using these menus, devised on a seasonal basis, and you will find that you can eat surprisingly well without breaking your diet. Friends will find the focus on fresh fruits, vegetables, fish and meat a refreshing change from the excesses too often associated with dining out.

Suitable wines, suggested at the beginning of each menu, should be served with the main course only – the first courses and desserts, being mainly composed of salads and fruits, are rather too acid to be accompanied with wine. Serve a sparkling mineral water instead and keep it on the table throughout the meal. The total calorie count given for each menu does not include any allowance for wine, so calculate this separately and add it on.

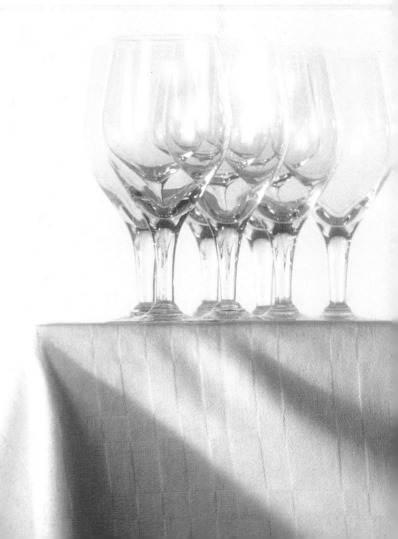

Ginger soup .... 10 Cal.
Tomato and mozzarella salad .... 140 Cal.
Poached goujons of sole .... 200 Cal.
Grapes in orange jelly .... 90-125 Cal.

Total Calories (approx): 440-475
Wines: Vouvray or Sancerre, chilled

Ginger Soup

This recipe needs to be started a day in advance.

METRIC/IMPERIAL	AMERICAN
1 pheasant, duck or chicken (or 1 carcase and 500 g/1 lb raw chicken joints)	1 pheasant, duck or chicken (or 1 carcase and 1 lb raw chicken joints)
1 onion, quartered	1 onion, quartered
1 leek, quartered	1 leek, quartered
1 large carrot, quartered	1 large carrot, quartered
2 sticks celery, halved	2 celery stalks, halved
3 stalks parsley	3 stalks parsley
1 small bay leaf	1 small bay leaf
salt and freshly ground black pepper	salt and freshly ground black pepper
Garnish:	**Garnish:**
1½ tbsp finely chopped ginger	1½ tbsp finely chopped ginger
12 sprigs watercress	12 sprigs watercress

Put the bird in a pressure cooker – a tough old game bird will do very well. Alternatively, you can use the carcase of a bird, adding some raw chicken joints for flavour. Add flavouring vegetables, herbs, salt and pepper. Cover with cold water and bring to the boil. Remove any scum that floats to the surface, then cover and cook on high pressure for 20 minutes. (If using an ordinary pan, allow 1 hour.) Reduce the pressure by running under cold water, and remove the bird. Remove the breasts and wings combined from the bird. (These can be eaten the same day, either hot or cold, with salad.) Put the bird back in the pot, cover and cook for another 40 minutes under high pressure (or 2 hours in an ordinary saucepan). Strain the stock and leave to cool, then chill overnight.

Next day, remove every scrap of fat from the surface and measure the stock. You only need 1.2 litres/2 pints (5 cups), so if you have more, reduce by fast boiling. Reheat and adjust the seasoning. Just before serving, bring back to the boil and drop in the chopped ginger. Simmer for 30 seconds, then add the watercress and turn off the heat. Stand, covered, for 5 minutes before serving in small cups.

Total Calories: 60
Calories per serving: 10

Tomato and Mozzarella Salad

METRIC/IMPERIAL	AMERICAN
1 kg/2 lb tomatoes, skinned and sliced	2 lb tomatoes, skinned and sliced
1 mozzarella, cut in 5 mm/¼ in cubes	1 mozzarella cut in ¼ in cubes
2 tbsp olive oil	2 tbsp olive oil
1 tbsp lemon juice	1 tbsp lemon juice
freshly ground black pepper	freshly ground black pepper

Lay the sliced tomatoes on a flat dish and scatter the little cubes of mozzarella over them. Dribble over the oil and lemon juice, and sprinkle with black pepper.

Total Calories: 840
Calories per serving: 140

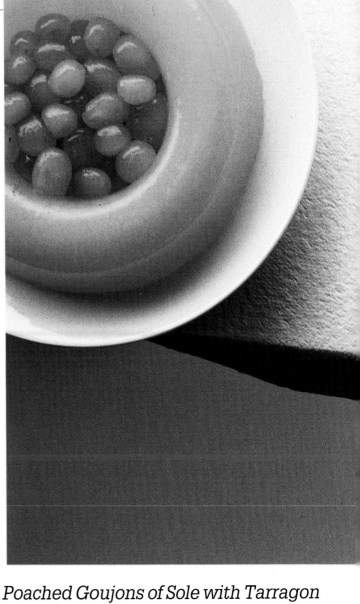

Poached Goujons of Sole with Tarragon

METRIC/IMPERIAL	AMERICAN
1 kg/2 lb fillets of Dover sole, skinned, with bones, etc.	2 lb fillets of sole, skinned, with bones, etc.
½ small onion	½ small onion
½ small carrot	½ small carrot
ends of leek and celery	ends of leek and celery
¼ tsp sea salt and 6 black peppercorns	¼ tsp coarse salt and 6 black peppercorns
15 g/½ oz butter	1 tbsp butter
1 tbsp sunflower seed oil	1 tbsp sunflower seed oil
3 shallots, finely chopped	3 shallots, finely chopped
150 ml/¼ pint dry white wine	⅔ cup dry white wine
5 tbsp single cream	⅓ cup light cream
4 tbsp chopped tarragon	¼ cup chopped tarragon

Cut the fish fillets into strips diagonally, about 6 cm × 1 cm (2½ ins × ½ in). Put the fish bones, skins, etc, in a pan with the onion, carrot, leek and celery, salt and peppercorns. Add 450 ml/¾ pint (2 cups) cold water, bring to the boil and simmer for 25 minutes. Strain, then reduce to 200 ml/⅓ pint (⅞ cup) by fast boiling.

Melt the butter and oil in a saucepan and cook the shallot until it softens and starts to change colour. Add the fish stock and the wine and bring to the boil, stirring. Drop in the strips of fish, a few at a time, and

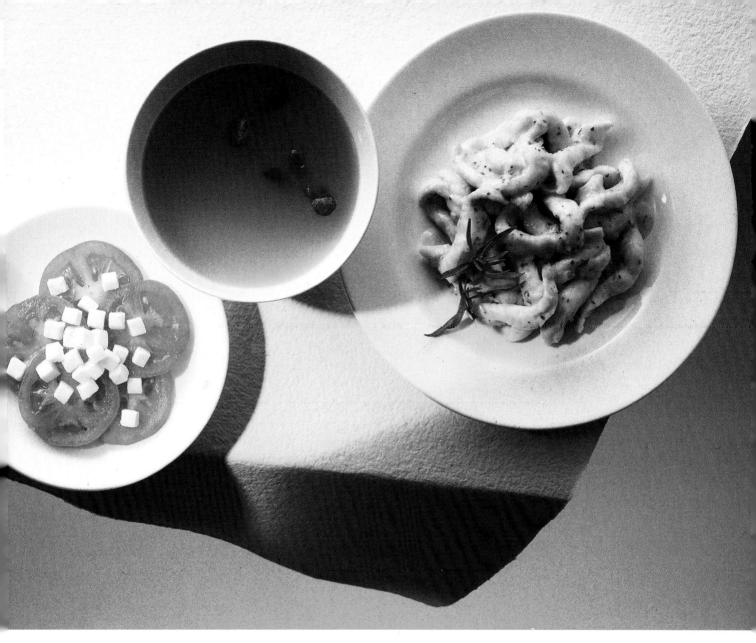

From the left: Poached Goujons of Sole with Tarragon, Ginger Soup, Tomato and Mozzarella Salad, Grapes in Orange Jelly

Grapes in Orange Jelly

METRIC/IMPERIAL	AMERICAN
8 large oranges or 12 small ones	8 large oranges or 12 small ones
25 g/1 oz sugar	2 tbsp sugar
1½ packets gelatine (¾ oz)	3 envelopes gelatine
350 g/12 oz white grapes, peeled and seeded	¾ lb white grapes, peeled and pitted

Start a day, or several hours, in advance. Pare the rind of 3 of the oranges and put in a bowl. Squeeze the juice of all the oranges. Measure the juice and pour it over the rind. Measure the amount of water needed to make the orange juice up to 900 ml/1½ pints (3¾ cups) and put it in a saucepan with the sugar. Bring to the boil and stir until all the sugar has dissolved, then add the fruit juice and rind. Bring back to the boil and skim until the surface is clear. Add 1 tablespoon cold water, bring back to the boil, and skim again. Remove from the heat and shake in the gelatine. Whisk with a fork until it has dissolved, then leave until cool.

When the liquid is cold, pour through a strainer and fill a 900 ml/1½ pint (3¾ cup) ring mould. Chill in the refrigerator overnight. Next day, turn out onto a flat plate and fill the centre with the grapes. (If you don't have a ring mould, make in a dish and serve without turning out. The grapes may be put in the bottom of the dish or omitted.)

Total Calories: 750, or 540 (without grapes)
Calories per serving: 125 or 90

adjust the heat so that the liquid barely simmers. Poach the fish for 1-2 minutes, then transfer to a dish, using a slotted spoon, and keep warm. When all are cooked, measure the liquid; if much more than 200 ml/ ⅓ pint (⅞ cup), reduce by fast boiling, then stir in the cream, adding salt and pepper to taste. Put the strips of fish back into the sauce, folding them in gently, with most of the tarragon, reserving a little for the garnish. Remove from the heat and stand, covered, for a couple of minutes to infuse the sauce with the flavour of tarragon, then pour into a clean dish and scatter the reserved tarragon over the top. Accompany with a lettuce salad dressed with lemon juice, and boiled or steamed potatoes for those who can afford the extra calories.

Total Calories: 1200 (without potatoes)
Calories per serving: 200

Artichokes with herb sauce .... 90 Cal.
Poached trout with watercress sauce .... 200–220 Cal.
Mixed red and green salad .... 70 Cal.
Raspberry jelly with foamy almond sauce .... 140 Cal.

Total Calories (approx): 500–520
Wines: Muscadet or Pouilly Fumé, chilled

Artichokes with Herb Sauce

METRIC/IMPERIAL	AMERICAN
6 globe artichokes, as fresh as possible	6 globe artichokes, as fresh as possible
Sauce:	**Sauce:**
40 g/1½ oz tofu (bean curd from health food stores)	1½ oz tofu (bean curd from health food stores)
150 ml/¼ pint plain yogurt	⅔ cup plain yogurt
3 tbsp sunflower seed oil	3 tbsp sunflower seed oil
3 tsp Dijon mustard	3 tsp Dijon-style mustard
6 tbsp freshly chopped herbs (chives, chervil, dill, tarragon, etc)	6 tbsp freshly chopped herbs (chives, chervil, dill, tarragon, etc)

Use the very freshest artichokes you can find, for their calorie content increases daily during storage, as the inulin is converted into sugar. Boil as usual; drain and leave to cool. Serve within 2 hours of cooking.

To make the sauce, put the tofu, yogurt, oil and mustard into a food processor and process until blended. Tip into a bowl and stir in the chopped herbs. Serve either in the centre of the artichokes, after removing the inner core of leaves and the choke, or in a separate bowl.

Total Calories: 550
Calories per serving: 90

Poached Trout with Watercress Sauce

METRIC/IMPERIAL	AMERICAN
6 rainbow trout (smallish)	6 rainbow trout (smallish)
few plaice bones, fish heads, etc.	few fish bones, heads, etc.
1 onion, halved	1 onion, halved
1 carrot, halved	1 carrot, halved
ends of leek and celery	ends of leek and celery
1 bay leaf	1 bay leaf
3 stalks parsley	3 stalks parsley
1 tsp salt	1 tsp salt
6 black peppercorns	6 black peppercorns
150 ml/¼ pint white wine	⅔ cup white wine
Watercress Sauce (optional):	**Watercress Sauce (optional):**
25 g/1 oz butter	2 tbsp butter
1½ tbsp flour	1½ tbsp flour
300 ml/½ pint fish stock (from poaching trout)	1¼ cups fish stock (from poaching trout)
5 tbsp single cream (for a hot sauce)	⅓ cup light cream (for a hot sauce)
2 tsp grated horseradish	2 tsp grated horseradish
2 tsp Dijon mustard	2 tsp Dijon-style mustard
1 tbsp orange juice	1 tbsp orange juice
salt and freshly ground black pepper	salt and freshly ground black pepper
1 tbsp finely chopped watercress, leaves only	1 tbsp finely chopped watercress, leaves only
5 tbsp plain yogurt (for a cold sauce)	⅓ cup plain yogurt (for a cold sauce)

Put the fish bones into a fish kettle with the flavouring vegetables, herbs and seasonings. Cover with cold water, add the white wine and bring slowly to the boil. Half cover the pot and simmer for 25 minutes, then remove the fish bones, vegetables and herbs. Bring back to the boil and drop in the trout. Adjust the heat so that it barely simmers, and poach for 5–7 minutes, depending on the size of the trout. Remove them and keep hot, or leave to cool. To avoid extra calories, simply boil up the stock until reduced slightly. Pour into a sauceboat and serve with the fish.

To serve with a hot sauce, boil up the stock till reduced to a good flavour, then strain and measure 300 ml/½ pint (1¼ cups). Melt the butter in a saucepan, stir in the flour and cook for 1 minute, stirring. Pour on the hot stock, stirring till smooth, and simmer for 3 minutes. Then add the cream, horseradish, mustard, orange juice, salt and pepper. Simmer for another minute, then stir in the chopped watercress. Pour into a sauceboat and serve with the trout. Accompany with steamed mange-touts and new potatoes for those who are not on a diet.

For a cold dish, make the sauce as above but omit the cream and watercress. Pour into a bowl and cool quickly in a sink half full of cold water, stirring to prevent a skin forming. When it is cold, stir in the yogurt, beating until smooth, and the chopped watercress. Pour into a sauceboat and serve with the cold trout, after removing the top skin. Accompany with a lettuce salad and steamed new potatoes, served warm, for those who are not dieting.

Calories per serving (with hot sauce): 220 (with cold sauce): 200
Total Calories (approx) (with hot sauce): 1320 (with cold sauce): 1200

Mixed Red and Green Salad

METRIC/IMPERIAL	AMERICAN
1 round lettuce, inner leaves only	1 round lettuce, inner leaves only
25 g (1 oz) tender spinach, cut in thinnest possible strips	1 oz tender spinach, cut in thinnest possible strips
1 small head radicchio, when available, cut in squares	1 small head radicchio, when available, cut in squares
25 g (1 oz) mâche (corn salad, lambs lettuce), trimmed	1 oz corn salad, trimmed
Dressing:	**Dressing:**
1 tbsp white wine vinegar	1 tbsp white wine vinegar
½ tbsp lemon juice	½ tbsp lemon juice
3 tbsp sunflower seed oil	3 tbsp sunflower seed oil
sea salt and freshly ground black pepper	sea salt and freshly ground black pepper

Lay the lettuce leaves in a salad bowl and scatter the strips of spinach over them. Lay the red squares of radicchio over the spinach, and the individual leaves of mâche (corn salad) over all. Mix the dressing in a small bowl. Before serving, mix the dressing again, pour over the salad, and toss lightly.

Total Calories: 400
Calories per serving: 70

Raspberry Jelly

METRIC/IMPERIAL	AMERICAN
500 g/1 lb raspberries, fresh or frozen	3 cups American raspberries, fresh or frozen
50 g/2 oz sugar	¼ cup sugar
1½ packets gelatine (¾ oz)	3 envelopes gelatine
2 ripe peaches	2 ripe peaches

Put the raspberries in a pan with the sugar. (If using frozen raspberries, thaw first.) Heat slowly until the juice runs, then increase the heat until it

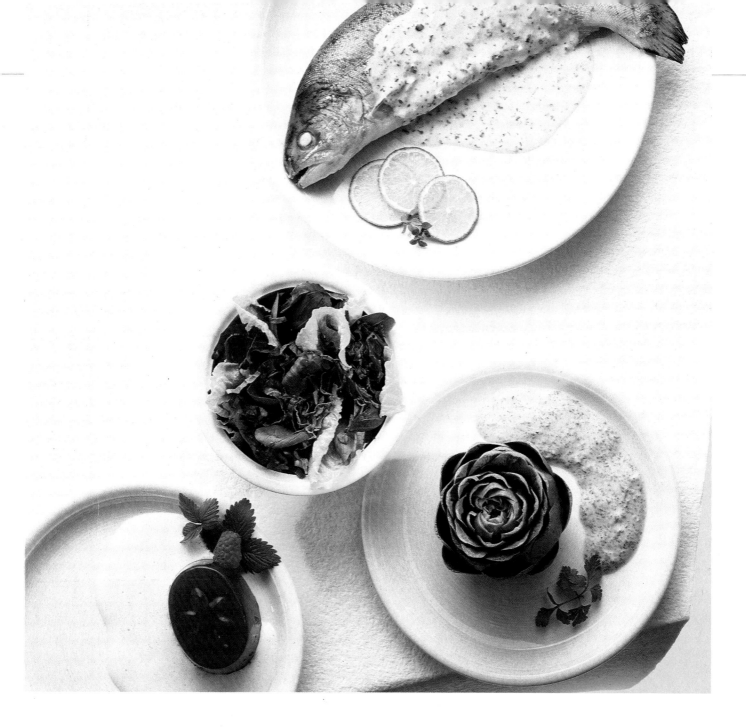

From the front: Raspberry Jellies with Foamy Almond Sauce, Artichokes with Herb Sauce, Mixed Red and Green Salad, Poached Trout

boils. Cook for 10 minutes, watching to see that the berries don't stick. Push through a coarse sieve (strainer) or fine food mill, pressing through everything except the seeds. Measure the juice and make up to 500 ml/ 18 fl oz (12¼ cups) with water. Soak the gelatine in a cup in 4 tablespoons water for 10 minutes, then stand in a small pan of very hot water until dissolved. Mix the gelatine with the juice, strain again, and cool.

Chill 6 small moulds in the freezer. Oval *oeuf en gelée* moulds are ideal. Peel the peaches and remove the stones (pits); cut them in quarters, then across in small slices. Pour a thin layer of liquid jelly into each mould and chill again until set. Arrange a layer of sliced peaches over the jelly, then add more liquid jelly to come level. Chill again and, when the second layer has set, fill up the moulds with remaining sliced peaches and liquid jelly. Chill in the refrigerator until completely set. Unmould onto small flat plates and serve with cream for those who are not on a diet.

Total Calories: 325
Calories per serving: 55

Foamy Almond Sauce

METRIC/IMPERIAL	AMERICAN
2 egg yolks	*2 egg yolks*
5 tbsp milk	*⅓ cup milk*
2 tbsp caster sugar	*2 tbsp sugar*
1 tbsp ground almonds	*1 tbsp ground almonds*

Have a china bowl standing over a saucepan of simmering water. Break the egg yolks into the bowl and beat with a wire whisk. After 2 minutes, start adding the milk, sugar and ground almonds, continuing to whisk steadily. Continue beating for about 5 minutes, until the sauce is light and foamy, and very slightly thickened. (It should just coat the back of a wooden spoon lightly.) Transfer the bowl to a sink half full of cold water and cool to luke-warm, stirring frequently to prevent a skin forming.

When the sauce has cooled sufficiently pour a little of it around each jelly on its plate, just before serving.

Total Calories: 500
Calories per serving: 85

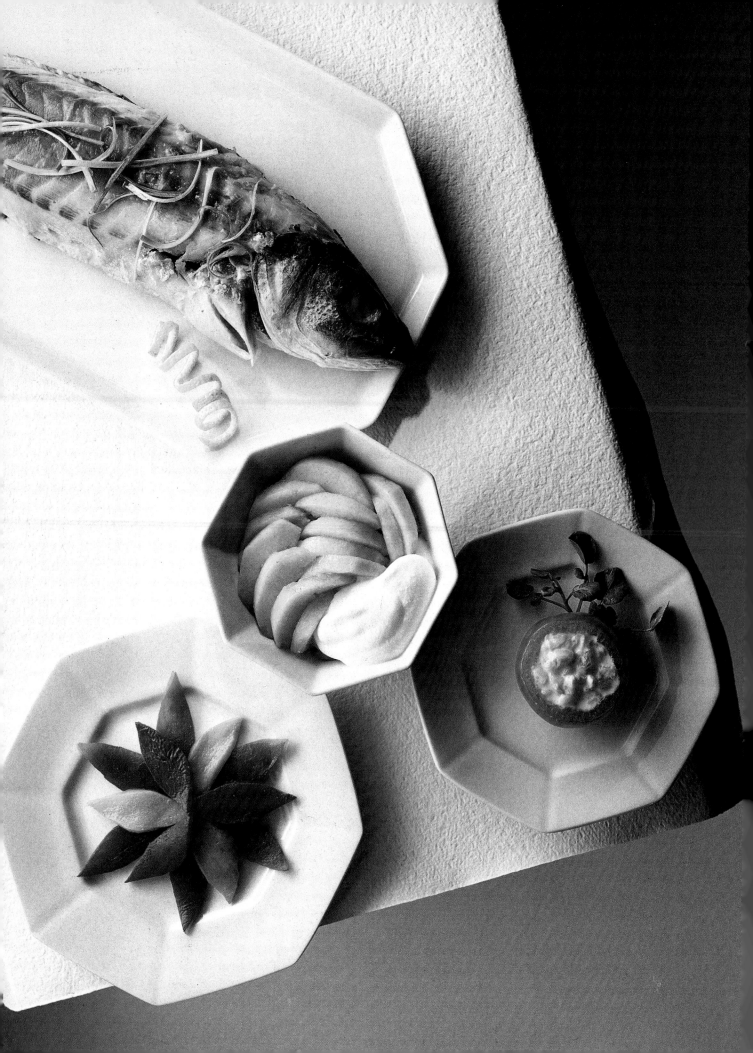

MENU III SPRING/SUMMER

Tomatoes stuffed with cucumber .... 40 Cal.
Grilled pepper salad .... 55 Cal.
Steamed bass, or salmon trout .... 175–260 Cal.
Sliced peaches, with yogurt cream .... 90 Cal.

Total Calories (approx): 360–445
Wine: Chablis, chilled

Tomatoes Stuffed with Cucumber

METRIC/IMPERIAL	AMERICAN
6 medium tomatoes	6 medium tomatoes
½ cucumber, peeled	½ cucumber, peeled
300 ml/½ pint plain yogurt	1¼ cups plain yogurt
1 clove garlic, crushed	1 clove garlic, crushed
sea salt and freshly ground black pepper	coarse salt and freshly ground black pepper
1–2 dashes Tabasco	1–2 dashes hot pepper sauce
2 tbsp chopped mint	2 tbsp chopped mint
1 bunch watercress	1 bunch watercress

Cut a slice off the tops of the tomatoes and scoop out the insides with a sharp-edged teaspoon. Drain away the seeds and juice and chop the flesh. Stand the tomatoes upside-down to drain for 30 minutes, then pat dry with absorbent kitchen paper towels. Grate the cucumber coarsely and mix into the yogurt with the garlic. Add the chopped tomato flesh, salt and pepper, and a couple of dashes of Tabasco (hot pepper sauce). Stir in the chopped mint and pile into the tomato cases. Serve on a bed of watercress, as a first course.

Total Calories: 240
Calories per serving: 40
NOTE: A grilled (broiled) pepper salad may be added, as another hors d'oeuvre. In this case omit the watercress.

Grilled Pepper Salad

METRIC/IMPERIAL	AMERICAN
6 medium peppers, preferably red, yellow and green, or just red and green	6 medium peppers, preferably red, yellow and green, or just red and green
2 tbsp olive oil	2 tbsp olive oil
sea salt and freshly ground black pepper	coarse salt and freshly ground black pepper

Preheat the grill (broiler), lay the peppers on the grill pan and cook as close to the heat as possible. Turn them over as the skin blisters, until they are evenly charred and blackened all over. Remove from the heat and leave to cool. Later, scrape away the skin with a small knife, and cut away the stalk and inner membrane, washing away the seeds under cold running water. Cut the flesh into petal shapes and lay on a flat dish. Sprinkle with olive oil, sea salt and black pepper. Serve as an hors d'oeuvre with stuffed tomatoes. A dish of hard-boiled eggs in mayonnaise may be added for those who are not dieting.

Total Calories: 340
Calories per serving: 55

Steamed Bass or Salmon Trout, Chinese Style

METRIC/IMPERIAL	AMERICAN
1 bass, or salmon trout, weighing 1.5 kg/3–3½ lb	1 bass, or salmon trout, weighing 1.5 kg/3–3½ lb
1 tsp sea salt	1 tsp coarse salt
1 tsp sugar	1 tsp sugar
½ tbsp sesame oil (from Chinese supermarket)	½ tbsp sesame oil (from Chinese supermarket)
½ tbsp soy sauce	½ tbsp soy sauce
8 thin slices root ginger	8 thin slices root ginger
2 large cloves garlic, peeled and thinly sliced	2 large cloves garlic, peeled and thinly sliced
4 spring onions, sliced lengthwise	4 scallions, sliced lengthwise
Sauce:	*Sauce:*
2 tbsp dry vermouth	2 tbsp dry vermouth
2 tbsp sunflower seed oil	2 tbsp sunflower seed oil
1 tbsp sesame oil	1 tbsp sesame oil
1 tbsp soy sauce	1 tbsp soy sauce
Garnish:	*Garnish:*
4 spring onions	4 scallions

Rub the fish inside and out with the salt, sugar, sesame oil and soy sauce. Lay a large piece of foil on a table and scatter half the sliced ginger, garlic and spring onions (scallions) over it. Lay the fish on them and scatter the remainder on top of it. Wrap the foil round the fish so that it is totally enclosed, and lay on the rack of a fish kettle. Bring about 1.5 cm/¾ in water to the boil in the kettle, then lower the rack into it and cover. Boil steadily for 30 minutes, then look to see if the fish is cooked. If the flesh comes away easily from the central bone, it is ready to serve.

While the fish cooks, make the sauce and prepare the garnish. Mix the sauce ingredients in a small bowl. Cut the spring onions (scallions) across into 3.5–5 cm (1½–2 in) lengths, then cut each piece into thin slivers. When the fish is ready, unwrap it and slide onto a platter. Strain the juices into the sauce and discard the garlic, ginger and spring onions (scallions). Remove the top skin from the fish, give the sauce a final whisk, and pour it over. Scatter with the slivers of spring onion (scallion) and serve. No vegetable is necessary, but you can accompany the fish with steamed mangetout if you like, and boiled or steamed new potatoes for those who can afford to eat them.

Total Calories: 1050
Calories per serving: 175 with mangetout

Sliced Peaches with Yogurt Cream

METRIC/IMPERIAL	AMERICAN
4 large peaches or 6 apricots	4 large peaches or 6 apricots
65 ml/2½ fl oz carton plain yogurt	¼ cup + 1 tbsp plain yogurt
2 tbsp whipped cream	2 tbsp whipped cream
1 egg white, beaten	1 egg white, beaten
½ tbsp vanilla sugar	½ tbsp vanilla sugar

Remove the stones (pits) from the peaches, skin them and slice. (Stone and slice apricots, if used.) Divide the slices between 6 glass bowls. Beat the yogurt until smooth, then fold in the whipped cream and the beaten egg white. Finally, fold in the vanilla sugar. Put a spoonful on the sliced fruit in each of the bowls.

Total Calories: 450
Calories per serving: 90

From the front: Grilled Pepper Salad, Tomatoes with Cucumber, Sliced Peaches with Yogurt Cream, Steamed Bass or Salmon Trout, Chinese Style

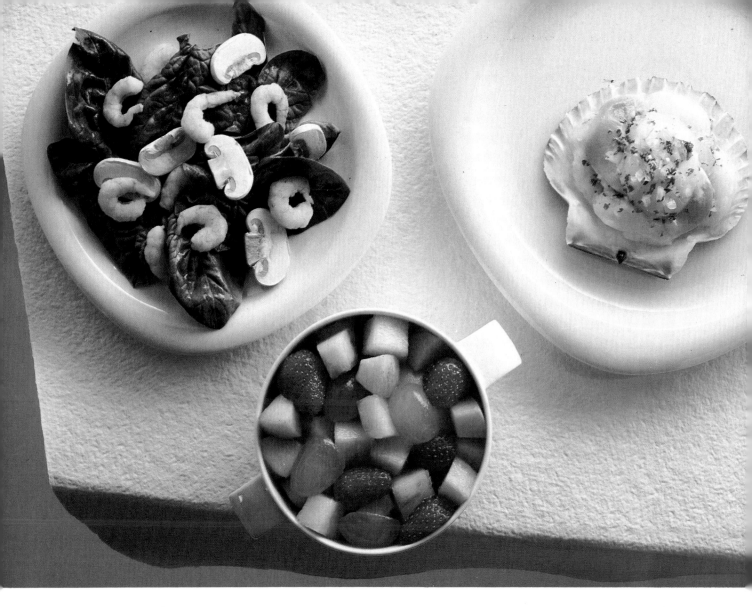

MENU IV SPRING/SUMMER

Ceviche of scallops .... 100 Cal.
(or Prawn, spinach & mushroom salad) .... 125 Cal.
Grilled chicken breasts with watercress .... 230–280 Cal.
Fresh fruit salad .... 70–90 Cal.

Total Calories (approx): 525–595
Wines: Beaujolais Villages or a dry rosé, lightly chilled

Ceviche of Scallops
This recipe must be started a day in advance.

METRIC/IMPERIAL	AMERICAN
12 large scallops, with 6 flat shells	*12 large scallops, with 6 flat shells*
250 ml/8 fl oz fresh lime or lemon juice or a mixture of the two	*1 cup fresh lime or lemon juice or a mixture of the two*
1½ tbsp finely chopped shallot	*1½ tbsp finely chopped shallot*
1½ tbsp finely chopped parsley	*1½ tbsp finely chopped parsley*
1½ tbsp olive oil	*1½ tbsp olive oil*

Start a day in advance. Clean the scallops, wash them and pat dry. Cut away the orange part and slice the white part into 1 cm/½ in slices. Put them in a bowl and pour the lime or lemon juice over them; chill for 24 hours. Just before serving, pour off the fruit juice and discard. Stir in the shallot, parsley and oil. Serve on the scallop shells.

Total Calories: 600
Calories per serving: 100

Prawn, Spinach & Mushroom Salad

METRIC/IMPERIAL	AMERICAN
250 g/8 oz tender spinach	*½ lb tender spinach*
250 g/8 oz button mushrooms	*½ lb button mushrooms*
250 g/8 oz peeled prawns	*½ lb shelled shrimp*
3 tbsp sunflower seed oil	*3 tbsp sunflower seed oil*
3 tbsp lemon juice	*3 tbsp lemon juice*
freshly ground black pepper	*freshly ground black pepper*

Pick the leaves off the washed spinach, discarding the stalks and pile loosely in a bowl. Wipe the mushrooms, trim the stalks level with the caps, and cut in halves or quarters, according to size. Scatter over the spinach. Lay the prawns (shrimp) over the mushrooms. Pour over the oil and lemon juice and toss well, sprinkling with freshly ground black pepper. Salt is not necessary.

Total Calories: 740
Calories per serving: 125

From the left: Prawn, Spinach & Mushroom Salad, Fresh Fruit Salad, Ceviche of Scallops, Grilled Chicken Breasts with Watercress

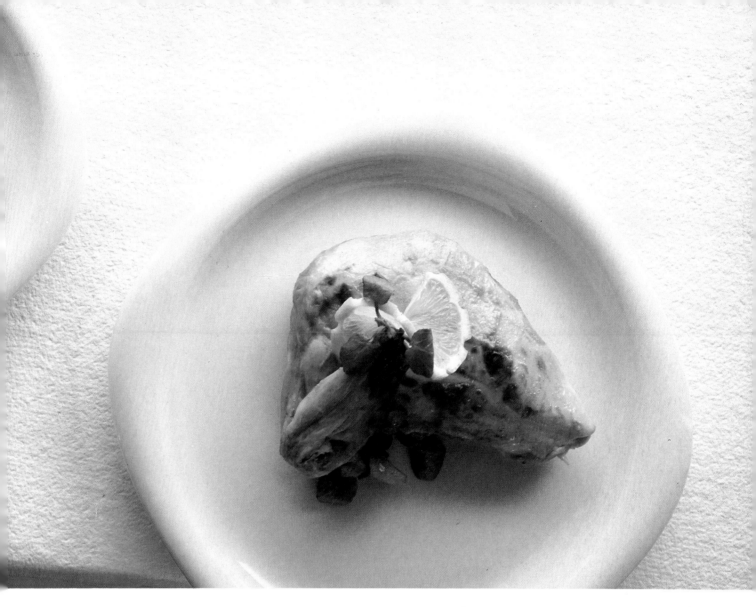

Grilled Chicken Breasts with Watercress

METRIC/IMPERIAL	AMERICAN
6 chicken breasts	*6 chicken breasts*
(skinned, optional)	*(skinned, optional)*
2 tbsp Dijon mustard	*2 tbsp Dijon-style mustard*
2 tbsp sunflower seed oil	*2 tbsp sunflower seed oil*
juice of 1 lemon	*juice of 1 lemon*
freshly ground black pepper	*freshly ground black pepper*
2 lemons, cut in quarters	*2 lemons, cut in quarters*

Watercress Salad: *Watercress Salad:*
2 bunches watercress   *2 bunches watercress*
1 tbsp olive oil   *1 tbsp olive oil*
juice of 1 lemon   *juice of 1 lemon*

Start 2 hours before serving. Paint the chicken joints with mustard. Lay them in a shallow dish and spoon over the oil and lemon juice. Grind some black pepper over them and leave for about 1 hour.

Later, heat the grill (broiler). Cook the chicken pieces until they are golden brown, allowing 8–10 minutes each side and basting with any oil and lemon juice in the pan. (Don't add more.) While they cook, trim the watercress using only the tender sprigs. Wash and shake dry, then pile in a bowl. Add oil and lemon juice and toss. Make a bed of watercress on a flat dish and serve the chicken joints on it, or serve the watercress in the bowl. Garnish the chicken with extra lemon quarters.

Total Calories: 1400
Calories per serving: 230 (without skin)

Fresh Fruit Salad

METRIC/IMPERIAL	AMERICAN
2 peaches, skinned and stoned	*2 peaches, skinned and pitted*
1 small melon, ogen	*1 small melon, ogen or*
or honeydew, or 1 wedge	*honeydew, or 1 wedge*
watermelon	*watermelon*
3 apricots or plums, stoned	*3 apricots or plums, pitted*
250 g/8 oz strawberries	*1¾ cups strawberries*
250 g/8 oz cherries, stoned, or	*2 cups pitted cherries or grapes*
grapes, seeded	*2 tbsp sugar*
2 tbsp caster sugar	*3 tbsp orange juice*
3 tbsp orange juice	*3 tbsp lime juice*
3 tbsp lime juice	

Cut the peaches, melon and apricots (or plums) into pieces about 1 cm/½ in square and pile in a glass bowl. Add the strawberries, halved, quartered or chopped, according to size, and the halved cherries (if using grapes, peel them if you have the time). Sprinkle with sugar and pour over the fruit juices. (When fresh limes are not available, use 4 tablespoons orange juice and 2 tablespoons lemon juice.) Serve with cream for those who are not dieting, or plain yogurt as an optional extra for those who are.

Total Calories: 420 (550 with yogurt)
Calories per serving: 70 (90 with 2 tbsp plain yogurt)

Smoked trout salad .... 175 Cal.
Boiled beef with horseradish sauce .... 495 Cal.
Sliced pink grapefruit with orange juice .... 75 Cal.
Total Calories: 745

Wines: Madiran or Cahors, at room temperature

Smoked Trout Salad

METRIC/IMPERIAL	AMERICAN
12 inner leaves batavia or curly endive	12 leaves chicory
12–14 leaves radicchio, when available	12–14 leaves radicchio, when available
18 tiny sprigs watercress or rosettes mâche	18 tiny sprigs watercress or lambs' lettuce (corn salad)
75 g/3 oz leek, or spring onions, white parts only	3 oz leek, or scallions, white parts only
75 g/3 oz carrot	3 oz carrot
75 g/3 oz fennel, when available	3 oz fennel, when available
2 × 6 oz smoked trout, skinned and filleted	2 × 6 oz smoked trout, skinned and filleted
75 g/3 oz button mushrooms, caps only, sliced	1 cup sliced button mushrooms

Dressing:

1 tbsp lemon juice	1 tbsp lemon juice
1 tbsp white wine vinegar	1 tbsp white wine vinegar
2 tbsp olive oil	2 tbsp olive oil
2 tbsp sunflower seed oil	2 tbsp sunflower seed oil
sea salt and freshly ground black pepper	sea salt and freshly ground black pepper

Wash all the leaves and shake dry. Cut the leek (or spring onions/ scallions), carrot and fennel into the thinnest possible slivers, like split matchsticks, about 3.5 cm/1½ in long. Put them in a small strainer and suspend in boiling water for exactly 1 minute, then drain and hold under cold running water. Drain again.

Cut each trout fillet across into 3 or 4 pieces. Using kitchen scissors, cut the salad leaves in pieces about 2.5 cm/1 in square and mix together. Divide them between 6 plates and scatter the sliced mushrooms over and among them. Lay the slivers of poached vegetables over all. Mix all the dressing ingredients together. Arrange the pieces of smoked trout round the edges of the plates. Just before serving, spoon a little of the dressing over each salad. Do not toss. Serve as a first course or as a very light main dish.

Total Calories: 1050
Calories per serving: 175

Boiled Beef with Horseradish Sauce

METRIC/IMPERIAL	AMERICAN
1.5 kg/3½ lb (unsalted) silverside of beef	3½ lb boneless rump
1 tsp sea salt	1 tsp coarse salt
12 black peppercorns	12 black peppercorns
1 large onion, halved	1 large onion, halved
1 large carrot, halved	1 large carrot, halved
1 leek, halved	1 leek, halved
1 stick celery, halved	1 celery stalk, halved
1 bay leaf	1 bay leaf
3 stalks parsley	3 stalks parsley

Horseradish sauce:

Horseradish sauce:	*Horseradish Sauce:*
150 ml/¼ pint plain yogurt	2/3 cup plain yogurt
2 tbsp grated horseradish	2 tbsp grated fresh horseradish
2 tsp lemon juice	2 tsp lemon juice

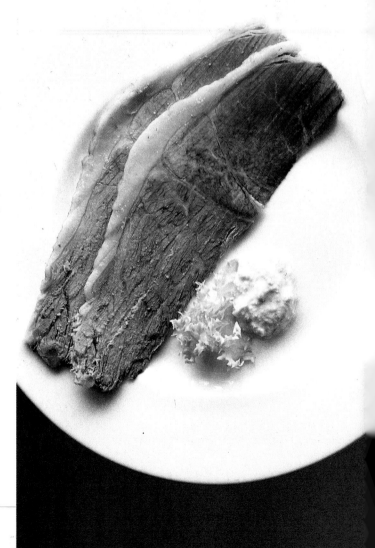

From the left: Boiled Beef with Horseradish Sauce, Sliced Grapefruit with Orange Juice, Smoked Trout Salad

Put the beef in a casserole and cover with cold water. Bring to the boil, removing any scum that rises to the surface. When it is quite clear, add salt and black peppercorns, onion, carrot, leek, celery, bay leaf and parsley. Simmer gently for 1½ hours, or 30 minutes per 500 g/lb if cooking a larger piece.

While the beef is cooking, make the sauce. Beat the yogurt until smooth, then stir in the grated horseradish and lemon juice. When the beef is cooked, carve it in thin slices and lay on a platter. Strain the stock into a bowl; allow it to settle for a few moments, then extract some of it from below the surface, using a bulb baster. Pour into a small jug. Serve the sliced beef with its stock accompanied by horseradish sauce and a dish of boiled carrots. (Boiled potatoes or even dumplings can be added for those who are not dieting.) The rest of the beef stock can be made into a delicious consommé for another meal. (See recipe for Ginger Soup p. 82 and substitute beef stock for game or poultry.) Any leftover beef can be eaten cold the following day with a salad.
Total Calories: 2780
Calories per serving: 495

Sliced Grapefruit with Orange Juice

METRIC/IMPERIAL	AMERICAN
3 pink grapefruit	3 pink grapefruit
juice of 2 oranges	juice of 2 oranges
1 tbsp caster sugar	1 tbsp sugar

Cut the peel off the grapefruit, taking the white pith with it, and cut in slices. Lay the grapefruit slices on a dish and sprinkle the sugar over them. Pour the fresh orange juice over and chill for an hour or two before serving.
Total Calories: 450
Calories per serving: 75

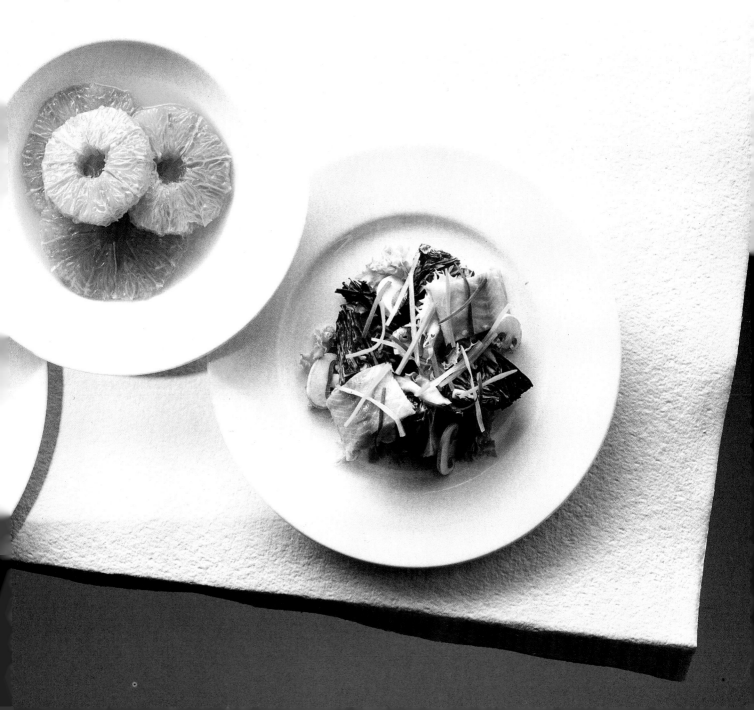

Vegetable terrine .... 50 Cal.
(or Prawn, spinach & mushroom salad) .... 90 Cal.
Calves' liver with orange juice .... 250–355 Cal.
Ricotta with herbs .... 60 Cal.

Total Calories: 360–505

Wines: Bourgeuil or Chinon, lightly chilled

Vegetable Terrine

This recipe needs to be started a day or two in advance.

METRIC/IMPERIAL	AMERICAN
Aspic:	**Aspic:**
750 g/1½ lb raw chicken joints or ½ raw chicken	1½ lb raw chicken joints or ½ raw chicken
½ calf's foot, or a pig's trotter, split	½ calf's foot, or a pig's foot, split
2 onions, halved, with extra onion skins	2 onions, halved, with extra onion skins
2 leeks, halved	2 leeks, halved
2 sticks celery, halved	2 celery stalks, halved
½ bay leaf	½ bay leaf
½ tsp salt	½ tsp salt
6 black peppercorns	6 black peppercorns
1 egg white, plus shell	1 egg white, plus shell
Vegetables:	**Vegetables:**
125 g/4 oz French beans	¼ lb green beans
125 g/4 oz carrots	¼ lb carrots
125 g/4 oz courgettes, unpeeled	¼ lb zucchini, unpeeled
125 g/4 oz broccoli	¼ lb broccoli
1 large bunch spring onions	1 large bunch scallions
Tomato Purée:	**Tomato Purée:**
500 g/1 lb ripe tomatoes, skinned and quartered	1 lb ripe tomatoes, skinned and quartered
1 tbsp orange juice	1 tbsp orange juice

Start 1–2 days in advance. Put the chicken and the calf's foot (or pig's trotter) in a deep pan and cover with cold water. Bring very slowly to the boil, skimming often as it approaches boiling point. When the surface is clear, add the halved vegetables, bay leaf, salt and peppercorns. Half cover the pan and simmer for 3 hours, skimming now and then. When the time is up, strain and cool. Throw away the meat and vegetables. Chill the stock overnight.

Next day, measure the stock. You only need about 1 litre/1¾ pints (4¼ cups), so if there is much more, reduce by fast boiling. Beat the egg white until foamy, but not stiff, and mix the crushed shell with it. Stir into the stock and reheat, beating with a whisk as it approaches boiling point. Let it boil up to the top of the pan, then remove from the heat and allow to settle. Replace over the heat and boil up once more, then pour through a strainer lined with a piece of muslin (cheesecloth). The strained aspic should be crystal clear. (If not, pour back into the pan, add the egg whites and boil up and strain once more.) Leave to cool, while you prepare the vegetables.

Trim the beans, cutting them in pieces about 3.5 cm/1½ in long. Cut the carrots and courgettes (zucchini) into similar strips. Divide the broccoli into sprigs. Trim the spring onions (scallions), leaving on the best part of the green leaves. Poach the vegetables separately in lightly salted water, keeping them quite crisp. Drain and cool in separate piles. To make the tomato purée, blend the tomatoes in a food processor, stir in the orange juice and chill.

Have 6 moulds chilling in the refrigerator. Oval *oeuf en gelée* tins are ideal, or small china dishes. (If you don't have 6 individual dishes, you can use a small loaf tin.) Pour a thin layer of aspic into each mould and put in the freezer for a few minutes to set. Then lay a few spring onions

(scallions) diagonally across each one. Pour in enough aspic to half cover them, and chill again. Once the second layer is set, you can fill the moulds with layers of different vegetables, pouring in the aspic to come level with the top. Chill in the refrigerator for 2–3 hours, until set, or overnight if more convenient. To serve, unmould onto small flat plates, and pour a little tomato purée around each one. Serve as a first course.

Total Calories: 300
Calories per serving: 50

Calves' Liver with Orange Juice

METRIC/IMPERIAL	AMERICAN
15 g/½ oz butter	1 tbsp butter
2 tbsp sunflower seed oil	2 tbsp sunflower seed oil
6 thin slices calves' liver (400 g/ 14 oz)	6 thin slices calf liver (14 oz)
4 shallots, chopped	4 small onions, chopped
8 tbsp freshly chopped parsley	½ cup freshly chopped parsley
sea salt and freshly ground black pepper	coarse salt and freshly ground black pepper
120 ml/4 fl oz orange juice	½ cup orange juice

Heat the butter with half the oil in a frying pan and cook the liver very briefly; 2 minutes on each side should be enough. Remove to a warm dish and put the remaining oil in the pan. Add the chopped shallots and cook for 1½–2 minutes, until golden. Add the parsley, sea salt and black pepper, and stir round until well mixed. Pour in the orange juice, swirl round once or twice, and pour over the liver. Serve with steamed broccoli and 150 g/5 oz new potatoes, or rice for those not on a diet.

Total Calories: 1500

Calories per serving: 250 with broccoli; 355 with potatoes

Ricotta with Herbs, Celery, and Water Biscuits

METRIC/IMPERIAL	AMERICAN
2 tbsp freshly chopped herbs (chives, dill, parsley, etc)	2 tbsp freshly chopped herbs (chives, dill, parsley, etc)
175 g/6 oz ricotta or low-fat curd cheese	¾ cup ricotta or low-fat curd cheese
sea salt and freshly ground black pepper	coarse salt and freshly ground black pepper
1 head celery, inner stalks only	1 bunch celery, inner stalks only
water biscuits	crackers

Stir a quarter of the chopped herbs into the ricotta, adding a little salt and freshly ground black pepper. Form the ricotta into a round and flatten the top. Sprinkle the remaining herbs over the disc, and press into a ramekin to shape it. Turn out on to a flat dish and serve, with the celery and water biscuits (crackers).

Total Calories: 350

Calories per serving: 60 with 2 biscuits (crackers).

From the front: Ricotta with Herbs, Celery and Water Biscuits, Vegetable Terrine, Calves' Liver with Orange Juice

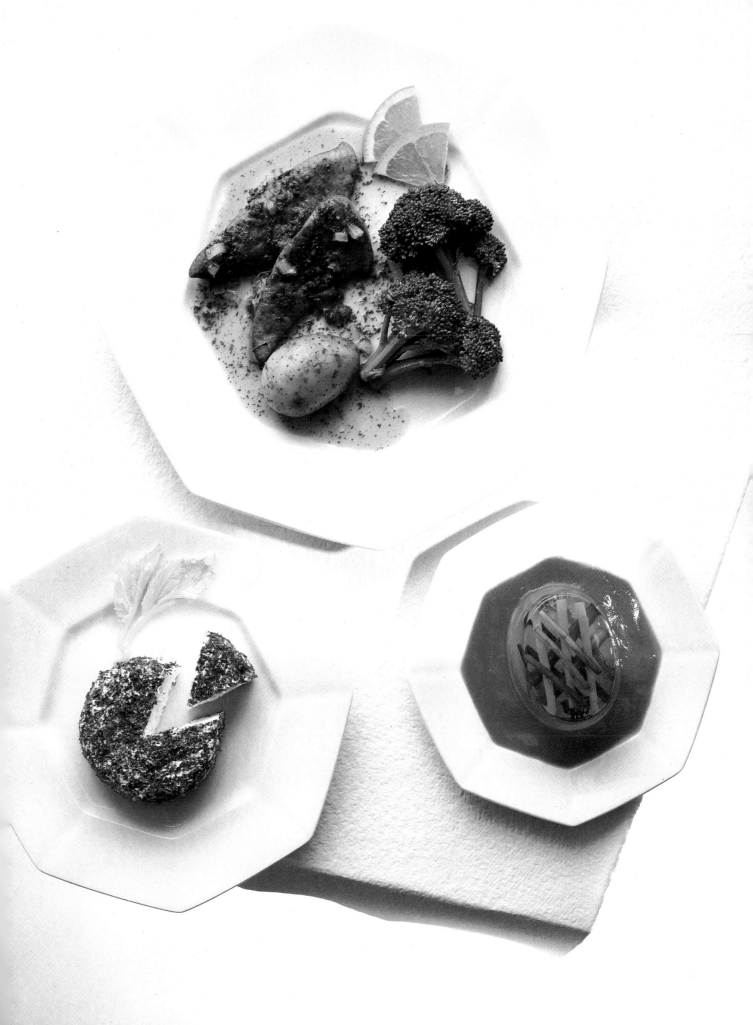

Recipe index

Use this alphabetical recipe reference section while following the diet, and afterwards too as a guide to a healthier style of eating – for these recipes not only save on calories but also on fat and sugar. The emphasis is on fresh, lightly cooked foods, fibre, wholegrains and an adventurous range of seasonings that helps make food appetizing while cutting down on salt. These are fundamental principles of good nutrition and worth carrying into your everyday diet whether you want to lose weight or not.

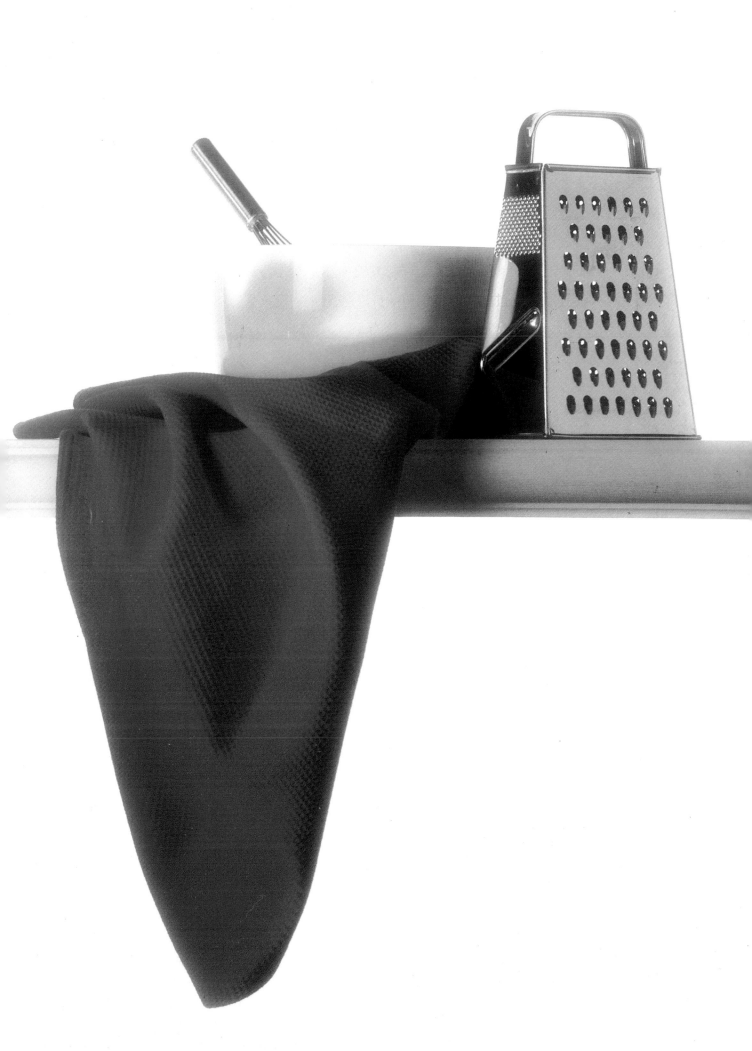

Americana Sauce

Metric/Imperial
1 tbsp olive oil
1 medium onion, chopped
1 clove garlic, crushed
1 tsp tomato purée
250 g/8 oz tomatoes, skinned,
    seeded and chopped (or canned)
salt and freshly ground black pepper
2 tbsp freshly chopped parsley

American
1 tbsp olive oil
1 medium onion, chopped
1 clove garlic, crushed
1 tsp tomato paste
1 cup skinned, seeded and chopped
    tomatoes (or canned)
salt and freshly ground black pepper
2 tbsp freshly chopped parsley

Heat the oil in a saucepan and lightly brown the onion with the garlic. Add the tomato purée (paste), tomatoes and seasoning. Simmer gently for about 15 minutes, stirring occasionally. Sprinkle with parsley before serving with pasta.
TOTAL CALORIES: 190
CALORIES PER SERVING: 95
SERVES 2

Artichoke Salad

Metric/Imperial
3 canned artichoke hearts, drained
    and sliced in half
1 tomato, sliced
few crisp lettuce leaves, shredded
1 tbsp Low Fat Dressing (page 110)
freshly chopped parsley

American
3 canned artichoke hearts, drained
    and sliced in half
1 tomato, sliced
few crisp lettuce leaves, shredded
1 tbsp Low Fat Dressing (page 110)
freshly chopped parsley

Arrange the artichoke hearts and the tomato slices on a bed of lettuce. Pour over the vinaigrette and toss lightly. Sprinkle with parsley.
TOTAL CALORIES: 65
SERVES 1

Variation

For a more substantial salad, add the following:
25 g/1 oz fresh green beans,
    blanched
50 g/2 oz tuna, drained
50 g/2 oz new potatoes, boiled in
    their skins and diced

Arrange these ingredients with the artichokes and tomatoes on the lettuce. Serve this salad as a light supper or lunch dish.
TOTAL CALORIES: 150

Aubergine Pie

Metric/Imperial
350 g/12 oz aubergines, trimmed and
    sliced
salt
Sauce:
500 g/1 lb tomatoes, skinned, seeded
    and chopped
1 bouquet garni
3 tbsp dry white wine
dash of Worcestershire sauce
1 clove garlic, crushed
1 large onion, finely chopped
salt and freshly ground black pepper
1 tbsp tomato purée
100 g/3½ oz Edam cheese, thinly
    sliced
25 g/1 oz fresh wholewheat
    breadcrumbs

American
¾ lb eggplant, trimmed and sliced
salt
Sauce:
2 cups skinned, seeded and chopped
    tomatoes
1 bouquet garni
3 tbsp dry white wine
dash of Worcestershire sauce
1 clove garlic, crushed
1 large onion, minced
salt and freshly ground black pepper
1 tbsp tomato paste
½ cup thinly sliced Edam cheese
½ cup soft wholewheat
    breadcrumbs

Arrange the aubergine (eggplant) in a colander, sprinkle with salt and leave for 1 hour. Rinse in cold water and dry on kitchen paper towels.

Put the tomatoes, bouquet garni, wine, Worcestershire sauce, garlic and onion into a saucepan and season well. Bring to the boil and simmer, uncovered, for 30–35 minutes. Remove the bouquet garni and stir in the tomato purée (paste). Adjust the seasoning, if necessary. Arrange a layer of aubergine (eggplant) in the bottom of an ovenproof dish. Spoon over a little tomato sauce, then arrange a little sliced cheese on top. Continue layering, finishing with cheese and breadcrumbs.

Bake in a preheated moderately hot oven, 200°C (400°F) or Gas Mark 6, for 35–40 minutes or until the aubergine (eggplant) is tender and the cheese topping golden brown.
TOTAL CALORIES: 360
CALORIES PER SERVING: 90
SERVES 4

Variation
Replace the aubergines (eggplant) with courgettes (zucchini).

TOTAL CALORIES: 300
CALORIES PER SERVING: 75

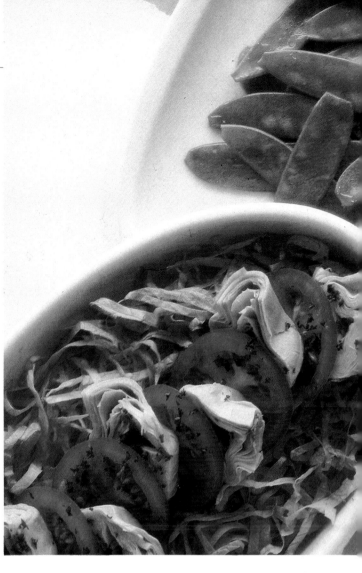

Baked Apple with Blackcurrant Sauce

Metric/Imperial
50 g/2 oz fresh blackcurrants
2 tbsp natural unsweetened apple
    juice
2 tsp thin honey
1 × 175 g/6 oz Bramley cooking
    apple, cored

American
½ cup fresh blackcurrants
2 tbsp natural unsweetened apple
    juice
2 tsp thin honey
1 × 6 oz tart apple, cored

Place the blackcurrants, apple juice and honey in a saucepan. Bring to the boil then simmer gently for 5 minutes until the currants are tender. Leave to cool, then purée.

Make a shallow cut around the middle of the apple. Place the apple in an ovenproof dish, pour the blackcurrant sauce into the centre and around the apple. Cover with a lid or foil and bake in a preheated moderate oven, 180°C (350°F) or Gas Mark 4, for 40–50 minutes until tender.
TOTAL CALORIES: 130
SERVES 1

Baked Apple with Plums and Red Wine

Metric/Imperial
1 × 175 g/6 oz Bramley cooking
    apple, cored
2 medium ripe plums, stoned
2 tsp thin honey
pinch of cinnamon
small pinch of ground cloves
1 tbsp dry red wine

American
1 × 6 oz tart apple, cored
2 medium ripe plums, pitted
2 tsp thin honey
pinch of cinnamon
small pinch of ground cloves
1 tbsp dry red wine

Make a shallow cut around the middle of the apple and place in an ovenproof dish. Chop the plums and mix with the honey, cinnamon and cloves. Fill the cavity in the apple with the mixture and pour over the wine. Cover with a lid or foil and bake in a preheated moderate oven, 180°C (350°F) or Gas Mark 4, for 40–50 minutes until the apple is tender. Serve hot or cold.
TOTAL CALORIES: 120
SERVES 1

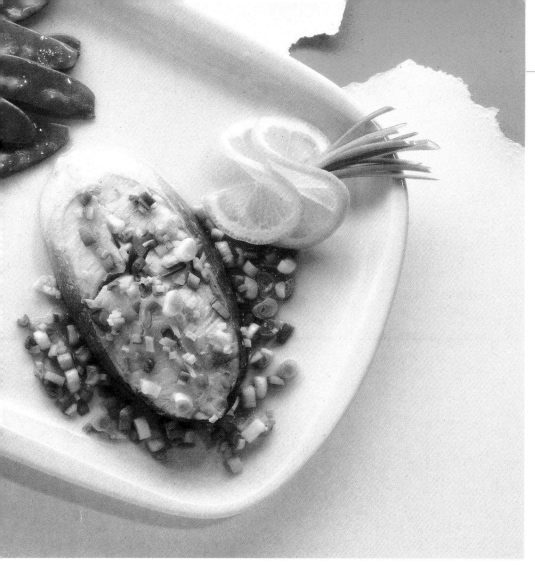

From the front: Artichoke Salad,
Baked Fish with Ginger

Barbecue Lamb

Metric/Imperial
pinch of garlic salt
pinch of dry mustard
pinch of sugar
pinch of ground ginger
freshly ground black pepper
1 × 175 g/6 oz lamb chop, fat removed
150 ml/¼ pint stock
2 tsp cornflour
1 tbsp water
freshly chopped parsley
Sauce:
2 tsp tomato ketchup
2 tsp Worcestershire sauce
1 tsp fruit sauce
½ tsp vinegar
dash of Tabasco

American
pinch of garlic salt
pinch of dry mustard
pinch of sugar
pinch of ground ginger
freshly ground black pepper
1 × 6 oz lamb chop, fat removed
⅔ cup stock
2 tsp cornstarch
1 tbsp water
freshly chopped parsley
Sauce:
2 tsp ketchup
2 tsp Worcestershire sauce
1 tsp fruit chutney
½ tsp vinegar
dash of hot pepper sauce

Mix the dry seasonings together and rub on both sides of the lamb. Cover and allow to stand for several hours.

Place in a non-stick frying pan (skillet) and fry quickly to brown both sides. Pour over the stock, bring to the boil and simmer gently for 30 minutes. Remove chop and keep warm. Blend the cornflour (cornstarch) with the water and pour into the hot cooking liquor. Bring to the boil stirring, until thickened. Mix the tomato ketchup and sauce ingredients together, stir into the cooking liquid. Boil to reduce slightly and return the chop to the pan. Cook for 20 minutes or until the meat is tender. Serve with parsley.
TOTAL CALORIES: 330
SERVES 1
Note: To barbecue the lamb chop, spread the chop with the dry seasoning and sprinkle with 1 tablespoon lemon or lime juice. Leave to stand (see recipe above). Place the chop on a barbecue and cook for 7–10 minutes each side, until browned and cooked through. Cook the sauce as directed.

Baked Egg

Metric/Imperial
1 tbsp cooked mixed vegetables
1 egg
salt and freshly ground black pepper
1 tbsp whipping cream

American
1 tbsp cooked mixed vegetables
1 egg
salt and freshly ground black pepper
1 tbsp whipping cream

Put the cooked vegetables into a small cocotte dish. Break in the egg and sprinkle with seasoning. Pour the whipping cream onto the egg. Bake in a preheated moderate oven, 180°C (350°F) or Gas Mark 4, for 7 minutes. Serve at once.
TOTAL CALORIES: 180
SERVES 1

Variations
Replace the mixed vegetables with: *25 g/1 oz peeled prawns (shrimp)* or *25 g/1 oz (2 tbsp) cooked ham, diced,* or *25 g/1 oz smoked salmon, diced*
TOTAL CALORIES:
with prawns (shrimp): 185
with ham: 230
with smoked salmon: 195

Baked Fish with Ginger

Metric/Imperial
1 × 175 g/6 oz cod cutlet
2 spring onions, finely chopped
small piece root ginger, finely chopped
grated rind of ½ lemon
1 tbsp dry sherry
spring onion and lemon slices

American
1 × 6 oz cod steak
2 scallions, minced
small piece ginger root, finely chopped
grated rind ½ lemon
1 tbsp dry sherry
scallion and lemon slices

Place the fish in an ovenproof dish. Sprinkle with the spring onion (scallion), ginger and lemon rind, then spoon over the sherry. Cover and chill for 2–3 hours.

Cook, covered, in a preheated moderate oven, 180°C (350°F) or Gas Mark 4, for 15 minutes or until the fish is tender and flakes easily. Serve garnished with the spring onion (scallion) and lemon slices.
TOTAL CALORIES: 150
SERVES 1

Banana, Honey and Nut Fool

Metric/Imperial
2 medium bananas (total weight 175 g/6 oz)
2 tsp thin honey
grated rind and juice of ½ lemon
15 g/½ oz hazelnuts, chopped and toasted
150 ml/¼ pint plain yogurt

American
2 medium bananas (total weight 6 oz)
2 tsp thin honey
grated rind and juice of ½ lemon
2 tbsp chopped hazelnuts, toasted
⅔ cup plain yogurt

Mash the bananas with the honey, lemon rind and juice. Stir in the hazelnuts and yogurt and mix well. Spoon the mixture into 2 individual glasses and serve at once.
TOTAL CALORIES: 320
CALORIES PER SERVING: 160
SERVES 2

Beef Carbonnade

Metric/Imperial
250 g/8 oz lean stewing steak, cubed
1 onion, chopped
pinch of grated nutmeg
pinch of sugar
freshly chopped mixed herbs or
    1 bouquet garni
150 ml/¼ pint brown ale
150 ml/¼ pint beef stock
salt and freshly ground black pepper
2 tsp cornflour
1 tbsp water
freshly chopped parsley

American
½ lb lean stewing steak, cubed
1 onion, chopped
pinch of grated nutmeg
pinch of sugar
freshly chopped mixed herbs or
    1 bouquet garni
⅔ cup brown ale
⅔ cup beef stock
salt and freshly ground black pepper
2 tsp cornstarch
1 tbsp water
freshly chopped parsley

Put the steak, onion, nutmeg, sugar, freshly chopped herbs or bouquet garni, ale and stock into a saucepan. Season and cover the pan, simmer gently for 1½–2 hours until the meat is tender. Mix the cornflour (cornstarch) with water. Stir into the casserole and bring to the boil, stirring constantly. Remove the bouquet garni, if using, and adjust the seasoning. Sprinkle with parsley before serving.
TOTAL CALORIES: 600
CALORIES PER SERVING: 300
SERVES 2

Variation
Substitute the brown ale with red wine and add 100 g/4 oz (1 cup) sliced mushrooms 30 minutes before the end of cooking time.
TOTAL CALORIES: 660
CALORIES PER SERVING: 330

Beef Goulash

Metric/Imperial
1 tsp oil
250 g/8 oz lean stewing beef, diced
1 medium onion, sliced
1 clove garlic, crushed
1 tbsp tomato purée
2 tsp paprika
1 tbsp flour
300 ml/½ pint beef stock
salt and freshly ground black pepper
1 bouquet garni
½ red pepper, seeded and sliced
3 tbsp plain yogurt

American
1 tsp oil
½ lb lean stewing beef, diced
1 medium onion, sliced
1 clove garlic, crushed
1 tbsp tomato paste
2 tsp paprika
1 tbsp flour
1¼ cups beef stock
salt and freshly ground black pepper
1 bouquet garni
½ red pepper, seeded and sliced
3 tbsp plain yogurt

Heat the oil in a heavy-based saucepan and brown the meat on all sides. Remove and keep warm. Fry (sauté) the onion and garlic until lightly browned. Add the tomato purée (paste), paprika and flour and cook for 1 minute, stirring. Add the stock and bring to the boil. Stir in the meat, seasoning, bouquet garni and red pepper. Cover and simmer gently for 1–1½ hours, stirring occasionally.

Discard the bouquet garni, adjust the seasoning and stir in the yogurt. Serve at once.
TOTAL CALORIES: 600
CALORIES PER SERVING: 300
SERVES 2
Note: If freezing, omit yogurt and add when re-heated, just before serving.

Left: Brown Rice and Nut Salad
Right: Carrot Soup

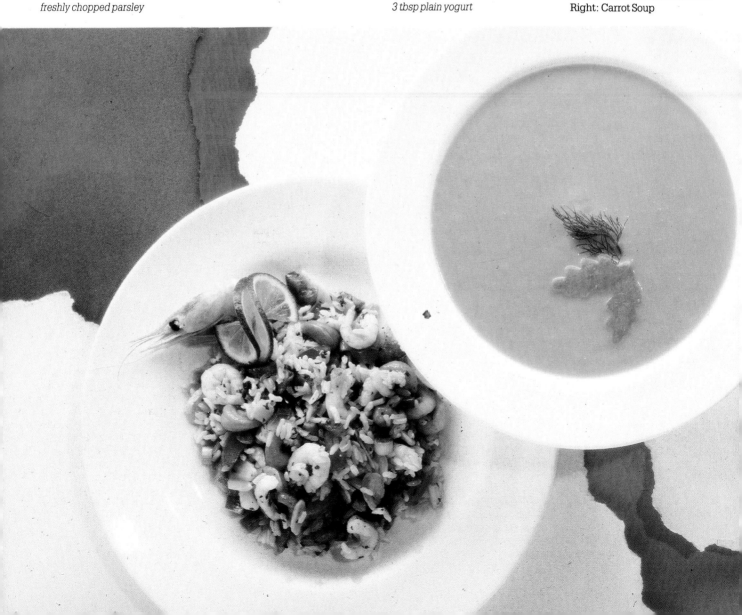

Bitkis

Metric/Imperial
250 g/8 oz lean minced beef
1 small onion, finely chopped
1 tbsp freshly chopped parsley
50 g/2 oz fresh wholewheat
 breadcrumbs
salt and freshly ground black pepper
flour
2 tsp oil
150 ml/¼ pint tomato sauce (see
 Gnocchi and Tomato Sauce recipe
 page 105)
4 tbsp plain yogurt

American
1 cup firmly packed lean ground beef
1 small onion, minced
1 tbsp freshly chopped parsley
1 cup soft fresh wholewheat bread
 crumbs
salt and freshly ground black pepper
flour
2 tsp oil
⅔ cup tomato sauce (see Gnocchi
 and Tomato Sauce page 105)
4 tbsp plain yogurt

Mix together the meat, onion, parsley, breadcrumbs and seasoning. Shape into 8 flat cakes, adding a little water if necessary to make the mixture hold together. Heat the oil in a non-stick frying pan until hot. Roll the cakes in flour and fry until brown on both sides. Arrange in a shallow ovenproof dish and pour over the tomato sauce. Bake in a preheated moderate oven, 180°C (350°F) or Gas Mark 4, for about 30 minutes. Heat the yogurt and pour over the Bitkis.
TOTAL CALORIES: 600
CALORIES PER SERVING: 150
SERVES 4

Braised Kidneys

Metric/Imperial
5 lambs' kidneys, halved, skinned
 and cored
1 small onion, chopped
1 carrot, sliced
1 tsp oil
2 tsp flour
175 ml/6 fl oz stock
1 tsp tomato purée
freshly chopped herbs (rosemary,
 sage, thyme)
salt and freshly ground black pepper
75 g/3 oz button mushrooms, sliced
freshly chopped parsley
25 g/1 oz brown rice, boiled, to serve

American
5 lamb kidneys, halved, skinned and
 cored
1 small onion, chopped
1 carrot, sliced
1 tsp oil
2 tsp flour
¾ cup stock
1 tsp tomato paste
freshly chopped herbs (rosemary,
 sage, thyme)
salt and freshly ground black pepper
¾ cup sliced button mushrooms
freshly chopped parsley
2 tbsp brown rice, boiled, to serve

Place the kidneys in a saucepan with the onion, carrot and oil. Cook gently for 5 minutes, then sprinkle in the flour and cook, stirring, for 1 minute. Add the stock, tomato purée (paste), herbs and seasoning. Simmer for a further 10 minutes, stirring in the mushrooms 5 minutes before the end of the cooking time. Serve at once, sprinkled with parsley and on a bed of brown rice.
TOTAL CALORIES: 420
CALORIES PER SERVING: 210
SERVES 2

Brown Rice and Nut Salad

Metric/Imperial
75 g/3 oz brown rice
salt and freshly ground black pepper
50 g/2 oz peeled prawns
2 spring onions, finely chopped
25 g/1 oz green pepper, seeded and
 thinly sliced
25 g/1 oz red pepper, seeded and
 thinly sliced
half quantity Lemon and Mustard
 Dressing (page 115)
15 g/½ oz cashew nuts
15 g/½ oz flaked almonds, toasted
2 tbsp freshly chopped parsley

American
⅓ cup brown rice
salt and freshly ground black pepper
⅓ cup shelled shrimp
2 scallions, finely chopped
1 oz green pepper, seeded and thinly
 sliced (about 1 tbsp)
1 oz red pepper, seeded and thinly
 sliced (about 1 tbsp)
half quantity Lemon and Mustard
 Dressing (page 115)
2 tbsp sliced almonds, toasted
1 tbsp cashew nuts
2 tbsp freshly chopped parsley

Cook the rice in boiling salted water for 30–35 minutes until tender, but still 'al dente'. Drain and cool.

Place the rice in a bowl and season. Add the prawns (shrimp), spring onions (scallions) and peppers. Pour over the dressing and stir in the nuts and parsley. Mix well until the rice, vegetables and nuts are coated in the dressing.
TOTAL CALORIES: 500
CALORIES PER SERVING: 250
SERVES 2

Cannelloni

Metric/Imperial
4 cannelloni
oil
350 g/12 oz spinach, chopped
salt and freshly ground black pepper
125 g/4 oz low fat curd cheese
pinch of grated nutmeg
Sauce:
150 ml/¼ pint stock
1 carrot, sliced
1 medium onion, sliced
1 stick celery, sliced
1 × 200 g/7 oz can tomatoes,
 chopped
1 bay leaf
1 tsp vinegar

American
4 cannelloni
oil
¾ lb spinach, chopped
salt and freshly ground black pepper
½ cup low fat small curd cottage
 cheese
pinch of grated nutmeg
Sauce:
⅔ cup stock
1 carrot, sliced
1 medium onion, sliced
1 celery stalk, sliced
1 can (8 oz) tomatoes, chopped
1 bay leaf
1 tsp vinegar

Place the cannelloni in boiling water with a few drops of oil and cook for 5 minutes until partially cooked. Drain and keep warm. Meanwhile, place the spinach in a saucepan with a little water and boil for 2–3 minutes. Drain very thoroughly. Mix with the seasoning, cheese and nutmeg, and fill the cannelloni. Set aside.

To make the sauce, place all the ingredients with seasoning in a saucepan and simmer for 10 minutes. Cool slightly, remove the bay leaf, and purée in a blender. Place the cannelloni in a shallow ovenproof dish and pour over the sauce. Bake in a preheated moderately hot oven, 200°C (400°F) or Gas Mark 6, for 5–10 minutes until the pasta is cooked. Serve at once.
TOTAL CALORIES: 645
CALORIES PER SERVING: 325
SERVES 2

Variation
Replace the spinach filling with the meat sauce in Lasagne and use to fill the cannelloni as above.
TOTAL CALORIES: 900
CALORIES PER SERVING: 450

Carrot Soup

Metric/Imperial
1 small onion, chopped
2 carrots, chopped
2 tsp flour
200 ml/⅓ pint stock
salt and freshly ground black pepper
5 tbsp skimmed milk
little crushed garlic (optional)
freshly chopped mint

American
1 small onion, chopped
2 carrots, chopped
2 tsp flour
⅞ cup stock
salt and freshly ground black pepper
⅓ cup skimmed milk
little crushed garlic (optional)
freshly chopped mint

Place the onion and carrots in a non-stick saucepan. Sprinkle on the flour and cook, stirring, for 1 minute. Pour on the stock, and adjust the seasoning. Bring to the boil and simmer for 30 minutes. Cool slightly, then purée the soup in a blender. Return the soup to the clean pan, add the milk and garlic (if using) and return to the boil. Serve sprinkled with freshly chopped mint.
TOTAL CALORIES: 190
SERVES 1

Celery Soup

Metric/Imperial
4 sticks celery, chopped
1 onion, chopped
150 ml/¼ pint stock
5 tbsp skimmed milk
salt and freshly ground black pepper
freshly chopped parsley
1 tsp cornflour

American
4 celery stalks, chopped
1 onion, chopped
⅔ cup stock
⅓ cup skimmed milk
salt and freshly ground black pepper
freshly chopped parsley
1 tsp cornstarch

Place the celery, onion, stock, milk and seasoning in a saucepan, bring to the boil and simmer for about 20 minutes. Cool slightly, then purée in a blender. Return to the clean saucepan and stir in the cornflour (cornstarch) mixed with 1 tablespoon of cold water. Bring to the boil, stirring constantly, until thickened. Sprinkle with parsley and serve with 40 g/1½ oz (1 slice) wholewheat bread and 25 g/1 oz Edam cheese.
TOTAL CALORIES: 80
SERVES 1

Chicken Florentine

Metric/Imperial
4 chicken breasts
450 ml/¾ pint chicken stock
1 bay leaf
salt and freshly ground black pepper
Spinach sauce:
100 g/4 oz frozen chopped spinach
1 bunch watercress, blanched
150 ml/¼ pint thin cream
1½ tbsp freshly chopped tarragon
1½ tbsp freshly chopped parsley

American
4 chicken breasts
2 cups chicken stock
1 bay leaf
salt and freshly ground black pepper
Spinach sauce:
¼ lb frozen chopped spinach
1 bunch watercress, blanched
⅔ cup light cream
1½ tbsp freshly chopped tarragon
1½ tbsp freshly chopped parsley

Bring the stock to the boil, add the chicken breasts, bay leaf and seasoning and simmer, covered, for 35 minutes. Remove the skin from the breasts, and keep them warm. Strain and reserve 150 ml/¼ pint (¾ cup) stock. Cook the spinach and drain well, then purée in a blender with the watercress, stock, cream and herbs. Pour into a saucepan and simmer for 3 minutes. Season, then pour the sauce over the chicken and serve at once.
TOTAL CALORIES: 1600
CALORIES PER SERVING: 400
SERVES 4

Chicken Salad with Curry Sauce

Metric/Imperial
250 g/8 oz boneless cooked chicken, skinned and diced
125 g/4 oz avocado flesh, diced
2 spring onions, chopped
curly endive leaves
25 g/1 oz cashew nuts or peanuts
Sauce:
1 tsp curry powder
1 clove garlic, crushed
3 tbsp plain yogurt
1 tbsp low calorie mayonnaise
2 tsp freshly chopped coriander or parsley

American
½ lb boneless cooked chicken, skinned and diced
¼ lb avocado flesh, diced
2 scallions, chopped
chicory leaves
2 tbsp cashew nuts or peanuts
Sauce:
1 tsp curry powder
1 clove garlic, crushed
3 tbsp plain yogurt
1 tbsp low calorie mayonnaise
2 tsp freshly chopped coriander or parsley

To make the sauce, put the curry powder and garlic into a bowl; gradually add the yogurt and mayonnaise, and mix well. Cover and refrigerate for 2–3 hours, then stir in the coriander or parsley.
Put the chicken, avocado and spring onion (scallion) into a bowl. Spoon over the sauce and mix well, until all the ingredients are coated in the sauce. Arrange the endive (chicory) leaves on a serving plate, pile the chicken mixture on top and sprinkle the cashew nuts or peanuts. Serve at once.
TOTAL CALORIES: 840
CALORIES PER SERVING: 420
SERVES 2

Chicken Veronique

Metric/Imperial
250 g/8 oz chicken joint
salt and freshly ground black pepper
sprig of fresh tarragon
stock (see method)
1 tsp cornflour
1 tbsp water
2 tsp lemon juice
8 grapes, pips removed and skinned

American
½ lb chicken joint
salt and freshly ground black pepper
sprig of fresh tarragon
stock (see method)
1 tsp cornstarch
1 tbsp water
2 tsp lemon juice
8 grapes, pitted and skinned

Skin the chicken joint and sprinkle with seasoning. Place on a piece of foil large enough to enclose it, lay the tarragon on top and fold up. Bake in a preheated moderate oven, 180°C (350°F) or Gas Mark 4, for about 1 hour. Remove the chicken and keep warm. Keep the juices and make up to 150 ml/¼ pint (⅔ cup) with stock, then pour into a saucepan. Mix the cornflour (cornstarch) with the water and stir into the stock. Bring to the boil, stirring, and add the lemon juice and seasoning. When the sauce is thickened, add the grapes and continue to cook for 5 minutes. Pour the sauce over the chicken before serving.
TOTAL CALORIES: 260
SERVES 1

Chicken with Almonds

Metric/Imperial
250 g/8 oz chicken joint
1 tsp oil
1 small onion, sliced
pinch of mixed dried herbs
salt and freshly ground black pepper
2 tbsp blanched almonds

American
½ lb chicken joint
1 tsp oil
1 small onion, sliced
pinch of mixed dried herbs
salt and freshly ground black pepper
2 tbsp blanched almonds

Remove the skin from the chicken and discard. Heat the oil in a non-stick frying pan (skillet) and add the onion, chicken, herbs and seasoning. Cook gently for 20–25 minutes, turning occasionally, until chicken is cooked through. Add the almonds and cook until golden brown.
TOTAL CALORIES: 350
SERVES 1

Chicken with Peach and Ginger

Metric/Imperial
250 g/8 oz chicken joint
salt and freshly ground black pepper
½ ripe peach, peeled
1 tsp ground ginger
1 tsp redcurrant jelly
watercress

American
½ lb chicken joint
salt and freshly ground black pepper
½ ripe peach, peeled
1 tsp ground ginger
1 tsp red currant jelly
watercress

Sprinkle the chicken with seasoning. Place in an ovenproof dish and bake in a preheated moderate oven, 180°C (350°F) or Gas Mark 4, for 30–35 minutes. About 10 minutes before the chicken is cooked, sprinkle the peach half with ginger and put in the oven to warm through. Spoon the redcurrant jelly into the hollow of the peach and serve at once with the

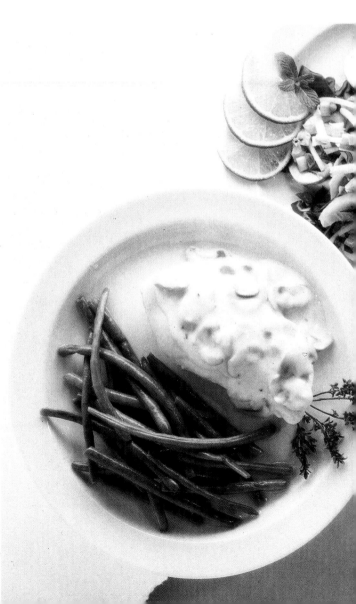

chicken and watercress. (Do not eat the skin.)

TOTAL CALORIES: 240
SERVES 1

Chilli con Carne

Metric/Imperial
200 g/7 oz very lean minced beef
1 large onion, finely chopped
1 tsp chilli powder
1 tsp paprika
salt and freshly ground black pepper
150 ml/¼ pint tomato juice
250 g/8 oz canned red kidney beans
freshly chopped parsley

American
1 cup very lean ground beef
1 large onion, finely chopped
1 tsp chili powder
1 tsp paprika
salt and freshly ground black pepper
⅔ cup tomato juice
¾ cup canned red kidney beans
freshly chopped parsley

From the left: Chinese Cabbage and Chicken Salad, Chicken with Peach and Ginger

Place the meat in a non-stick saucepan and fry (sauté) quickly, stirring constantly, until browned. Drain off excess fat and pat the meat with kitchen paper towel. Add the onion to the meat in the pan, sprinkle over the spices and seasoning and cook for 1 minute before pouring in the tomato juice. Bring to the boil, cover and simmer gently for 1 hour or until the beef is tender. Moisten with a little water during cooking if necessary. Add the beans, adjust the seasoning and heat through before serving. Garnish with the parsley.

TOTAL CALORIES: 700
CALORIES PER SERVING: 350
SERVES 2

Chinese Cabbage and Chicken Salad

Metric/Imperial
50 g/2 oz Chinese cabbage, thinly sliced
50 g/2 oz red cabbage, thinly sliced
2 spring onions
50 g/2 oz fresh beansprouts
25 g/1 oz button mushrooms, sliced
2 tsp soy sauce
juice and grated rind of 2 limes
25 g/1 oz cucumber, cut into julienne strips
2 medium carrots, cut into julienne strips
250 g/8 oz lean boneless chicken, cooked and cut into julienne strips
2 sticks celery, cut into julienne strips

American
¾ cup thinly sliced Chinese cabbage
¾ cup thinly sliced red cabbage
2 scallions
1 cup fresh beansprouts
¼ cup sliced button mushrooms
2 tsp soy sauce
juice and grated rind of 2 limes
1 oz cucumber, cut into matchstick strips
2 medium carrots, cut into matchstick strips
½ lb lean boneless chicken, cooked and cut into matchstick strips
2 celery stalks, cut into matchstick strips

Place the cabbage in a bowl and add the spring onions (scallions), beansprouts and mushrooms. Mix together the soy sauce, lime juice and rind, pour over the cabbage mixture and toss well. Pile onto a serving dish and arrange the strips of cucumber, carrot, chicken and celery in a lattice pattern on top.

TOTAL CALORIES: 420
CALORIES PER SERVING: 210
SERVES 2

Chinese Stuffed Pepper

Metric/Imperial
1 large green or red pepper
Filling:
25 g/1 oz brown rice
1 stick celery, finely chopped
1 clove garlic, crushed
25 g/1 oz flat mushrooms, chopped
1 tomato, skinned, seeded and chopped
1 small leek, finely chopped
150 ml/¼ pint dry white wine
½ tsp mixed dried herbs
little salt
freshly ground black pepper
little stock (see method)
25 g/1 oz sweetcorn
2 tsp soy sauce
chopped fresh coriander

American
1 large green or red pepper
Filling:
2 tbsp brown rice
1 celery stalk, finely chopped
1 clove garlic, crushed
¼ cup chopped flat mushrooms
1 tomato, skinned, seeded and chopped
1 small leek, finely chopped
⅔ cup dry white wine
½ tsp mixed dried herbs
little salt
freshly ground black pepper
little stock (see method)
1 tbsp whole kernel corn
2 tsp soy sauce
chopped fresh coriander

Remove the top of the pepper by cutting through just below the stem. Discard the seeds and white pith and blanch in boiling water for 2 minutes. Drain well.

Place the rice, celery, garlic, mushrooms, tomato and leek in a saucepan. Pour over the wine and add the herbs and seasoning. Bring to the boil, half cover, and simmer gently for 25 minutes or until the rice is almost tender. Add a little stock if the mixture becomes too dry, stirring occasionally. Mix in the corn and soy sauce.

Stand the pepper in an ovenproof dish and spoon the rice mixture into the centre. Spoon any remaining mixture around the pepper. Cover with foil and cook in a preheated moderate oven, 180°C (350°F) or Gas Mark 4, for 15–20 minutes or until the pepper is tender. Serve hot, sprinkled with chopped coriander.

TOTAL CALORIES: 170
SERVES 1

Note: If liked, the pepper can be sprinkled with toasted sesame seeds.

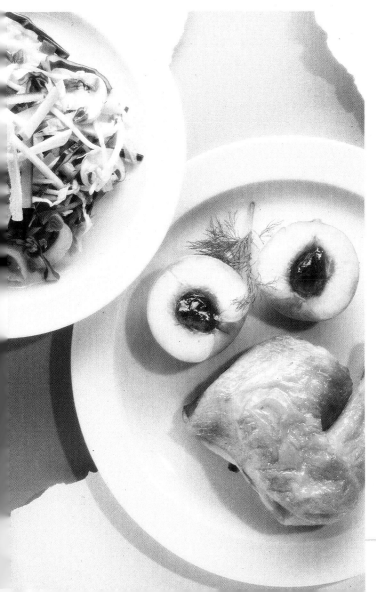

Corn and Fish Chowder

Metric/Imperial
25 g/1 oz lean bacon, diced
½ onion, chopped
1 stick celery, sliced
½ green pepper, chopped
2 tsp flour
150 ml/¼ pint light stock
salt and freshly ground black pepper
75 g/3 oz cooked white fish, diced
50 g/2 oz cooked sweetcorn
150 ml/¼ pint skimmed milk

American
1 tbsp diced lean bacon
½ onion, chopped
1 celery stalk, sliced
½ green pepper, chopped
2 tsp flour
⅔ cup light stock
salt and freshly ground black pepper
3 oz cooked white fish, diced
⅓ cup cooked kernel corn
⅔ cup skimmed milk

Brown the bacon in a non-stick pan, then add the onion, celery and pepper. Cook for 2–3 minutes, stirring. Sprinkle over the flour and continue stirring for 1 minute. Add the stock and seasoning, bring to the boil and simmer for 5 minutes. Stir in the fish, sweetcorn (kernel corn) and milk. Simmer for 4 minutes and serve.
TOTAL CALORIES: 250
SERVES 1

Cottage Pie

Metric/Imperial
125 g/4 oz very lean minced beef or veal
1 small onion, chopped
1 small carrot, diced
2 tomatoes, chopped
pinch of mixed dried herbs
1 tsp tomato purée
salt and freshly ground black pepper
1–2 tbsp stock
150 g/5 oz freshly mashed potato

American
½ cup very lean ground beef or veal
1 small onion, chopped
1 small carrot, diced
2 tomatoes, chopped
pinch of mixed dried herbs
1 tsp tomato paste
salt and freshly ground black pepper
1–2 tbsp stock
⅔ cup freshly mashed potato

Put the meat, onion, carrot, tomatoes, herbs, tomato purée (paste) and seasoning into a non-stick frying pan (skillet). Pour over the stock, bring to the boil and then simmer gently, stirring often, until the meat is cooked. Pour off any fat and transfer the meat mixture to an ovenproof dish. Cover with the potato; place in a moderate oven, 180°C (350°F) or Gas Mark 4, for about 20 minutes.
TOTAL CALORIES: 390
SERVES 1

Courgette and Tomato Pie

Metric/Imperial
1 × 397 g/14 oz can tomatoes
50 g/2 oz onions, sliced
1 or 2 cloves garlic, crushed
1 tsp mixed dried herbs
salt and freshly ground black pepper
2 tsp freshly chopped basil
2 tbsp dry white wine
500 g/1 lb courgettes, sliced diagonally
Topping:
500 g/1 lb potatoes
50 g/2 oz low fat cream cheese with herbs
2 tbsp skimmed milk
2 spring onions, chopped
freshly ground black pepper
grated nutmeg
25 g/1 oz Edam cheese, grated

American
1 can (16 oz) tomatoes
½ cup sliced onions
1 or 2 cloves garlic, crushed
1 tsp mixed dried herbs
salt and freshly ground black pepper
2 tsp freshly chopped basil
2 tbsp dry white wine
1 lb zucchini, sliced diagonally
Topping:
1 lb potatoes
¼ cup low fat cream cheese with herbs
2 tbsp skimmed milk
2 scallions, chopped
freshly ground black pepper
grated nutmeg
¼ cup grated Edam cheese

Place the tomatoes and juice in a saucepan. Add the onions, garlic, herbs, and season well. Bring to the boil and add the wine. Cook, uncovered, for 20 minutes, then add the courgettes (zucchini). Reduce the heat and cook for a further 2–3 minutes. Spoon the mixture into 4 individual ovenproof dishes.
Boil the potatoes until soft, then drain and mash until smooth. Mix in the cream cheese, skimmed milk, spring onions (scallions), black pepper and a little nutmeg. Spoon on top of the courgettes (zucchini) mixture and press the top with a fork. Sprinkle over the grated cheese. Place in a preheated moderately hot oven, 200°C (400°F) or Gas Mark 6, for 20–25 minutes or until brown.
TOTAL CALORIES: 860
CALORIES PER SERVING: 215
SERVES 4

Cream of Onion Soup

Metric/Imperial
600 ml/1 pint skimmed milk
1 bay leaf
15 g/½ oz butter
2 onions, sliced
2 tsp flour
salt and freshly ground black pepper
1 egg, beaten

American
2½ cups skimmed milk
1 bay leaf
1 tbsp butter
2 onions, sliced
2 tsp flour
salt and freshly ground black pepper
1 egg, beaten

Heat the milk and bay leaf until scalded, then set aside. Melt the butter in a saucepan and add the onion. Cook without browning until the onion is soft, then stir in the flour. Continue cooking for 1 minute, stirring well. Strain the milk onto the mixture and bring to the boil, stirring constantly. Simmer for 10 minutes and add seasoning. Cool the soup slightly, then purée in a blender until smooth. Return the soup to the clean pan and gradually stir in the beaten egg – do not allow to boil. Sprinkle with parsley and serve.
TOTAL CALORIES: 445
CALORIES PER SERVING: 225
SERVES 2

Crêpes
Makes 8

Metric/Imperial
125 g/4 oz plain flour
pinch of salt
1 egg
300 ml/½ pint skimmed milk

American
1 cup all-purpose flour
pinch of salt
1 egg
1¼ cups skimmed milk

Sift the flour and salt into a mixing bowl and make a well in the centre. Beat the egg and half the milk together and pour into the well. Using a wooden spoon, gradually stir the mixture until all the flour has been drawn in from the sides. Then beat well until the mixture is smooth. Stir in the remaining milk and set aside in a cool place for several hours before using.
Wipe a little oil around a non-stick frying pan (skillet). Heat the pan and when the oil is almost smoking, pour in a little crêpe mixture to cover the pan. When the bubbles begin to rise on the surface the crêpe should be golden underneath, so turn it over, cooking until golden on that side. Remove and store in a warm place.
TOTAL CALORIES: 600
CALORIES PER CREPE: 75
SERVES 4

Crêpe Fillings
Make the fillings, as below, and divide into eight. Spread a spoonful of filling on each pancake, and roll up. Arrange on an ovenproof dish, cover with foil and bake in a preheated moderately hot oven, 200°C (400°F) or Gas Mark 6, for 20 minutes.
SERVES 4

Mixed vegetables: mix together 175 g/6 oz low fat cheese with herbs and garlic, a dash of Tabasco (hot pepper sauce) and 1 tbsp plain yogurt. Stir in 1 × 250 g/8 oz packet mixed vegetables, cooked and cooled, 1 tbsp freshly chopped parsley, seasoning and mix well.
TOTAL CALORIES FOR FILLING: 395

Prawn and chive: mix together 250 g/8 oz peeled prawns (shrimp), 2 tbsp freshly chopped chives, 150 ml/¼ pint (⅔ cup) plain yogurt, grated rind and juice of 1 lemon, and a dash of Tabasco (hot pepper sauce).
TOTAL CALORIES FOR FILLING: 330

Smoked haddock: mix together 250 g/8 oz poached, cooled and flaked smoked haddock, 15 g/½ oz (1 tbsp) butter, grated rind and juice of 1 lemon, 2 tbsp plain yogurt, 2 tbsp parsley, pepper.
TOTAL CALORIES FOR FILLING: 415

Crunchy Salad

Metric/Imperial
2 crisp apples, cored and diced
juice of 1 lemon
2 sticks celery, chopped
25 g/1 oz walnuts
75 g/3 oz white cabbage, finely sliced
50 g/2 oz Gouda cheese, diced
75 g/3 oz green pepper, seeded and diced
25 g/1 oz cucumber, diced
half quantity Blue Cheese Dressing (page 115)
1 tbsp sunflower seeds, toasted

American
2 crisp apples, cored and diced
juice of 1 lemon
2 celery stalks, chopped
¼ cup walnuts
1¼ cups finely sliced white cabbage
⅓ cup diced Gouda cheese
3 oz green pepper, seeded and diced
¼ cup diced cucumber
half quantity Blue Cheese Dressing (page 115)
1 tbsp sunflower seeds, toasted

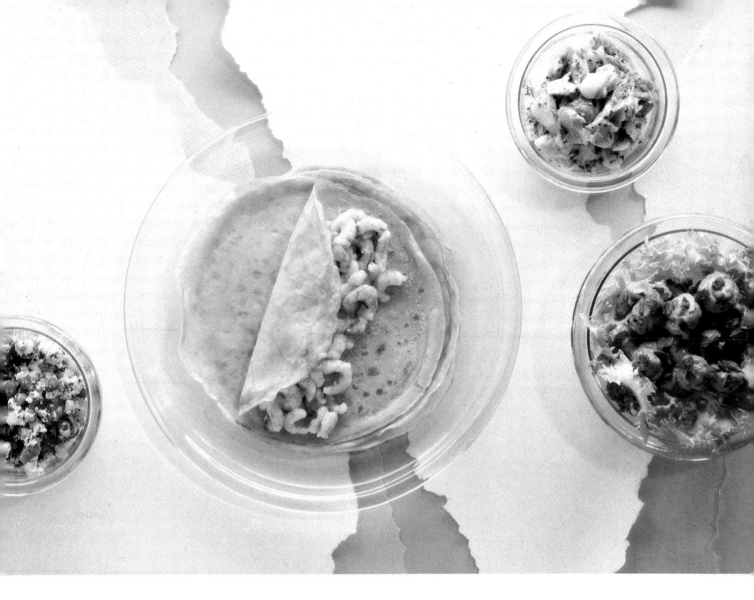

Toss the apples in the lemon juice. Add the celery, walnuts and cabbage and mix well. Stir in the cheese, green pepper and cucumber and spoon over the dressing.

TOTAL CALORIES: 610
CALORIES PER SERVING: 305
SERVES 2

Cucumber Appetizer

Metric/Imperial
6 cm/2½ in length of cucumber
25 g/1 oz cottage cheese
25 g/1 oz peeled prawns, chopped
freshly chopped parsley

American
2½ in length of cucumber
1 tbsp cottage cheese
1 tbsp shelled shrimp, chopped
freshly chopped parsley

Halve the cucumber lengthwise and scoop out the seeds. Mix together the cottage cheese and prawns (shrimp) and season. Fill the cucumber slices and sprinkle with parsley.

TOTAL CALORIES: 55
SERVES 1

Cucumber and Mint Soup

Metric/Imperial
175 g/6 oz cucumber, peeled and diced
300 ml/½ pint consommé
150 ml/¼ pint tomato juice
150 ml/¼ pint cold water
150 ml/¼ pint plain yogurt
125 g/4 oz peeled prawns
few drops of Tabasco
1–2 tbsp roughly chopped mint
1–2 cloves garlic, roughly chopped
salt and freshly ground black pepper
juice and grated rind of 1 lemon
few cucumber slices

American
1½ cups peeled and diced cucumber
1¼ cups consommé
⅔ cup tomato juice
⅔ cup cold water
⅔ cup plain yogurt
⅔ cup shelled shrimp
few drops of hot pepper sauce
1–2 tbsp roughly chopped mint
1–2 cloves garlic, roughly chopped
salt and freshly ground black pepper
juice and grated rind of 1 lemon
few cucumber slices

Place all the ingredients, except the cucumber slices, in a blender. Blend until smooth. Chill for 2–3 hours in the refrigerator. Adjust the seasoning and serve garnished with the cucumber slices.

TOTAL CALORIES: 250
CALORIES PER SERVING: 65
SERVES 4

Curried Mushroom Salad

Metric/Imperial
2 tsp curry powder
1 clove garlic, crushed
2 tbsp plain yogurt
1 tbsp low calorie mayonnaise
1 tbsp freshly chopped parsley
1 tbsp chopped chives
300 g/10 oz button mushrooms
175 g/6 oz endive
25 g/1 oz lean back bacon, grilled until crisp
1 tbsp sunflower seeds, toasted

American
2 tsp curry powder
1 clove garlic, crushed
2 tbsp plain yogurt

Crêpes with Prawn Filling, Mixed Vegetable Filling and Smoked Haddock Filling. Right: Curried Mushroom Salad

1 tbsp low calorie mayonnaise
1 tbsp freshly chopped parsley
1 tbsp chopped chives
2½ cups button mushrooms
6 oz chicory
1 slice lean bacon, broiled until crisp
1 tbsp sunflower seeds, toasted

Place the curry powder and garlic in a bowl. Stir in the yogurt and mayonnaise and mix well. Cover and leave in the refrigerator for 4-6 hours.

Add the parsley and chives to the dressing, then stir in the mushrooms and leave to chill for a further 1 hour.

Arrange the endive (chicory) on a serving dish and spoon the mushroom mixture into the centre. Crumble the bacon over the top and sprinkle with sunflower seeds.

TOTAL CALORIES: 400
CALORIES PER SERVING: 200
SERVES 2

Fennel and Orange Salad

Metric/Imperial

175 g/6 oz plaice or sole fillets,
 skinned
3 tbsp dry white wine
1 bouquet garni
salt and freshly ground black pepper
2 heads fennel, thinly sliced
2 medium oranges, peeled and cut
 into segments
half quantity Avocado Salad Cream
 (page 115)
1 head endive

American

6 oz flounder or sole fillets, skinned
3 tbsp dry white wine
1 bouquet garni
salt and freshly ground black pepper
2 heads fennel, thinly sliced
2 medium oranges, peeled and cut
 into segments
half quantity Avocado Salad Cream
 (page 115)
1 head chicory

Place the fish in a non-stick frying
pan. Pour over the wine, add the
bouquet garni and season well.
Slowly bring to the boil and simmer
for 2–3 minutes until the fish is just
tender. Turn off the heat and leave
the fish to cool in the liquor. When
cool, drain and flake the flesh.

Place the fennel, orange segments and fish in a bowl. Spoon over
the salad cream and toss lightly.

Arrange the endive (chicory) on a
serving plate and spoon the salad
into the centre. Serve at once.
TOTAL CALORIES: 420
CALORIES PER SERVING: 210
SERVES 2

Fillet Steak with Green Peppercorns and Herbs

Metric/Imperial

1 × 150 g/5 oz fillet steak, trimmed of
 all fat
2 tsp green peppercorns, drained if
 necessary
1 tsp freshly chopped thyme
25 g/1 oz button mushrooms, sliced
2 tbsp dry red wine
dash of Worcestershire sauce
½ tsp French mustard
1 spring onion, chopped
extra chopped thyme, to serve

American

1 × 5 oz fillet steak, trimmed of all fat
2 tsp green peppercorns, drained if
 necessary
1 tsp freshly chopped thyme
¼ cup sliced button mushrooms
2 tbsp dry red wine
dash of Worcestershire sauce
½ tsp Dijon-style mustard

1 scallion, chopped
extra chopped thyme, to serve

Season the steak with salt and press
the peppercorns into both sides.
Heat a non-stick or dry frying pan
(skillet) and add the steak. Cook for
2–3 minutes on each side until
browned, then add the remaining
ingredients. Bring to the boil and
cook for a further 1 minute. Remove
the steak from the pan (skillet), place
on a hot serving plate and keep
it warm.

Increase the heat and boil the pan
mixture rapidly for 1–2 minutes, until it has reduced slightly. Spoon over
the steak and serve at once,
sprinkled with thyme.
TOTAL CALORIES: 290
SERVES 1

Fish Pie

Metric/Imperial

175 g/6 oz cod or other white fish
 fillet, skinned
150 ml/¼ pint dry white wine
1 tsp mixed dried herbs
small strip of lemon rind
125 g/4 oz peeled prawns
300 ml/½ pint white sauce (page
 123), using fish liquor and milk
 (see below)
175 g/6 oz mashed potato
1 tbsp freshly chopped parsley
2 tsp freshly chopped chives
1 tomato, sliced

American

6 oz cod or other white fish fillet,
 skinned
⅔ cup dry white wine
1 tsp mixed dried herbs
small strip of lemon rind
¼ lb peeled shrimp
1¼ cups white sauce (page 123),
 using fish liquor and milk (see
 below)
¾ cup mashed potato
1 tbsp freshly chopped parsley
2 tsp freshly chopped chives
1 tomato, sliced

Put the fish in a frying pan (skillet)
and add the wine, dried herbs and
lemon rind. Gradually bring to the
boil, then simmer for 5–7 minutes
until the fish is tender. Remove the
fish from the pan and flake the flesh.
Strain the cooking liquid and reserve
for the white sauce.

Put the fish and prawns (shrimp)
into a shallow ovenproof dish and
spoon over the sauce. Mix the
mashed potato and fresh herbs
together and spoon or pipe the mixture over the fish. Arrange tomato
slices on top and bake in a preheated
moderate oven, 200°C (400°F) or Gas

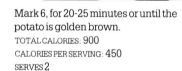

Mark 6, for 20-25 minutes or until the
potato is golden brown.
TOTAL CALORIES: 900
CALORIES PER SERVING: 450
SERVES 2

Fish Stuffed with Prawns and Lemon

Metric/Imperial

175 g/6 oz plaice fillets or haddock
 fillet, skinned
100 g/3½ oz peeled prawns
grated rind of ½ lemon
2 tsp fresh dill
salt and freshly ground black pepper
6 tbsp dry white wine
1 bouquet garni
1 tbsp toasted sesame seeds

American

6 oz flounder fillet or haddock fillet,
 skinned
½ cup shelled shrimp
grated rind of ½ lemon
2 tsp fresh dill
salt and freshly ground black pepper
6 tbsp dry white wine
1 bouquet garni
1 tbsp toasted sesame seeds

Clockwise from the front: Fennel
and Orange Salad, French
Vegetable Quiche, Fillet Steak with
Green Peppercorns and Herbs

Lay the fish fillets on a board. Mix the
prawns (shrimp), lemon rind and dill
together and season well. Arrange
the prawns (shrimp) in the centre of
the fish and roll them up. Place in an
ovenproof dish and pour over the
wine. Add the bouquet garni, cover
and cook in a preheated moderate
oven, 180°C (350°F) or Gas Mark 4,
for 12–15 minutes until the fish is
cooked and tender. Drain the fish
and arrange on a hot serving dish.
Remove the bouquet garni and boil
the liquor for 5–10 minutes until reduced and thickened. Spoon over
the fish, sprinkled with the sesame
seeds and serve at once.
TOTAL CALORIES: 480
SERVES 1

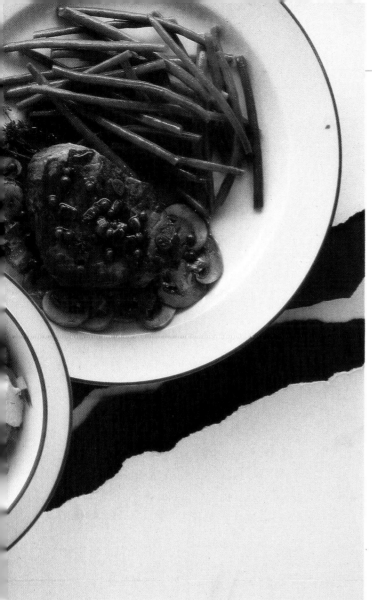

French Onion Soup

Metric/Imperial
1 tsp butter
110 g/4 oz onion, chopped
150 ml/¼ pint beef stock
salt and freshly ground black pepper
50 g/2 oz French bread slices
25 g/1 oz hard cheese, grated

American
1 tsp butter
¼ lb onion, chopped
⅔ cup beef stock
salt and freshly ground black pepper
2 oz French bread slices
¼ cup grated hard cheese

Melt the butter in a saucepan and cook the onion gently for 5 minutes until soft. Add the stock, simmer for 20 minutes and adjust the seasoning. Pour into a flameproof soup bowl, place the bread slices on top and sprinkle with cheese. Place under a preheated grill (broiler) until the cheese is bubbling and lightly browned on top. Serve at once.

TOTAL CALORIES: 280
SERVES 1

French Vegetable Quiche

Metric/Imperial
50 g/2 oz plain flour
50 g/2 oz wholemeal flour
pinch of salt
pinch of cayenne pepper
50 g/2 oz margarine
ice-cold water
Filling:
2 eggs
150 ml/¼ pint skimmed milk
100 g/3½ oz low fat cream cheese with garlic and herbs
2 tomatoes, skinned, seeded and chopped
1 onion, finely chopped
1 clove garlic, crushed
1 courgette, diced
½ green or red pepper, diced
½ tsp mixed dried herbs
salt and freshly ground black pepper
25 g/1 oz Edam cheese, thinly sliced

American
½ cup all-purpose flour
½ cup wholewheat flour
pinch of salt
pinch of cayenne

¼ cup margarine
ice-cold water
Filling:
2 eggs
⅔ cup skimmed milk
½ cup low fat cream cheese with garlic and herbs
2 tomatoes, skinned, seeded and chopped
1 onion, minced
1 clove garlic, crushed
1 zucchini, sliced
½ green or red pepper, diced
½ tsp mixed dried herbs
salt and freshly ground black pepper
¼ cup thinly sliced Edam cheese

Place the flours in a bowl with the salt and cayenne. Rub (cut) the margarine into the flour until the mixture resembles fine breadcrumbs. Stir in 2 teaspoons of cold water at a time, until the dough is firm. Lightly knead the dough on a floured board, roll out and use to line 4 7.5 cm (3 in) tins.

Beat the eggs, milk and cream cheese together. Place the prepared vegetables in a saucepan with the herbs and season well. Bring to the boil and simmer, uncovered, for 10 minutes or until the vegetables are softened and the mixture is reduced. Cool, then spoon into the pastry cases (pie shells). Spoon over the egg mixture and arrange the sliced cheese on top. Bake in a preheated oven, 190°C (375°F) or Gas Mark 5, for 20-25 minutes until set and golden brown. Serve hot or cold.

TOTAL CALORIES: 1040
CALORIES PER SERVING: 260
SERVES 4

Gazpacho

Metric/Imperial
350 g/12 oz fresh tomatoes, skinned and roughly chopped
2 cloves garlic, crushed
2 spring onions, chopped
¼ cucumber, chopped
1 red pepper, seeded and chopped
1 green pepper, seeded and chopped
1 sprig of thyme
1 sprig of parsley
1 sprig of basil
2 tbsp lemon juice
300 ml/½ pint tomato juice
few drops of Tabasco
salt and freshly ground black pepper
freshly chopped parsley

American
1½ cups skinned and roughly chopped tomatoes
2 cloves garlic, crushed
2 scallions, chopped
¼ cucumber, chopped
1 red pepper, seeded and chopped
1 green pepper, seeded and chopped
1 sprig of thyme
1 sprig of parsley
1 sprig of basil
2 tbsp lemon juice
1¼ cups tomato juice
few drops of hot pepper sauce
salt and freshly ground black pepper
freshly chopped parsley

Place all the ingredients, except the chopped parsley, in a blender and blend until very smooth. Chill in the refrigerator. Adjust the seasoning and serve sprinkled with parsley.

TOTAL CALORIES: 140
CALORIES PER SERVING: 70
SERVES 2

Gazpacho Garnishes
Arrange the following in small dishes to accompany the soup: 1 tomato, diced; 1 green pepper, seeded and finely diced; 1 small courgette (zucchini), finely diced; 1 slice bread, toasted and cut into small pieces.

Gnocchi with Tomato Sauce

Metric/Imperial
250 g/8 oz potato, boiled and mashed
1 egg
15 g/½ oz flour
salt and freshly ground black pepper
20 g/¾ oz Edam cheese. grated, to serve
Tomato Sauce:
1 tbsp oil
50 g/2 oz onion, chopped
250 g/8 oz canned tomatoes
freshly chopped basil or parsley

American
½ lb potato, boiled and mashed
1 egg
½ oz flour
salt and freshly ground black pepper
¾ oz Edam cheese. grated, to serve
Tomato Sauce:
1 tbsp oil
2 oz onion, chopped
½ lb canned tomatoes
freshly chopped basil or parsley

Place the mashed potato in a bowl, add the egg, flour and seasoning and mix well. Mould into small walnut-sized balls and place in a sieve (strainer). Lower into a saucepan of boiling water and cook until gnocchi rise to surface. Drain and keep warm.

Heat the oil in a saucepan and fry (sauté) the onion gently until soft. Add the tomatoes and seasoning. Simmer until the liquid has reduced, then stir in the herbs. Pour the sauce over and sprinkle with cheese.

TOTAL CALORIES: 550
SERVES 1

Green Fruit Salad

Metric/Imperial
125 g/4 oz ogen melon
125 g/4 oz honeydew melon
2 kiwi fruit, peeled and sliced
50 g/2 oz green grapes, pipped
175 g/6 oz pear, peeled, cored and chopped
juice and grated rind of 1 orange
125 g/4 oz banana

American
¼ lb cantaloupe melon
¼ lb honeydew melon
2 kiwi fruit, peeled and sliced
½ cup pitted green grapes
6 oz pear, peeled, cored and chopped
juice and grated rind of 1 orange
4 oz banana

Cube the melon or shape into balls, using a melon baller. Place in a bowl with the kiwi fruit and grapes. Add the pear to the other fruit with the orange rind and juice. Lastly, slice and add the banana just before serving.

TOTAL CALORIES: 340
CALORIES PER SERVING: 85
SERVES 4

Ham and Cider Sauce

Metric/Imperial
250 g/8 oz gammon joint
1 bay leaf
few peppercorns
few whole cloves
120 ml/4 fl oz cider
Cider Sauce:
2 tsp brown sugar
1 tbsp raisins
4 tbsp cider
salt and freshly ground black pepper
1 tsp cornflour

American
½ lb fresh ham (rump portion)
1 bay leaf
few peppercorns
few whole cloves
½ cup cider
Cider Sauce:
2 tsp brown sugar
1 tbsp raisins
4 tbsp cider
salt and freshly ground black pepper
1 tsp cornstarch

Place the gammon (ham) in a large saucepan with the bay leaves and peppercorns, with enough water to cover. Bring to the boil and simmer for 1–1½ hours until tender. Drain the gammon (ham) and remove the skin and most of the fat. Stud with cloves and place in a roasting pan with 120 ml/4 fl oz (½ cup) cider. Bake in a preheated moderate oven, 180°C (350°F) or Gas Mark 4, for 15 minutes, basting occasionally with the cider. Remove the meat and keep warm while making the sauce.

Place the brown sugar, raisins, cider and seasoning in a saucepan. Add the cider and meat juices from the roasting pan. Mix the cornflour (cornstarch) with a little water and stir into the sauce. Bring to the boil, then simmer, stirring. Serve the sauce with the sliced gammon (ham).

TOTAL CALORIES: 680
CALORIES PER SERVING: 340
SERVES 2

Herb Chicken

Metric/Imperial
4 × 100 g/3½ oz chicken breasts
50 g/2 oz low fat cream cheese with garlic and herbs
1–2 cloves garlic, crushed
25 g/1 oz button mushrooms, very finely chopped
2 tsp freshly chopped thyme
salt and freshly ground black pepper
grated rind of ½ lemon
150 ml/¼ pint dry white wine
1 fresh bouquet garni (parsley, rosemary, thyme and sage)

American
4 × 3½ oz chicken breasts
¼ cup low fat cream cheese with garlic and herbs
1–2 cloves garlic, crushed
¼ cup very finely chopped button mushrooms
2 tsp freshly chopped thyme
salt and freshly ground black pepper
grated rind of ½ lemon
⅔ cup dry white wine
1 fresh bouquet garni (parsley, rosemary, thyme and sage)

Make a horizontal cut into each chicken breast to make a pocket (make sure not to cut right through). Mix together the cream cheese, garlic, mushrooms and thyme. Season well and stir in the grated lemon rind. Divide the mixture into 4 and spoon into the chicken breast pockets. Sew up the chicken neatly using string and a trussing needle.

Place the chicken breasts in a nonstick frying pan and pour over the wine. Add the bouquet garni and season well. Bring to the boil, then cover the pan and simmer for 20–25 minutes or until tender. Arrange the chicken on a hot serving dish and keep warm. Discard the bouquet garni and boil the juices for 5–10 minutes or until reduced by about half. Spoon the juices over the chicken and serve at once.

TOTAL CALORIES: 720
CALORIES PER SERVING: 180
SERVES 4

Herring with Mustard Sauce

Metric/Imperial
1 × 150 g/5 oz herring
150 ml/¼ pint White Sauce (page 123)
1 tsp dry mustard
1 tsp wine vinegar

American
1 × 5 oz herring
⅔ cup white sauce (page 123)
1 tsp dry mustard
1 tsp wine vinegar

Place the herring under a preheated grill (broiler) and cook for 5–7 minutes on each side until the flesh is tender. Meanwhile, prepare the white sauce and stir in the mustard and vinegar. Serve the fish at once with the sauce.

TOTAL CALORIES: 365
SERVES 1

Hot Crab

Metric/Imperial
1 × 500 g/1 lb cooked crab, cleaned
2 spring onions, finely chopped
grated rind and juice of ½ lemon
pinch of cayenne pepper
salt
½ tbsp fresh brown breadcrumbs
½ tbsp freshly grated Parmesan cheese
fresh thyme and lemon wedges

American
1 × 1 lb cooked crab, cleaned
2 scallions, finely chopped
grated rind and juice of ½ lemon
pinch of cayenne
salt
½ tbsp soft fresh brown bread crumbs
½ tbsp freshly grated Parmesan cheese
fresh thyme and lemon wedges

Remove the crabmeat from the shell and reserve the shell. Flake the crabmeat in a bowl and add the spring onion (scallion), lemon rind and juice, cayenne and salt. Pile this mixture into the crab shell and sprinkle over the breadcrumbs and Parmesan cheese.

Place on a baking sheet and cook in a preheated moderate oven, 180°C (350°F) or Gas Mark 4, for 20 minutes until heated through and golden brown. Serve at once with fresh thyme and lemon wedges.

TOTAL CALORIES: 250
SERVES 1

Indian Chicken

This recipe needs to be prepared the day before.

Metric/Imperial
175 g/6 oz boneless chicken breast
lemon wedges and shredded lettuce
Marinade:
¼ tsp chilli powder
small piece root ginger, finely chopped
1 clove garlic, crushed
¼ tsp ground coriander
¼ tsp ground cumin
½ tsp paprika
4 tbsp plain yogurt
squeeze of lemon juice
½ tsp grated lemon rind

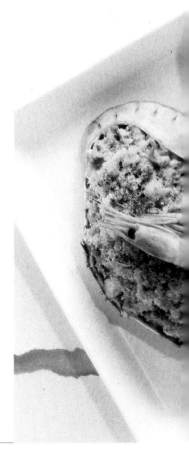

American

6 oz boneless chicken breast
lemon wedges and shredded lettuce
Marinade:
1/4 tsp chili powder
small piece ginger root, minced
1 clove garlic, crushed
1/4 tsp ground coriander
1/4 tsp ground cumin
1/2 tsp paprika
4 tbsp plain yogurt
squeeze of lemon juice
1/2 tsp grated lemon rind

To make the marinade, mix the chilli powder, ginger, garlic, coriander, cumin, paprika, yogurt, lemon juice and rind in a bowl. Score the chicken on both sides and place in the marinade. Chill overnight.

Remove the chicken from the marinade and place on a piece of foil large enough to completely cover it. Place in a roasting tin (pan), spoon over the marinade and seal the foil. Bake in a preheated moderate oven, 180°C (350°F) or Gas Mark 4, for 30 minutes, basting occasionally. Open the foil and return the chicken to the oven for a further 5–7 minutes.

Remove the chicken, drain off the marinade and place on a serving plate. Serve at once with lemon wedges and shredded lettuce.
TOTAL CALORIES: 270
SERVES 1

Irish Stew

Metric/Imperial

250 g/8 oz lean lamb, diced
2 medium onions, sliced
250 g/8 oz potato, sliced
salt and freshly ground black pepper
300 ml/1/2 pint beef stock
4 tsp tomato purée
freshly chopped parsley

American

1 cup diced lean lamb
2 medium onions, sliced
1 1/3 cups sliced potato
salt and freshly ground black pepper
1 1/4 cups beef stock
4 tsp tomato paste
freshly chopped parsley

Place the lamb, onion and potato in layers in a casserole dish with plenty of seasoning. Finish with a layer of potatoes. Mix the stock and tomato purée (paste) together and pour over the ingredients. Cover and cook in a preheated moderate oven, 180°C (350°F) or Gas Mark 4, for 1–1 1/2 hours. Reduce the oven temperature to 150°C (300°F) or Gas Mark 2 and take the top off the casserole for the last 30 minutes to brown the potatoes. Serve sprinkled with chopped parsley.
TOTAL CALORIES: 770
CALORIES PER SERVING: 385
SERVES 2

Jacket Potatoes

1 × 175 g/6 oz potato, scrubbed

Fillings

1 Boursin cheese and chives: *mix together 25 g/1 oz (2 tbsp) soft low fat cheese with herbs and garlic, 1 tbsp freshly chopped chives and a dash of Tabasco.*
TOTAL CALORIES: 110

2 Cottage cheese, spring onion (scallion) and curry powder: *mix together 50 g/2 oz (1/4 cup) sieved cottage cheese, 2 finely chopped spring onions (scallions) and 1/4 tsp curry powder.*
TOTAL CALORIES: 80

3 Ham and sweetcorn (kernel corn): *mix together 25 g/1 oz (2 tbsp) diced, cooked ham, 25 g/1 oz drained sweetcorn (kernel corn), 1 tsp grated onion and 1 tsp chopped parsley.*
TOTAL CALORIES: 100

4 Prawn (shrimp) and tuna: *mix together 25 g/1 oz drained and flaked tuna, 25 g/1 oz peeled prawns (shelled shrimp), 1 chopped spring onion (scallion) and 2 tsp finely chopped parsley.*
TOTAL CALORIES: 115

Prick the potato and bake in a preheated moderately hot oven, 200°C (400°F) or Gas Mark 6, for about 1 hour, until soft.

Cut the potato in half lengthwise. Scoop out the flesh and mash until smooth. Add any of the above fillings to the potato and mix well. Spoon the mixture back into the potato shells. Place on a baking sheet and return to the oven for 12–15 minutes until hot. Serve at once.
TOTAL CALORIES PER 1 × 175 g/6 oz POTATO: 180 (plus filling)

From the front: Hot Crab, Green Fruit Salad, Jacket Potatoes

Kidneys in Red Wine

Metric/Imperial
1 tsp oil
1 small onion, chopped
1 small carrot, sliced
1 stick celery, sliced
6 lambs' kidneys, halved, skinned and cored
2 tsp tomato purée
300 ml/½ pint stock
4 tbsp red wine
salt and freshly ground black pepper
freshly chopped parsley

American
1 tsp oil
1 small onion, chopped
1 small carrot, sliced
1 celery stalk, sliced
6 lambs' kidneys, halved, skinned and cored
2 tsp tomato paste
1¼ cups stock
4 tbsp red wine
salt and freshly ground black pepper
freshly chopped parsley

Heat the oil in a heavy saucepan and gently cook the onion, carrot and celery for 10 minutes. Add the kidneys and cook until browned. Mix together the tomato purée (paste), stock and wine, pour over the kidneys and season well. Cover and simmer gently for 12–15 minutes. Remove the kidneys and keep warm. Boil the sauce rapidly until reduced and thickened. Add the kidneys and heat through. Adjust the seasoning and serve sprinkled with parsley.
TOTAL CALORIES: 340
CALORIES PER SERVING: 170
SERVES 2

Lamb Kebab

Metric/Imperial
2 small tomatoes
3 squares red or green pepper, blanched
75 g/3 oz marinated lamb, sliced
4 button onions or quarters of a large onion

American
2 small tomatoes
3 squares red or green pepper, blanched
3 oz marinated lamb, sliced
4 pearl onions or quarters of a large onion

Thread the tomatoes, pepper, lamb and onions alternately onto a skewer. Grill (broil) for 7–8 minutes each side, turning once, until all the ingredients are cooked and tender.
TOTAL CALORIES: 160
SERVES 1

Lamb Noisette with Garlic and Rosemary

Metric/Imperial
1 × 100 g/3½ oz lamb noisette, trimmed of all fat
1 clove garlic, thinly sliced
few sprigs fresh rosemary
½ tsp French mustard with herbs or coarse grain mustard
salt and freshly ground black pepper
juice of ½ lemon

American
1 × 3½ oz lamb noisette, trimmed of all fat
1 clove garlic, thinly sliced
few sprigs fresh rosemary
½ tsp Dijon-style mustard with herbs, or coarse grain mustard
salt and freshly ground black pepper
juice of ½ lemon

Make small incisions all over the lamb and insert the slices of garlic and a few sprigs of rosemary. Spread the mustard on both sides of the meat, season with a little salt and pepper, and sprinkle over the lemon juice.

Leave to marinate for about 30 minutes. Preheat the grill (broiler) and cook the lamb for 4–6 minutes each side or until cooked as preferred.
TOTAL CALORIES: 220
SERVES 1

Lamb with Apricot Stuffing

Metric/Imperial
1 × 1.5 kg/3½ lb leg of lamb, boned
thyme sprigs
parsley sprigs
Stuffing:
6 dried apricots, chopped
½ tsp thyme
2 tbsp freshly chopped parsley
50 g/2 oz walnuts, chopped
1 small onion, chopped
75 g/3 oz wholewheat breadcrumbs
salt and freshly ground black pepper
2 sticks celery, chopped
beaten egg, to bind

American
1 × 3½ lb leg of lamb, boned
thyme sprigs
parsley sprigs
Stuffing:
6 dried apricots, chopped
½ tsp thyme
2 tbsp freshly chopped parsley
½ cup chopped walnuts
1 small onion, chopped
1½ cups soft fresh wholewheat bread crumbs
salt and freshly ground black pepper
2 celery stalks, chopped
beaten egg, to bind

Clockwise: Lamb Kebab, Lentil Soup, Liver Provençal

Mix all the stuffing ingredients together using only just enough egg to bind. Fill the leg of lamb with the mixture and sew or tie firmly using a trussing needle and string. Place in a roasting pan and sprinkle with some thyme sprigs. Place in a preheated moderately hot oven, 200°C (400°F) or Gas Mark 6, for 1½–1¾ hours. Serve sliced, with parsley sprigs.
TOTAL CALORIES: 2350
CALORIES PER SERVING: 590
SERVES 4

Lasagne

Metric/Imperial
25 g/1 oz lasagne (about 2 sheets)
150 ml/¼ pint white sauce (page 123)
15 g/½ oz grated Parmesan cheese
Meat sauce:
200 g/7 oz lean minced beef
2 tomatoes, skinned and chopped
1 onion, chopped
2 tsp tomato purée
1 tsp mixed dried herbs
salt and freshly ground black pepper
150 ml/¼ pint beef stock

American
1 oz lasagne (about 2 sheets)
⅔ cup white sauce (page 123)
2 tbsp grated Parmesan cheese
Meat sauce:
1 cup lean ground beef
2 tomatoes, skinned and chopped
1 onion, chopped
2 tsp tomato paste
1 tsp mixed dried herbs
salt and freshly ground black pepper
⅔ cup beef stock

Put the beef, tomatoes and onion in a saucepan and cook gently for 5 minutes, stirring. Stir in the tomato purée (paste) to the beef mixture, then add the herbs, seasoning and stock. Simmer for 20 minutes. Meanwhile, cook the lasagne in boiling salted water, then drain well. Put a layer of lasagne in an ovenproof dish, cover with half the meat sauce and white sauce, then repeat the layers, finishing with the white sauce. Sprinkle over the Parmesan and place in a preheated moderate oven, 180°C (350°F) or Gas Mark 4, for 25–30 minutes, until browned and heated through.
TOTAL CALORIES: 700
CALORIES PER SERVING: 350
SERVES 2

Note: For a quicker recipe, buy lasagne that does not need pre-cooking and layer it as directed.

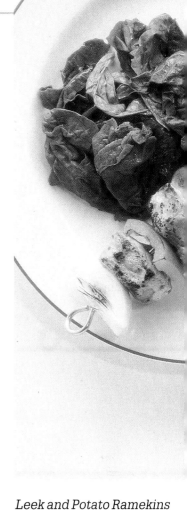

Leek and Potato Ramekins

Metric/Imperial
175 g/6 oz potato, roughly chopped
125 g/4 oz potato, diced
2 eggs
8 tbsp single cream
2 tbsp skimmed milk
125 g/4 oz leeks, thinly sliced, blanched and drained
freshly grated nutmeg

American
6 oz potato, roughly chopped
¼ lb potato, diced
2 eggs
8 tbsp light cream
2 tbsp skimmed milk
¼ lb leeks, thinly sliced, blanched and drained
freshly grated nutmeg

Boil the chopped potatoes, then drain and mash. Mix with the diced potato, eggs, cream and skimmed milk. Stir in the leeks, nutmeg and seasoning. Grease 4 ramekin dishes and spoon in the mixture. Bake in a preheated moderate oven, 180°F (350°F) Gas Mark 5, for 20–25 minutes until golden brown.

TOTAL CALORIES: 950
CALORIES PER SERVING: 240
SERVES 4

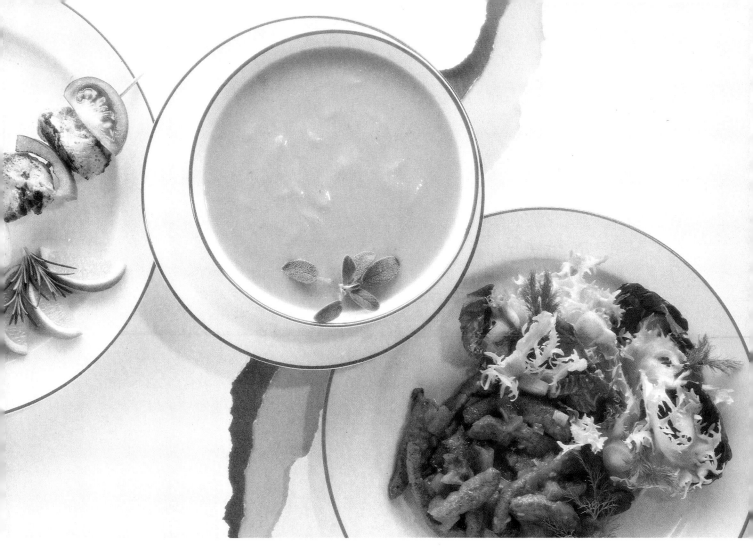

Leek and Thyme Quiche

Metric/Imperial
50 g/2 oz plain flour
50 g/2 oz wholemeal flour
pinch of salt
pinch of cayenne pepper
50 g/2 oz margarine
ice-cold water
Filling:
200 g/7 oz leeks, trimmed and thinly
    sliced
3 eggs
150 ml/¼ pint skimmed milk
50 g/2 oz Cheddar cheese, finely
    grated
salt and cayenne pepper
2 tsp freshly chopped thyme

American
½ cup all-purpose flour
½ cup wholewheat flour
pinch of salt
pinch of cayenne
¼ cup margarine
ice-cold water
Filling:
1½ cups thinly sliced leeks
3 eggs
⅔ cup skimmed milk
⅔ cup freshly grated Cheddar
    cheese
salt and cayenne
2 tsp freshly chopped thyme

Place the flours in a bowl with the salt and cayenne. Rub (cut) the margarine into the flour until the mixture resembles fine breadcrumbs. Stir in 2 teaspoons of cold water at a time until the dough is firm.

Lightly knead the pastry on a floured board. Roll out and use to line 4 individual tins (pans), 7.5 cm (3 in) in diameter. Chill for 20 minutes while making the filling.

Blanch the leeks in boiling salted water for 2 minutes, then drain and dry on kitchen paper towels. Mix the eggs, milk, cheese, salt, cayenne and thyme together. Divide the leeks into 4 portions and arrange in the bottom of the pastry cases (pie shells). Spoon over the egg mixture.

Bake in a preheated moderately hot oven, 200°C (400°F) or Gas Mark 6, for 20-25 minutes or until set and golden brown. Serve hot or cold.
TOTAL CALORIES: 1230
CALORIES PER SERVING: 310
SERVES 4
※*Note: If frozen, allow to thaw, then place in a moderate oven, 180°C (350°F) or Gas Mark 4, for 10–12 minutes until heated through. Do not re-freeze.*

Lentil Soup

Metric/Imperial
25 g/1 oz lentils, soaked overnight
1 onion, chopped
2 sticks celery, chopped
1 carrot, sliced
300 ml/½ pint stock
salt
grated nutmeg
freshly chopped parsley and mint

American
2 tbsp lentils, soaked overnight
1 onion, chopped
2 celery stalks, chopped
1 carrot, sliced
1¼ cups stock
salt
grated nutmeg
freshly chopped parsley and mint

Place the lentils, onion, celery, carrot and stock in a saucepan. Bring to the boil and simmer for 20–30 minutes or until the lentils are quite soft. Cool slightly, then purée in a blender. Season with salt and nutmeg, and adjust the consistency with a little more stock, if necessary. Serve sprinkled with parsley and mint.
TOTAL CALORIES: 130
SERVES 1

Liver Provençal

Metric/Imperial
200 g/7 oz calves' or lambs' liver
seasoned wholemeal flour
2 tsp oil
150 g/5 oz onion, chopped
200 g/7 oz tomatoes, skinned and
    chopped
½ tsp mixed dried herbs
salt and freshly ground black pepper

American
7 oz calf or lamb liver
seasoned wholewheat flour
2 tsp oil
1¼ cups chopped onion
¾ cup skinned and chopped
    tomatoes
½ tsp mixed dried herbs
salt and freshly ground black pepper

Cut the liver into thin strips and coat lightly in the seasoned flour. Heat the oil in a frying pan (skillet) and cook the onion gently for about 5 minutes until soft. Add the liver, tomatoes and herbs and season well. Simmer very gently for 5 minutes, taking care not to overcook the liver. Serve at once.
TOTAL CALORIES: 460
CALORIES PER SERVING: 230
SERVES 2

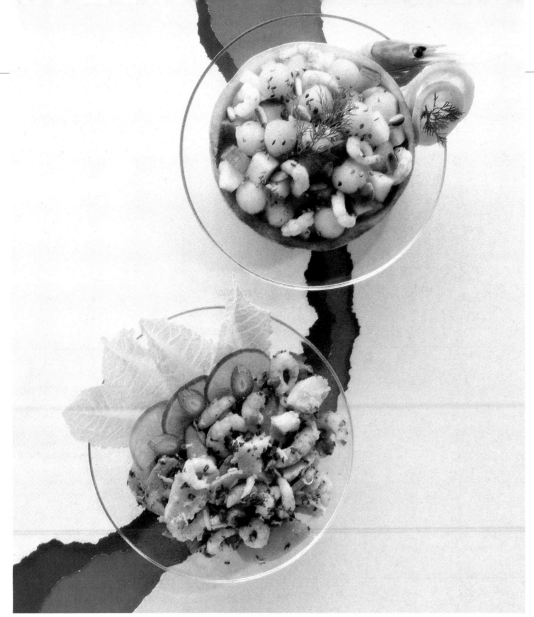

Low Fat Dressing

Metric/Imperial
4 tbsp plain yogurt
2 tbsp sunflower seed oil
1 tbsp lemon juice
2 tbsp freshly chopped herbs
(chervil, dill, chives, etc)
dash of Tabasco

American
4 tbsp plain yogurt
2 tbsp sunflower seed oil
1 tbsp lemon juice
2 tbsp freshly chopped herbs
(chervil, dill, chives, etc)
dash of hot pepper sauce .

Using a small whisk, beat the yogurt until smooth, then add the other ingredients and beat until well mixed. This can be served over any salad, either mixed green or *salades composés*.

TOTAL CALORIES: 50 per tbsp

Low Fat Gravy

This recipe may be used to serve with roasted meat, or when a dry frying pan is used to cook steaks and chops.

Metric/Imperial
sediment from the pan
150 ml/¼ pint dry white or red wine
pinch of mixed dried herbs
dash of Worcestershire sauce or
Tabasco
salt and freshly ground black pepper

American
sediment from the pan
⅔ cup dry white or red wine
pinch of mixed dried herbs
dash of Worcestershire sauce or hot
pepper sauce
salt and freshly ground black pepper

Drain any fat from the pan, or use a special fat-removing brush to do this. Place the pan over a low heat and cook until it becomes 'sticky'. Add the wine (use red wine for red meat and white wine for pork, veal and poultry), stirring constantly. Add a little Worcestershire sauce or Tabasco (hot pepper sauce) and seasoning. Serve at once.

TOTAL CALORIES: 100
CALORIES PER SERVING: 50
SERVES 2

Liver Stroganoff

Metric/Imperial
250 g/8 oz calves' liver
salt and freshly ground black pepper
2 tsp oil
50 g/2 oz onions, sliced
125 g/4 oz button mushrooms, sliced
3 tbsp sherry or dry white wine
5 tbsp soured cream
freshly chopped parsley

American
½ lb calf liver
salt and freshly ground black pepper
2 tsp oil
½ cup sliced onions
1 cup chopped button mushrooms
3 tbsp sherry or dry white wine
5 tbsp sour cream
freshly chopped parsley

Cut the liver into thin strips and season with salt and pepper. Heat the oil in a non-stick frying pan (skillet), add the onions and fry (sauté) until lightly browned. Add the liver, mushrooms and sherry or wine and simmer for 5 minutes. Season and stir in the soured cream and sprinkle with parsley just before serving.

TOTAL CALORIES: 630
CALORIES PER SERVING: 315
SERVES 2

Note: If freezing, omit the soured cream and parsley and add when reheated, just before serving.

Liver with Orange

Metric/Imperial
1 small onion, sliced
2 tsp butter
125 g/4 oz calves' or lambs' liver,
thinly sliced
2 tsp flour
150 ml/¼ pint stock
salt and freshly ground black pepper
¼ tsp French mustard
1 tbsp red wine
2 slices of orange
25 g/1 oz brown rice, boiled in stock,
to serve

American
1 small onion, sliced
2 tsp butter
¼ lb calf or lamb liver, thinly sliced
2 tsp flour
⅔ cup stock
salt and freshly ground black pepper
¼ tsp Dijon-style mustard
1 tbsp red wine
2 slices of orange
2 tbsp brown rice, boiled in stock, to
serve

Place the onion and butter in a frying pan (skillet) and cook gently for 5 minutes until the onion is soft. Add the liver and cook for a further 7 minutes, turning once. Remove the liver and keep warm. Add the flour to the pan and cook for 1 minute, stirring. Stir in the stock and bring to the boil. Add seasoning with the mustard, red wine and orange slices. Simmer for 1 minute, then pour over the liver and serve with rice.

TOTAL CALORIES: 430
SERVES 1

Mediterranean Seafood Sauce

Metric/Imperial

100 g/3½ oz onion, finely chopped
150 ml/¼ pint dry white wine
100 g/3½ oz tomatoes, skinned,
    seeded and chopped
1 or 2 cloves garlic, crushed
1 fresh bouquet garni (thyme,
    rosemary and parsley)
1 tsp French mustard
dash of Worcestershire sauce
pinch of cayenne pepper
100 g/3½ oz crabmeat
200 g/7 oz peeled prawns
100 g/3½ oz scallops, cleaned and
    quartered
salt and freshly ground black pepper
freshly chopped parsley

American

¾ cup minced onion
⅔ cup dry white wine
½ cup skinned, seeded and chopped
    tomatoes
1 or 2 cloves garlic, crushed
1 bouquet garni (thyme, rosemary
    and parsley)
1 tsp Dijon-style mustard
dash of Worcestershire sauce
pinch of cayenne
½ cup crab meat
1 generous cup shelled shrimp
3½ oz scallops, cleaned and
    quartered
salt and freshly ground black pepper
freshly chopped parsley

Place the onion, wine, tomatoes garlic, bouquet garni, mustard, Worcestershire sauce and cayenne into a saucepan. Bring to the boil and cook rapidly for 15-20 minutes, stirring occasionally, until thickened and reduced. Add the shellfish and seasoning, then simmer for 5 minutes. Serve sprinkled with parsley.
TOTAL CALORIES: 580
CALORIES PER SERVING: 145
SERVES 4

Melon, Pear and Cucumber Salad

Metric/Imperial

1 ripe ogen melon
1 ripe comice pear
¼ cucumber, diced
125 g/4 oz peeled prawns
Lemon Dressing (page 115)
salt and freshly ground black pepper
15 g/½ oz pinenuts, toasted
1 tbsp sesame seeds, toasted
2 whole prawns and lemon twists

American

1 small ripe honeyball melon
1 ripe comice pear
¼ cucumber, diced
½ cup shelled shrimp
Lemon Dressing (page 115)
salt and freshly ground black pepper
2 tbsp pine nuts
·1 tbsp sesame seeds, toasted
2 whole shrimp and lemon twists

Halve the melon, remove seeds and scoop out the flesh. Peel, core and dice the pear and add to the melon flesh with the cucumber and prawns (shrimp). Add the dressing, seasoning and pinenuts and spoon into the shells. Garnish with sesame seeds, whole prawns (shrimp) and lemon.
TOTAL CALORIES: 390
CALORIES PER SERVING: 200
SERVES 2

Middle Eastern Rice

Metric/Imperial

25 g/1 oz butter
25 g/1 oz flaked almonds
25 g/1 oz cashew nuts
1 medium onion, thinly sliced
2 carrots, coarsely grated
175 g/6 oz brown rice
2 cloves garlic, thinly sliced
1 tsp ground cumin
1 tsp ground coriander
1 tsp turmeric
½ tsp ground cinnamon
¼ tsp ground cloves
salt and freshly ground black pepper
3 tbsp raisins
1 medium eating apple, peeled,
    cored and chopped
300 ml/½ pint consommé, diluted to
    make 600 ml/1 pint
150 ml/¼ pint dry white wine
100 g/3½ oz frozen peas

American

2 tbsp butter
¼ cup flaked almonds
¼ cup cashew nuts
1 medium onion, thinly sliced
2 carrots, coarsely grated
¾ cup brown rice
2 cloves garlic, thinly sliced
1 tsp ground cumin
1 tsp ground coriander
1 tsp turmeric
½ tsp ground cinnamon
¼ tsp ground cloves
salt and freshly ground black pepper
3 tbsp raisins
1 medium eating apple, peeled,
    cored and chopped
1¼ cups consommé, diluted to make
    2½ cups
⅔ cup dry white wine
½ cup frozen peas

Melt the butter in a large saucepan and fry (sauté) the nuts for 1–2 minutes until brown. Add the carrots, rice, garlic, spices and seasoning and fry for 2 minutes. Stir in the raisins, apple, consommé and wine, and simmer for 30–35 minutes. Add the peas and cook for 1 minute, then sprinkle with the nuts.
TOTAL CALORIES: 1380
CALORIES PER SERVING: 345
SERVES 4

Minestrone

Metric/Imperial

1 rasher streaky bacon, chopped
1 medium onion, chopped
75 g/3 oz green cabbage, chopped
2 tomatoes, skinned and chopped
2 tsp tomato purée
1 carrot, diced
150 ml/¼ pint stock
salt and freshly ground black pepper
75 g/3 oz canned haricot beans,
    drained

American

1 slice bacon, chopped
1 medium onion, chopped
1 cup chopped green cabbage
2 tomatoes, skinned and chopped
2 tsp tomato paste
1 carrot, diced
⅔ cup stock
salt and freshly ground black pepper
3 oz canned haricot beans, drained

Cook the bacon and onion in a heavy saucepan until the onion is soft. Add the cabbage, tomatoes, tomato purée (paste), carrot, stock and seasoning. Simmer for 20 minutes, then stir in the haricot beans. Adjust the seasoning before serving. Serve with 40 g/1½ oz (1 slice) wholewheat bread and 25 g/1 oz grated Edam cheese.
TOTAL CALORIES: 240
SERVES 1

Mixed Seafood Salad

Metric/Imperial

100 g/3½ oz scallops, cleaned
100 g/3½ oz peeled prawns
100 g/3½ oz crabmeat
25 g/1 oz button mushrooms, sliced
2 spring onions, chopped
grated rind and juice of 1 lime
2 tsp freshly chopped parsley
2 tsp freshly chopped thyme
1 clove garlic, crushed (optional)
salt and freshly ground black pepper
2 large Spanish tomatoes, each
    weighing 200 g/7 oz
few crisp lettuce leaves
2 whole prawns and lime slices

American

3½ oz scallops, cleaned
½ cup shelled shrimp
½ cup crab meat
¼ cup sliced button mushrooms
2 scallions, chopped
grated rind and juice of 1 lime
2 tsp freshly chopped parsley
2 tsp freshly chopped thyme
1 clove garlic, crushed (optional)
salt and freshly ground black pepper
2 large tomatoes, each weighing 7 oz
few crisp lettuce leaves
2 whole shrimp and lime slices

Wash the scallops and pat dry. Poach them in simmering water for 1–2 minutes until cooked and tender. Drain and cool.

Mix the scallops, prawns (shrimp) and crabmeat together; add the mushrooms, spring onions (scallions), lime juice and rind and mix well. Stir in the herbs, garlic (if using) and seasoning.

Cut the tomatoes in half, scoop out the seeds and carefully remove the flesh, leaving a little around the skin so that the tomato does not collapse. Chop up the tomato flesh and fold into the fish mixture. Pile the mixture into the four tomato shells.

Arrange the lettuce leaves on a serving dish and put the tomato shells on top. Spoon any remaining mixture around the tomatoes and serve with the whole prawns (shrimp) and slices of lime.
TOTAL CALORIES: 400
CALORIES PER SERVING: 200
SERVES 2

Orange and Pear Fruit Salad

Metric/Imperial

175 g/6 oz dried pears
150 ml/¼ pint natural unsweetened
    orange juice
1 tbsp brandy
15 g/½ oz raisins
3 oranges, cut into segments
1 tbsp pistachio nuts

American

6 oz dried pears
⅔ cup natural unsweetened orange
    juice
1 tbsp brandy
1½ tbsp raisins
3 oranges, cut into segments
1 tbsp pistachio nuts

Soak the pears in the orange juice and brandy for 2 hours. Transfer to a saucepan, bring to the boil, add the raisins and simmer, covered, for 20–25 minutes until the pears are tender. Leave to cool in a serving dish. Mix the orange segments and pistachios together, and spoon over the pears. Chill before serving.
TOTAL CALORIES: 500
CALORIES PER SERVING: 125
SERVES 4

Orange and Tomato Soup

Metric/Imperial
4 tomatoes, skinned and chopped
1 carrot, sliced
3 peppercorns
300ml/½ pint stock
1 small onion, chopped
pinch of salt
1 rounded tsp arrowroot
juice of ½ orange
shredded orange rind

American
4 tomatoes, skinned and chopped
1 carrot, sliced
3 peppercorns
1¼ cups stock
1 small onion, chopped
pinch of salt
1 rounded tsp arrowroot
juice of ½ orange
shredded orange rind

Place the tomatoes, carrots, peppercorns, stock and seasoning in a saucepan and simmer for 30 minutes. Cool slightly, remove the peppercorns, then purée in a blender or rub through a sieve (strainer). Mix the arrowroot with 1 tablespoon of cold water and stir into the soup. Return to the clean saucepan and bring to the boil, stirring constantly. Add the orange juice and reheat. Garnish with shredded orange rind and serve with 40g/1½oz (1 slice) wholewheat bread.

TOTAL CALORIES: 100
SERVES 1

Oriental Red Mullet

Metric/Imperial
1 × 175g/6oz red mullet, gutted
2 spring onions. chopped
50g/2oz button mushrooms, thinly
    sliced
small piece root ginger, cut into
    julienne strips
1 tbsp soy sauce
lemon slices or wedges and fresh
    coriander leaves

American
1 × 6oz red mullet, cleaned
2 scallions, chopped
½ cup thinly sliced button
    mushrooms
small piece ginger root, cut into
    matchstick strips
1 tbsp soy sauce
lemon slices or wedges and fresh
    coriander leaves

Wash the fish and dry well. Mix the spring onions (scallions), mushrooms, ginger and soy sauce together. Place the fish in an ovenproof dish, spoon the mushroom mixture into the cavity of the fish and the remaining mixture around it. Cook in a preheated moderate oven, 180°C (350°F) or Gas Mark 4, for 12–15 minutes until tender. Serve, covered, with lemon and coriander.

TOTAL CALORIES: 220
SERVES 1
Note: If mullet is unavailable, use trout of the same weight. Total calories will then be 150.

Clockwise from the front: Oriental Red Mullet, Poached Salmon Steak, Peach and Orange Sorbet

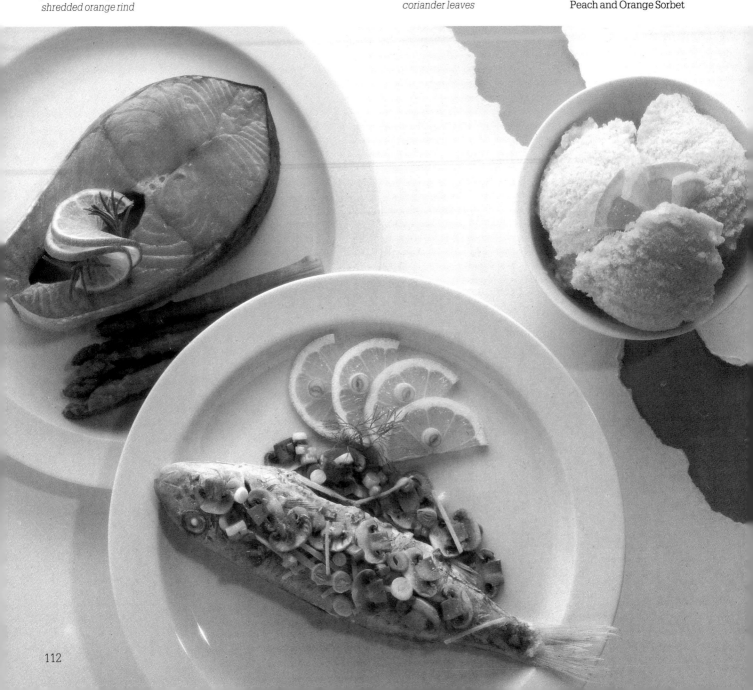

Peach and Orange Sorbet

Metric/Imperial
75 g/3 oz sugar
250 ml/8 fl oz water
350 g/12 oz peaches, skinned and stones removed
3 tbsp unsweetened orange
1 egg white
1½ tbsp icing sugar

American
⅓ cup sugar
1 cup water
¾ lb peaches, skinned and pits removed
3 tbsp unsweetened orange juice
1 egg white
1½ tbsp confectioners' sugar

Dissolve the sugar in the water in a heavy-based saucepan over a low heat. Gradually bring to the boil and boil rapidly for 3 minutes, then allow to cool. Place the peaches in a blender with the sugar syrup and purée. Add to the orange juice and mix well. Pour the mixture into a plastic freezer container with lid. Freeze until the mixture is half frozen.

Whisk the egg white until stiff, then gradually whisk in the icing (confectioners') sugar. Then whisk in the semi-frozen peach and orange purée until smooth and combined. Pour the mixture back into the freezer container and freeze until set. When serving, spoon or scoop into bowls and serve at once.
TOTAL CALORIES: 670
CALORIES PER SERVING: 170
SERVES 4

Pepperoni

Metric/Imperial
2 tsp butter
½ small green pepper, cored, seeded and sliced
½ small red pepper, cored, seeded and sliced
1 small onion, sliced
½ clove garlic, crushed (optional)
salt and freshly ground black pepper

American
2 tsp butter
½ small green pepper, cored, seeded and sliced
½ small red pepper, cored, seeded and sliced
1 small onion, sliced
½ clove garlic, crushed (optional)
salt and freshly ground black pepper

Melt the butter in a small saucepan and add the peppers, onion and garlic (if using). Cook gently for about 15 minutes until soft. Season lightly.
TOTAL CALORIES: 120
SERVES 1

Piperade

Metric/Imperial
25 g/1 oz butter
4 spring onions, chopped
1 green pepper, seeded and sliced
1 red pepper, seeded and sliced
2 courgettes, sliced
1 clove garlic, crushed
100 g/3½ oz very lean rashers bacon, chopped
2 tomatoes, skinned, seeded and chopped
½ tsp mixed dried herbs
4 eggs, beaten
chopped parsley and chives

American
2 tbsp butter
4 scallions, chopped
1 green pepper, seeded and sliced
1 red pepper, seeded and sliced
2 zucchini, sliced
1 clove garlic, crushed
4 very lean bacon slices, chopped
2 tomatoes, skinned, seeded and chopped
½ tsp mixed dried herbs
4 eggs, beaten
chopped parsley and chives

Heat the butter in a non-stick frying pan and gently fry (sauté) the spring onions (scallions), green and red pepper for 2 minutes, stirring occasionally. Add the courgettes (zucchini) and garlic, then increase the heat, add the bacon, and cook for 2 minutes. Stir in the tomatoes and herbs and cook, uncovered, for 5 minutes. Stir in the eggs and cook until just scrambled. Pile onto a warmed serving dish. Sprinkle with the parsley and chives and serve at once.
TOTAL CALORIES: 750
CALORIES PER SERVING: 190
SERVES 4

Poached Salmon Steak

Metric/Imperial
few peppercorns
1 bay leaf
juice of ½ lemon
½ medium onion, sliced
½ carrot, sliced
1 × 150 g/5 oz salmon steak

American
few peppercorns
1 bay leaf
juice of ½ lemon
½ medium onion, sliced
½ carrot, sliced
1 × 5 oz salmon steak

Place the peppercorns, bay leaf, lemon juice, onion and carrot in a saucepan and add sufficient water to just cover the vegetables. Place the salmon on top, cover the pan and poach gently for 10–12 minutes until the flesh is cooked and tender. Drain the salmon, discarding the vegetables, and serve at once.
TOTAL CALORIES: 200
SERVES 1

Pork Casserole

Metric/Imperial
175 g/6 oz pork fillet, cubed
1 small onion, chopped
3 tsp tomato purée
2 tsp soy sauce
1 tsp sugar
200 ml/⅓ pint stock
salt and freshly ground black pepper
1 tsp cornflour

American
6 oz pork tenderloin, cubed
1 small onion, chopped
3 tsp tomato paste
2 tsp soy sauce
1 tsp sugar
⅞ cup stock
salt and freshly ground black pepper
1 tsp cornstarch

Place the pork, onion, tomato purée (paste), soy sauce, sugar, stock and seasoning in a saucepan. Stir well, bring to the boil and simmer for about 45 minutes or until the meat is tender. Mix the cornflour (cornstarch) with a little water and stir into the casserole. Bring to the boil, stirring, and adjust the seasoning.
TOTAL CALORIES: 460
CALORIES PER SERVING: 230
SERVES 2

Pork Chop with Cider

Metric/Imperial
1 small onion, sliced
1 × 175 g/6 oz pork chop, trimmed of all fat
150 ml/¼ pint stock
150 ml/¼ pint dry cider
salt and freshly ground black pepper
50 g/2 oz cooking apple, sliced
freshly chopped parsley

American
1 small onion, sliced
1 × 6 oz centre cut pork chop, trimmed of all fat
⅔ cup stock
⅔ cup hard cider
salt and freshly ground black pepper
½ cup sliced apple
freshly chopped parsley

Put the onion in a small flameproof casserole and place the chop on top. Add the stock, cider and seasoning. Cover and place in a preheated moderately hot oven, 190°C (375°F) or Gas Mark 5, for about 1 hour.

Remove the chop to a serving dish and keep warm. Place the casserole on top of the stove, add the apple and bring to the boil, stirring. Adjust the seasoning and simmer for 15 minutes until the sauce is thickened and reduced. Spoon the sauce over the chop and serve sprinkled with parsley.
TOTAL CALORIES: 500
SERVES 1

Pork Curry

Metric/Imperial
1 tbsp oil
100 g/3½ oz onions, sliced
1½ tsp ground coriander
½ tsp ground turmeric
1 tsp ground cumin
¼ tsp ground ginger
½–1 tsp chilli powder
500 g/1 lb very lean pork fillet, diced
small piece root ginger, finely chopped
2–3 cloves garlic, crushed
1 × 397 g/14 oz can tomatoes
salt and freshly ground black pepper
1 tbsp freshly grated coconut

American
1 tbsp oil
¾ cup sliced onions
1½ tsp ground coriander
½ tsp ground turmeric
1 tsp ground cumin
¼ tsp ground ginger
½–1 tsp chili powder
1 lb very lean pork tenderloin, diced
small piece ginger root, minced
2–3 cloves garlic, crushed
1 can (16 oz) tomatoes
salt and freshly ground black pepper
1 tbsp freshly grated coconut

Heat the oil in a pan, add the onions and fry (sauté) until lightly browned. Add the spices and cook for a further 2 minutes. Add the pork and brown on all sides (do not allow the onion and spices to burn). Pour off any excess fat, then add the ginger, garlic, tomatoes with their juice and season well. Bring to the boil, cover and simmer for 30 minutes. Sprinkle over the coconut and simmer, uncovered, for a further 30 minutes, stirring occasionally, until the meat is tender and the sauce thickened. Serve immediately.
TOTAL CALORIES: 1280
CALORIES PER SERVING: 320
SERVES 4

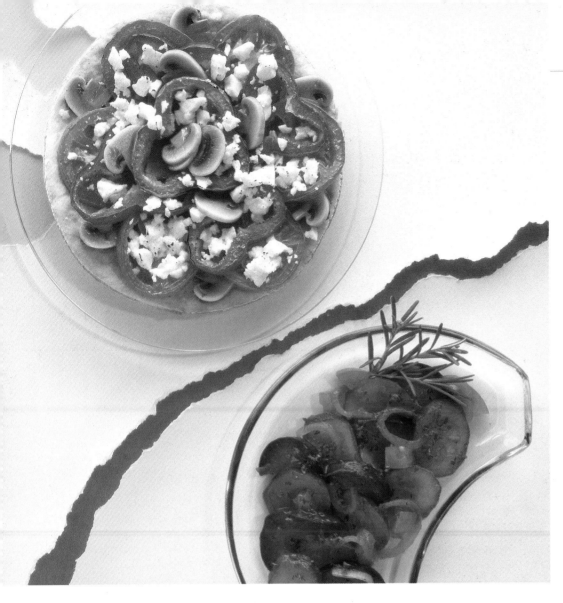

resembles fine breadcrumbs. Then add just enough milk to mix into a soft dough. Knead well until thoroughly mixed. Flatten into 2 rounds about 13 cm (5 in) in diameter and place on a greased baking sheet. Season.

Top with remaining ingredients finishing with cheese. Bake in a preheated hot oven, 220°C (425°F) or Gas Mark 7, for 15–20 minutes.

TOTAL CALORIES: 900

CALORIES PER SERVING: 450

SERVES 2

Ratatouille

Metric/Imperial
1 courgette, sliced
2 tomatoes, skinned, seeded and chopped
½ small onion, sliced
¼ small aubergine, sliced
150 ml/¼ pint stock or tomato juice
½ clove garlic, crushed
salt and freshly ground black pepper

American
1 zucchini, sliced
2 tomatoes, skinned, seeded and chopped
½ small onion, sliced
¼ small egg plant, sliced
⅔ cup stock or tomato juice
½ clove garlic, crushed
salt and freshly ground black pepper

Put all the ingredients in a saucepan and season well. Bring to the boil, stirring occasionally, for 15–20 minutes until the vegetables are soft and the liquid reduced.

TOTAL CALORIES: 35

SERVES 1

Ratatouille Pies

Metric/Imperial
50 g/2 oz wholemeal flour
50 g/2 oz plain flour
pinch of salt
ice-cold water
Filling:
15 g/½ oz butter
1 medium onion, thinly sliced
1 small aubergine, diced
1 courgette, thinly sliced
2 tomatoes, skinned, seeded and chopped
1 tbsp tomato purée
salt and freshly ground black pepper
2 tsp coriander seeds

American
½ cup wholewheat flour
½ cup all-purpose flour
pinch of salt
ice-cold water

Pork Fillet with Prunes

Metric/Imperial
150 g/5 oz pork fillet
salt and freshly ground black pepper
5 prunes, soaked and stoned
150 ml/¼ pint dry white wine

American
5 oz pork tenderloin
salt and freshly ground black pepper
5 prunes, soaked and pitted
⅔ cup dry white wine

Cut a pocket in the pork, sprinkle with salt and pepper and fill with the prunes. Tie up securely with string and place on a rack in a roasting pan with the wine. Roast in a preheated moderately hot oven, 190°C (375°F) or Gas Mark 5, for about 35 minutes, basting occasionally with the wine. When cooked, remove the meat from the pan, remove string, and keep warm. Strain the juices into a saucepan and bring to the boil, stirring. Continue boiling until reduced by half. Pour the juices over the meat and serve immediately.

TOTAL CALORIES: 305

SERVES 1

Front: Ratatouille
Back: Quick Pizza

Potato, Carrot and Onion Soup

Metric/Imperial
110 g/4 oz potato, sliced
½ onion, chopped
1 carrot, diced
1 leek, sliced
150 ml/¼ pint skimmed milk
salt and freshly ground black pepper

American
¼ lb potato, sliced
½ onion, chopped
1 carrot, diced
1 leek, sliced
⅔ cup skimmed milk
salt and freshly ground black pepper

Place all the ingredients in a saucepan, bring to the boil and simmer for 30 minutes. Cool slightly, then purée the soup in a blender or press through a sieve (strainer). Reheat in the clean saucepan and serve with 75 g/3 oz French bread.

TOTAL CALORIES: 175

SERVES 1

Quick Pizza

Metric/Imperial
Pizza Base:
125 g/4 oz self-raising flour
pinch bicarbonate of soda
25 g/1 oz butter
4–5 tbsp skimmed milk
Topping:
salt and freshly ground black pepper
50 g/2 oz cooked peas
4 tomatoes, sliced
75 g/3 oz mushrooms, sliced
50 g/2 oz feta cheese, crumbled

American
Pizza Base:
1 cup self-rising flour
pinch of baking soda
2 tbsp butter
4–5 tbsp skimmed milk
Topping:
salt and freshly ground black pepper
½ cup cooked peas
4 sliced tomatoes
1 cup sliced mushrooms
¼ cup feta cheese, crumbled

First make the base: sift the flour and soda into a large mixing bowl. Rub (cut) in the butter until the mixture

Filling:
1 tbsp butter
1 medium onion, thinly sliced
1 small eggplant, diced
1 zucchini, thinly sliced
2 tomatoes, skinned, seeded and
    chopped
½ green pepper, seeded and
    chopped
1 tbsp tomato paste
salt and freshly ground black pepper
2 tsp coriander seeds

Place the flours in a bowl and mix together with the salt. Add 2 tsp cold water at a time to give a firm dough. Knead lightly. Roll out and use to line 4 × 7.5 cm (3 in) individual flan tins (pie pans). Prick the bottoms and chill for 30 minutes.

Melt the butter in a saucepan, add the onion and aubergine (eggplant) and cook gently for 10 minutes. Stir in the courgette (zucchini), tomatoes, pepper and tomato purée (paste). Add seasoning and the coriander seeds. Bring to the boil, cover and simmer for 2 minutes.

Line the pastry cases (pie shells) with foil or greaseproof (waxed) paper and beans and bake in a preheated moderately hot oven, 200°C (400°F) or Gas Mark 6, for 12–15 minutes until golden brown. Remove the foil or paper and cook for a further 2–3 minutes. Spoon in the filling and serve hot or cold.

TOTAL CALORIES: 580
CALORIES PER SERVING: 145
SERVES 4

Red Cabbage with Apple

Metric/Imperial
75 g/3 oz apple, sliced
75 g/3 oz red cabbage, sliced
50 g/2 oz onion, chopped
15 g/½ oz raisins
¼ tsp freshly grated nutmeg
2 tsp cider or wine vinegar
salt and freshly ground black pepper

American
3 oz apple, sliced
3 oz red cabbage, sliced
2 oz onion, chopped
½ oz raisins
¼ tsp freshly grated nutmeg
2 tsp cider or wine vinegar
salt and freshly ground black pepper

Arrange the apple slices, cabbage, onion and raisins in layers in a small ovenproof dish, sprinkling with nutmeg and vinegar, and seasoning to taste. Place in a moderate oven, 180°C (350°F) or Gas Mark 4, and bake for 1 hour. Adjust the seasoning before serving.

TOTAL CALORIES: 90
SERVES 1

Red Fruit Salad

Metric/Imperial
125 g/4 oz redcurrants
25 g/1 oz thin honey
grated rind of 1 lemon
250 g/8 oz strawberries
250 g/8 oz raspberries
50 g/2 oz cherries, stoned and halved

American
1 cup redcurrants
1½ tbsp thin honey
grated rind of 1 lemon
1½ cups strawberries
1½ cups raspberries
½ cup cherries, pitted and halved

Place the redcurrants in a saucepan with the honey and lemon rind. Stew for 3–4 minutes until tender. Cool, then rub through a strainer.

Halve the strawberries, if large, and put into a bowl with the raspberries and cherries. Pour over the redcurrant sauce, mix and chill.

TOTAL CALORIES: 240
CALORIES PER SERVING: 60
SERVES 4

Salad Dressings

Avocado Salad Cream

Place ½ avocado in a blender with 2 roughly chopped spring onions (scallions), juice of ½ lemon, a pinch of ground ginger, 15 g/½ oz (¼ cup) skimmed milk powder, 5 tbsp (⅓ cup) warm water, a dash of Tabasco (hot pepper sauce) and salt and freshly ground black pepper. Blend until smooth. Add a little cold water if the dressing is too thick. Use at once, as avocado discolours.

TOTAL CALORIES: 250

Blue Cheese Dressing

Chop 100 g/3½ oz (about ½ cup) blue brie cheese and place in a blender with 2 tbsp plain yogurt. Add freshly ground black pepper, a dash of Tabasco (hot pepper sauce) and 1 tbsp chives and blend until smooth. Store in the refrigerator for up to 1 week.

TOTAL CALORIES: 325

Cottage Cheese and Chive Dressing

Sieve (strain) 50 g/2 oz (¼ cup) cottage cheese. Stir in the juice of 1 lemon, 1 crushed clove garlic, a pinch of cayenne pepper, salt and 2–3 tbsp warm water. Mix until smooth. Store in the refrigerator for up to 1 week.

TOTAL CALORIES: 65

Cucumber and Yogurt Dressing

Put 175 g/6 oz (1½ cups) roughly chopped cucumber into a blender with 150 ml/¼ pint (⅔ cup) plain yogurt. Add 5 tbsp (⅓ cup) warm water, the juice and grated rind of 1 lemon, 1 crushed clove garlic, a bunch of mint leaves and salt and freshly ground black pepper. Blend until smooth. Store in the refrigerator for a few days.

TOTAL CALORIES: 100

Egg and Caper Dressing

Place a roughly chopped hard-boiled egg in a blender with ¼ tsp French (Dijon-style) mustard, 1 clove garlic, 2 tsp lemon juice and 1 tbsp capers. Gradually add 2 tbsp olive oil, drop by drop, and blend until smooth. Store in the refrigerator for up to about 1 week.

TOTAL CALORIES: 325

Egg Dressing

Remove the shell from 1 hard-boiled egg while it is still warm. Put the egg into a blender with 3 tbsp plain yogurt, ½ tsp French (Dijon-style) mustard, 1 crushed clove garlic, dash of Worcestershire sauce, a small bunch of parsley and salt and freshly ground black pepper. Blend until smooth and use at once as this dressing will not keep.

TOTAL CALORIES: 125

French Dressing

Mix together 2 tbsp lemon juice and 4 tbsp olive oil (preferably green) or walnut oil in a bowl. Add ½–1 tsp thin honey, ¼ tsp mixed dried herbs, ¼ tsp French (Dijon-style) mustard and salt and freshly ground black pepper. Mix well and store in the refrigerator.

TOTAL CALORIES: 600

Herb Dressing

Place 200 ml/½ pint (⅞ cup) plain yogurt in a bowl and add 1 crushed clove garlic, a dash of Worcestershire sauce, salt and freshly ground black pepper and 1 tbsp each of freshly chopped parsley, mint, chives and thyme. Stir in 2 tsp grated lemon rind and 1 tsp lemon juice. Store tightly covered in the refrigerator.

TOTAL CALORIES: 105

Lemon and Mustard Dressing

Grate the rind from a medium-sized lemon and squeeze the juice. Mix the juice and rind with 1 tsp French (Dijon-style) mustard and stir in 1 tsp each of freshly chopped parsley, chives and thyme. Mix thoroughly. Store in the refrigerator for up to 2 weeks.

TOTAL CALORIES: 20

Lemon and Tarragon Dressing

Place 2 tbsp lemon juice in a bowl, stir in ½ tsp thin honey, 1 tbsp finely chopped tarragon and ½ tsp grated lemon rind. Season with salt and freshly ground black pepper. Use at once.

TOTAL CALORIES: 30

Thousand Island Dressing

Place a roughly chopped hard-boiled egg in a blender with ½ canned pimento, 4 stuffed olives, 1 roughly chopped shallot, a squeeze of lemon juice and 7 tbsp plain yogurt. Season with salt and freshly ground black pepper and blend until smooth. Store in the refrigerator for 1 week.

TOTAL CALORIES: 155

Tomato Dressing

Place 150 ml/¼ pint (⅔ cup) tomato juice into a screw-topped jar with 1 crushed clove garlic (or 1 tbsp minced onion), a dash of Worcestershire sauce and ½ tsp grain mustard. Add salt and freshly ground black pepper and shake well. Store in the refrigerator and use within 3–4 days.

TOTAL CALORIES: 30

Scampi Provençal

Metric/Imperial
150 ml/¼ pint water
1 slice of onion
few peppercorns
2 tbsp dry white wine
250 g/8 oz fresh scampi
1 onion, chopped
1 clove garlic, crushed
2 tsp tomato purée
2 tomatoes, chopped
75 g/3 oz mushrooms, sliced

American
⅔ cup water
1 slice of onion
few peppercorns
2 tbsp dry white wine
½ lb jumbo shrimp
1 onion, chopped
1 clove garlic, crushed
2 tsp tomato paste
2 tomatoes, chopped
¾ cup sliced mushrooms

Put the water, onion slice, peppercorns and white wine in a saucepan, add the scampi (shrimp) and poach for 5–10 minutes. Drain, reserving the stock, and keep the scampi (shrimp) warm.

Place the chopped onion, garlic, tomato purée (paste), tomatoes and 150 ml/¼ pint (⅔ cup) of the reserved stock in a saucepan. Bring to the boil, then simmer for a few minutes until slightly thickened. Stir the scampi (shrimp) into the sauce with the mushrooms and cook for a further 1 minute. Adjust the seasoning and serve.

TOTAL CALORIES: 350
CALORIES PER SERVING: 175
SERVES 2

Skewered Chicken

This recipe needs to be made the day before.

Metric/Imperial
175 g/6 oz boneless chicken breast
1 tsp French mustard with herbs
1 tsp freshly chopped thyme
grated rind and juice of 2 limes or 1 lemon
6 sage leaves
lime wedges

American
6 oz boneless chicken breast
1 tsp Dijon-style mustard with herbs
1 tsp freshly chopped thyme
grated rind and juice of 2 limes or 1 lemon
6 sage leaves
lime wedges

Cut the chicken into cubes. Place the mustard, thyme, lime or lemon juice and rind in a bowl. Add the chicken and toss well until it is coated with the marinade. Chill overnight.

Thread the chicken and sage leaves alternately onto a skewer. Place under a preheated grill (broiler) for 10-12 minutes, turning occasionally and basting. Serve at once with lime wedges.
TOTAL CALORIES: 230
SERVES 1

Smoked Haddock Roulade

Metric/Imperial
4 eggs, separated
salt
pinch of cayenne pepper
pinch of grated nutmeg
Filling:
175 g/6 oz fresh smoked haddock
175 g/6 oz cottage cheese, sieved
2 tbsp freshly chopped chives
grated rind of ½ lemon
1 tbsp freshly grated Parmesan cheese

American
4 eggs, separated
salt
pinch of cayenne
pinch of grated nutmeg
Filling:
6 oz fresh smoked haddock
¾ cup strained cottage cheese
2 tbsp freshly chopped chives
grated rind of ½ lemon
1 tbsp freshly grated Parmesan cheese

Place the egg yolks, salt, cayenne and nutmeg in a bowl and mix well. Whisk the egg whites until stiff, then carefully fold them into the yolk mixture. Spread evenly in a lined and greased 30 × 20 cm (12 × 8 in) Swiss roll tin (jelly roll pan). Bake in a preheated moderately hot oven, 200°C (400°F) or Gas Mark 6, for 10-15 minutes until well risen and brown.

Meanwhile, make the filling. Poach the haddock in water for 8-10 minutes, drain well and remove the skin and bones. Flake the fish and add the cottage cheese, chives and lemon rind. Heat together in a saucepan, stirring for 2-3 minutes.

Turn the roulade onto a piece of waxed paper sprinkled with the Parmesan cheese. Carefully peel off the lining paper, spread with the filling and roll up like a Swiss (jelly) roll. Serve immediately.
TOTAL CALORIES: 740
CALORIES PER SERVING: 185
SERVES 4

Smoked Salmon Quiche

Metric/Imperial
50 g/2 oz plain flour
50 g/2 oz wholemeal flour
pinch of salt
pinch of cayenne pepper
50 g/2 oz margarine
ice-cold water
Filling:
3 eggs
150 ml/¼ pint skimmed milk
100 g/3½ oz cottage cheese, sieved
2 tbsp freshly chopped chives
salt and freshly ground black pepper
½ tsp grated lemon rind
150 g/5 oz smoked salmon

American
½ cup all-purpose flour
½ cup wholewheat flour
pinch of salt
pinch of cayenne
¼ cup margarine
ice-cold water
Filling:
3 eggs
⅔ cup skimmed milk
½ cup strained cottage cheese
2 tbsp freshly chopped chives
salt and freshly ground black pepper
½ tsp grated lemon rind
5 oz smoked salmon

Place the flours in a bowl and add the salt and cayenne. Rub (cut) the margarine into the flour until the mixture resembles fine breadcrumbs. Stir in 2 teaspoons of water at a time, until the dough is firm. Lightly knead the dough on a floured board, roll out and use to line 4 individual tins (pans), 7.5 cm (3 in) in diameter. Chill for 20 minutes.

Beat the eggs, milk and cottage cheese together. Add the chives, seasoning and lemon rind. Roughly chop the smoked salmon and arrange in the bottom of the pastry cases (pie shells). Spoon over the egg and cheese mixture.

Bake in a preheated moderately hot oven, 200°C (400°F) or Gas Mark 6, for 20-25 minutes until set and golden brown. Serve hot or cold.
TOTAL CALORIES: 920
CALORIES PER SERVING: 230
SERVES 4
Note: If frozen, allow to thaw, then place in a moderate oven, 180°C (350°F) or Gas Mark 4, for 10-12 minutes until heated through. Do not re-freeze.

Smoked Trout and Bean Salad

Metric/Imperial
200 g/7 oz canned red kidney beans, drained
250 g/8 oz smoked trout fillets
50 g/2 oz leek, thinly sliced
50 g/2 oz cauliflower florets
15 g/½ oz shelled pistachio nuts
25 a/1 oz cucumber, diced
half quantity Cottage Cheese and Chive Dressing (page 115)
crisp lettuce leaves
small bunch watercress

American
7 oz canned red kidney beans, drained
½ lb smoked trout fillet
½ cup thinly sliced leek
½ cup cauliflower florets
1 tbsp shelled pistachio nuts
¼ cup diced cucumber
half quantity Cottage Cheese and Chive Dressing (page 115)
crisp lettuce leaves
small bunch watercress

Wash the kidney beans in a colander and drain well. Flake the smoked trout and put into a bowl with the beans, leek, cauliflower, pistachios and cucumber. Spoon over the dressing and mix well. Arrange the lettuce and watercress in a bowl and spoon the salad into the centre.
TOTAL CALORIES: 680
CALORIES PER SERVING: 340
SERVES 2

Sole Florentine

Metric/Imperial
175 g/6 oz lemon sole fillets, rolled up
120 ml/4 fl oz dry white wine
1 bouquet garni
175 g/6 oz fresh spinach
salt and freshly ground black pepper
freshly grated nutmeg
2 tbsp plain yogurt

American
6 oz sole fillets, rolled up
½ cup dry white wine
1 bouquet garni
6 oz fresh spinach
salt and freshly ground black pepper
freshly grated nutmet
2 tbsp plain yogurt

Place the sole in a non-stick saucepan with the wine and bouquet garni and poach for 2-3 minutes until tender. Drain and keep hot. Cook the spinach in the water left on the leaves after washing. Drain well and season with salt, pepper and a little nutmeg. Return to the clean pan and heat through, then remove from the heat and stir in the yogurt. Serve the sole on a bed of sauce.
TOTAL CALORIES: 320
SERVES 1

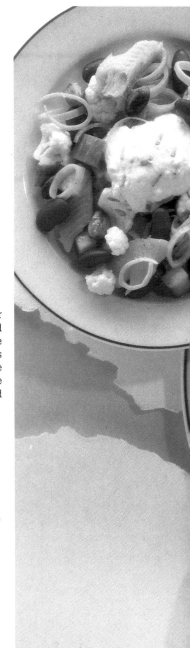

Sole with Herbs and Wine

Metric/Imperial
2 × 150 g/5 oz lemon or Dover sole
    fillets
1 tbsp freshly chopped dill
1 tbsp freshly chopped parsley
1 tsp freshly chopped lemon thyme
grated rind of ½ lemon
5 tbsp dry white wine
salt and freshly ground black pepper
750 g/1½ lb chopped cooked
    spinach

American
2 × 5 oz sole fillets
1 tbsp freshly chopped dill
1 tbsp freshly chopped parsley
1 tsp freshly chopped lemon thyme
grated rind of ½ lemon
5 tbsp dry white wine
salt and freshly ground black pepper
3 cups chopped cooked spinach

Put the fish into a large ovenproof dish. Sprinkle with the herbs and lemon rind and spoon over the wine. Season well and leave to marinate for 1 hour.

Cook in a preheated moderate oven, 180°C (350°F) or Gas Mark 4, for 12–15 minutes or until the fish is tender. Serve at once on a bed or chopped cooked spinach.
TOTAL CALORIES: 540
CALORIES PER SERVING: 270
SERVES 2

Sole with Lemon and Prawns

Metric/Imperial
150 g/5 oz lemon or Dover sole fillets
25 g/1 oz peeled prawns
grated rind and juice of ½ lemon
2 tsp freshly chopped parsley
1 tsp freshly chopped chives
salt and freshly ground black pepper

American
5 oz sole fillets
2 tbsp shelled shrimp
grated rind and juice of ½ lemon
2 tsp freshly chopped parsley
1 tsp freshly chopped chives
salt and freshly ground black pepper

Place the sole fillets on a board. Divide the prawns (shrimp) into 2 portions and arrange down the centre of each fillet. Sprinkle over the lemon rind and herbs, and season well. Roll up the fish and place in an ovenproof dish. Pour over the lemon juice and cover with foil. Place in a preheated moderately hot oven, 190°C (375°F) or Gas Mark 5, for 10–15 minutes until the fish is tender and flakes easily. Serve at once.
TOTAL CALORIES: 160
SERVES 1

Soufflé Cheese Omelette

Metric/Imperial
2 eggs, separated
1 tbsp cold water
25 g/1 oz hard cheese, grated
pinch of mixed dried herbs
salt and freshly ground black pepper

American
2 eggs, separated
1 tbsp cold water
¼ cup grated hard cheese
pinch of mixed dried herbs
salt and freshly ground black pepper

Place the egg yolks and water in a bowl and mix well. Stir in the cheese, herbs and seasoning. Whisk the egg whites until stiff and fold into the yolk mixture. Heat an 18–20 cm (7–8 in) non-stick omelette pan, pour in the egg mixture and cook over a low heat until the mixture is almost set and the underneath is light golden brown. Place the pan under a preheated hot grill (broiler) for about a minute to cook the top. Fold the omelette in half, slide onto a warmed plate and serve immediately.
TOTAL CALORIES: 250
SERVES 1

Clockwise from the front: Smoked Salmon Quiche, Smoked Trout and Bean Salad, Skewered Chicken

Spinach and Cottage Cheese Quiche

Metric/Imperial
50 g/2 oz plain flour
50 g/2 oz wholemeal flour
pinch of salt
pinch of cayenne pepper
50 g/2 oz margarine
ice-cold water
Filling:
2 eggs
150 ml/¼ pint skimmed milk
2 spring onions, chopped
100 g/3½ oz cottage cheese, sieved
50 g/2 oz Camembert cheese, finely
    chopped
pinch of cayenne pepper
1 tsp freshly chopped parsley
100 g/3½ oz cooked spinach,
    drained and finely chopped

American
½ cup all-purpose flour
½ cup wholewheat flour
pinch of salt
pinch of cayenne
¼ cup margarine
ice-cold water
Filling:
2 eggs
⅔ cup skimmed milk
2 scallions, chopped
½ cup strained cottage cheese
½ cup finely chopped Camembert
    cheese
pinch of cayenne
1 tsp freshly chopped parsley
½ cup cooked and finely chopped
    spinach

Place the flours in a bowl and add the salt and cayenne. Rub (cut) the margarine into the flour until the mixture resembles fine breadcrumbs. Stir in 2 teaspoons of water at a time until the dough is firm.

Lightly knead the dough on a floured board. Roll it out and use to line 4 individual tins (pans), 7.5 cm (3 in) in diameter. Chill for 20 minutes while making the filling.

Mix together the eggs, milk, spring onion (scallion), cheeses, cayenne, parsley and spinach. Spoon the mixture into the pastry cases (pie shells). Bake in a preheated moderately hot oven, 190°C (375°F) or Gas Mark 5, for 20–25 minutes until set and golden brown. Serve hot or cold.
TOTAL CALORIES: 800
CALORIES PER SERVING: 200
SERVES 4

Note: If frozen, allow to thaw, then place in a moderate oven, 180°C (350°F) or Gas Mark 4, for 10–12 minutes until heated through. Do not re-freeze.

Spinach Roulade

Metric/Imperial
300 g/10 oz fresh spinach
4 eggs, separated
salt
pinch of cayenne pepper
pinch of grated nutmeg
Filling:
100 g/3½ oz low fat cream cheese
    with herbs and garlic
25 g/1 oz mature Cheddar cheese,
    grated

American
10 oz fresh spinach
4 eggs, separated
salt
pinch of cayenne
pinch of grated nutmeg
Filling:
½ cup low fat cream cheese with
    herbs and garlic
¼ cup grated sharp Cheddar cheese

Steam the spinach for 3 minutes, drain well and chop finely.

Place half the spinach in a bowl and mix with the egg yolks, salt, cayenne and nutmeg. Whisk the egg whites until very stiff and fold into the spinach mixture. Spread the mixture evenly in a lined and greased 30 × 20 cm (12 × 8 in) Swiss roll tin (jelly roll pan). Bake in a preheated moderately hot oven, 200°C (400°F) or Gas Mark 6, for 10–15 minutes.

Meanwhile put the remaining spinach, cream cheese and grated cheese into a small pan. Heat through until the cheese has melted and the mixture is hot. Season with salt and cayenne.

Turn the roulade onto a piece of waxed paper and carefully peel off the paper. Spread with the filling and roll up like a Swiss (jelly) roll. Serve immediately.
TOTAL CALORIES: 680 (980)
CALORIES PER SERVING: 170(245)
SERVES 4

Spinach Soufflé

Metric/Imperial
25 g/1 oz butter
50 g/2 oz wholemeal flour
300 ml/½ pint skimmed milk
pinch of mixed dried herbs
salt and cayenne pepper
¼ tsp dry mustard
3 eggs, separated
100 g/3½ oz fresh spinach,
    blanched, drained and finely
    chopped
100 g/3½ oz mature Cheddar
    cheese, grated

American
2 tbsp butter
½ cup wholewheat flour

1¼ cups skimmed milk
pinch of mixed dried herbs
salt and cayenne
¼ tsp dry mustard
3 eggs, separated
½ cup blanched, drained and
    chopped fresh spinach
¾ cup grated sharp Cheddar cheese

Melt the butter in a saucepan, stir in the flour and cook for 1 minute. Gradually stir in the milk; bring to the boil, stirring constantly, and cook for 2 minutes. Add the herbs, salt, cayenne and mustard. Stir until mixed together, then remove from the heat and quickly mix in the egg yolks, spinach and cheese.

Whisk the egg whites until very stiff. Fold into the spinach mixture and divide between 4 individual, greased, soufflé dishes. Bake in a preheated moderately hot oven, 190°C (375°F) or Gas Mark 5, for 20–25 minutes. Serve immediately.
TOTAL CALORIES: 1100
CALORIES PER SERVING: 275
SERVES 4

Steak and Kidney Casserole

Metric/Imperial
250 g/8 oz lean stewing steak, cubed
2 lamb's kidneys, halved, cored and
    diced
1 medium onion, chopped
200 g/7 oz tomatoes, chopped
150 ml/¼ pint beef stock
salt and freshly ground black pepper
2 tsp cornflour
1 tbsp water

American
½ lb lean stewing steak, cubed
2 lamb kidneys, halved, cored and
    diced
1 medium onion, chopped
¾ cup chopped tomatoes
⅔ cup beef stock
salt and freshly ground black pepper
2 tsp cornstarch
1 tbsp water

Put the steak, kidneys, onion, tomatoes and stock into a small flameproof casserole dish. Season and cook in a preheated moderate oven, 180°C (350°F) or Gas Mark 4, for about 1½ hours or until meat is tender. Mix the cornflour (cornstarch) with the water, add a little hot stock and stir into the casserole. Place the casserole on top of the stove, bring to the boil, stirring, and cook for a further 2 minutes. Adjust the seasoning and serve.
TOTAL CALORIES: 610
CALORIES PER SERVING: 305
SERVES 2

Strawberry Sorbet

Metric/Imperial
75 g/3 oz sugar
250 ml/8 fl oz water
grated rind of 1 lemon
2 tsp lemon juice
300 g/10 oz strawberries, puréed
1 egg white
1½ tbsp icing sugar

American
⅓ cup sugar
1 cup water
grated rind of 1 lemon
2 tsp lemon juice
2 cups strawberries, puréed
1 egg white
1½ tbsp confectioners' sugar

Dissolve the sugar in the water in a heavy-based saucepan over a low heat. Gradually bring to the boil and boil rapidly for 3 minutes, then allow to cool. Add the lemon rind and juice and strawberries. Mix well and pour into a plastic freezer container with a lid. Freeze until half frozen.

Whisk the egg white until stiff, then gradually whisk in the icing (confectioners') sugar. Then whisk in the semi-frozen strawberry purée until smooth and combined. Pour the mixture into a freezer container and freeze until set. When serving, scoop into bowls and serve at once.
Note: It is best to remove the sorbet from the freezer 30 minutes before required so that it is not too hard.
TOTAL CALORIES: 480
CALORIES PER SERVING: 120
SERVES 4

Stuffed Aubergine

Metric/Imperial
1 × 200 g/7 oz aubergine
2 tomatoes, chopped
50 g/2 oz mushrooms, chopped
1 small onion, chopped
75 g/3 oz cooked chicken, diced
salt and freshly ground black pepper
300 ml/½ pint stock

American
1 × 7 oz (medium) eggplant
2 tomatoes, chopped
½ cup chopped mushrooms
1 small onion, chopped
⅓ cup diced cooked chicken
salt and freshly ground black pepper
1¼ cups stock

Halve the aubergine (eggplant) and scoop out most of the flesh. Chop the flesh and mix about half with the tomatoes, mushrooms, onion, chicken and seasoning. Pile the mixture back into the aubergine (eggplant) shells and place them in an ovenproof dish. Pour the stock

around the aubergine (eggplant), cover and cook in a preheated moderate oven, 180°C (350°F) or Gas Mark 4, for about 1 hour or until tender.
TOTAL CALORIES: 180
SERVES 1

Stuffed Pepper with Tomato Sauce

Metric/Imperial
1 large green pepper
75 g/3 oz lean minced beef
1 tsp flour
1 tomato, skinned and chopped
1 small onion, chopped
1 tsp tomato purée
pinch of mixed dried herbs
salt and freshly ground black pepper
little stock
Tomato Sauce:
2 tomatoes, chopped
1 small onion, chopped
1 tsp wine vinegar
1 tsp sugar
150 ml/¼ pint stock
1 bay leaf
salt and freshly ground black pepper

American
1 large green pepper
½ cup loosely packed, lean ground
    beef
1 tsp flour
1 tomato, skinned and chopped
1 small onion, chopped
1 tsp tomato paste
pinch of mixed dried herbs
salt and freshly ground black pepper
little stock
Tomato Sauce:
2 tomatoes, chopped
1 small onion, chopped
1 tsp wine vinegar
1 tsp sugar
⅔ cup stock
1 bay leaf
salt and freshly ground black pepper

Cut a slice from the stalk end of the pepper and discard the seeds and white pith. Place the beef in a bowl and sprinkle with the flour, then mix in the tomato, onion, tomato purée (paste), herbs and seasoning. Place the meat mixture in a non-stick frying pan and cook gently until the meat is browned, stirring constantly. Add a little stock, if necessary.

Fill the pepper, replace the top slice and place in a small ovenproof dish. Bake in a preheated moderately hot oven, 190°C (375°F) or Gas Mark 5, for 25 minutes.

Meanwhile prepare the tomato sauce by placing the tomatoes, onion, vinegar, sugar, stock, bay leaf and seasoning in a saucepan. Bring to the boil and simmer, uncovered, for about 15 minutes. Remove the bay leaf, adjust the seasoning and pour the sauce over the pepper. Serve at once.

TOTAL CALORIES: 280
SERVES 1

Stuffed Roast Shoulder of Lamb

Metric/Imperial
1 × 1 kg/2 lb boned shoulder of lamb
Stuffing:
150 g/5 oz sausagemeat
250 g/8 oz chestnut purée
1 tbsp freshly chopped parsley
1 tsp freshly chopped rosemary
1 small onion, finely chopped
salt and freshly ground black pepper
rosemary sprigs
parsley sprigs

American
1 × 2 lb boneless lamb shoulder
Stuffing:
⅔ cup sausage meat
1 cup chestnut purée
1 tbsp freshly chopped parsley
1 tsp freshly chopped rosemary
1 small onion, minced
salt and freshly ground black pepper
rosemary sprigs
parsley sprigs

First, make the stuffing. Mix together the sausagemeat, chestnut purée, parsley, rosemary, onion and seasoning. Stuff the lamb, roll up and tie securely with string. Place in a roasting pan and strew with rosemary sprigs. Roast in a preheated moderate oven, 180°C (350°F) or Gas Mark 4, for 1½–2 hours, basting occasionally. Turn oven up to 200°C (400°F) or Gas Mark 6 for about 15 minutes to crisp the outside. Serve sliced with parsley sprigs and gravy (see page 110).

TOTAL CALORIES: 2380
CALORIES PER SERVING: 400–595
SERVES 4–6

Stuffed Veal (Veal Olives)

Metric/Imperial
2 × 125 g/4 oz veal escalopes, beaten flat
1 tsp oil
1 stick celery, sliced
1 carrot, sliced
2 tsp tomato purée
150 ml/¼ pint light stock
Marinade:
2 tsp lemon juice
grated rind of ½ lemon
freshly ground black pepper
pinch of mace
2 tbsp dry white wine
Stuffing:
1 small onion, chopped
2 bacon rashers, grilled and chopped
25 g/1 oz wholewheat breadcrumbs
2 tsp mixed dried herbs
beaten egg

American
2 × ¼ lb veal scaloppini, beaten flat
1 tsp oil
1 celery stalk, sliced
1 carrot, sliced
2 tsp tomato paste
⅔ cup light stock
Marinade:
2 tsp lemon juice
grated rind of ½ lemon
freshly ground black pepper
pinch of mace
2 tbsp dry white wine
Stuffing:
1 small onion, chopped
2 bacon slices, broiled and chopped
½ cup soft fresh wholewheat bread crumbs
2 tsp mixed dried herbs
beaten egg

Place the escalopes (scaloppini) in a flat dish, mix the marinade ingredients, pour over the veal and leave to marinate for several hours.

To make the stuffing, place all the dry ingredients in a bowl, season well and mix with just enough egg to bind. Divide between the escalopes (scaloppini) and roll them into olive shapes. Tie securely with string.

Heat the oil in a heavy-based saucepan and brown the olives on all sides. Add the marinade and remaining ingredients. Bring to the boil, cover and simmer gently for about 30–35 minutes or until tender. Remove the veal olives, cut off the string, and keep warm. Boil the sauce until reduced by half. Strain and pour over the veal.

TOTAL CALORIES: 580
CALORIES PER SERVING: 290
SERVES 2

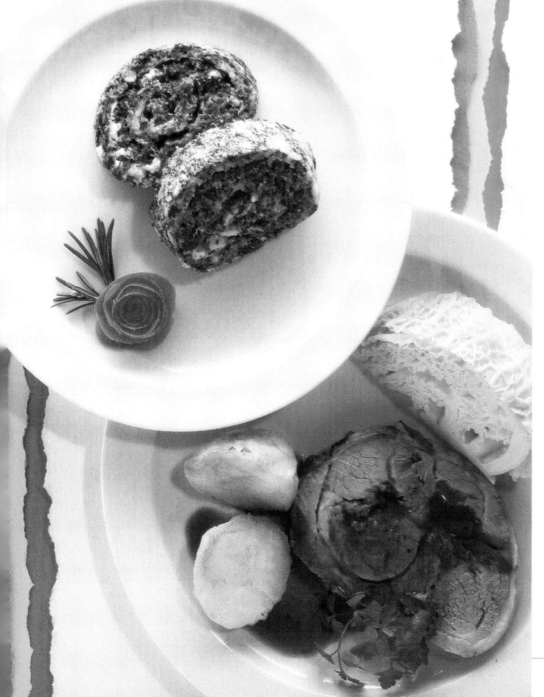

Front: Stuffed Roast Shoulder of Lamb   Back: Spinach Roulade

Sweet and Sour Chicken

Metric/Imperial
1 tsp oil
50 g/2 oz onion, chopped
2 tsp flour
200 ml/⅓ pint stock
2 tsp dark brown sugar
2 tsp soy sauce
2 tsp vinegar
salt and freshly ground black pepper
175 g/6 oz cooked, diced chicken
1 carrot, cut into fine strips
3 water chestnuts, sliced
6 spring onions, sliced

American
1 tsp oil
½ cup chopped onion
2 tsp flour
⅞ cup stock
2 tsp dark brown sugar
2 tsp soy sauce
2 tsp vinegar
salt and freshly ground black pepper
⅔ cup cooked diced chicken
1 carrot, cut into fine strips
1 celery stalk, cut into fine strips
3 water chestnuts, sliced
6 scallions, sliced

Heat the oil in a saucepan, add the onions and fry (sauté) lightly until browned. Add the flour, cook for 1 minute and gradually stir in the stock. Bring to the boil and then add the sugar, soy sauce, vinegar and seasoning. Simmer for about 5 minutes, then add the chicken. Continue simmering for 10 minutes before adding the carrot, celery and water chestnuts. Keep over the heat for 1 minute longer, then sprinkle with the spring onions (scallions).
TOTAL CALORIES: 440
CALORIES PER SERVING: 220
SERVES 2

Swiss Steak

Metric/Imperial
250 g/8 oz lean stewing steak
1 medium onion, sliced
200 g/7 oz tomatoes, skinned and chopped
freshly chopped herbs
salt and freshly ground black pepper
200 ml/⅓ pint beef stock
1 tsp cornflour
75 g/3 oz button mushrooms, sliced
freshly chopped basil or parsley

American
½ lb lean stewing steak
1 medium onion, sliced
⅞ cup skinned and chopped tomatoes
freshly chopped herbs
salt and freshly ground black pepper
⅞ cup beef stock
1 tsp cornstarch

Clockwise from the front: Three Bean Salad, Vegetable Curry, Swiss Steak

¾ cup sliced button mushrooms
freshly chopped basil or parsley

Cut the steak into 4 pieces. Place in a small saucepan with the onion, tomatoes, herbs and seasoning. Cover with the stock and simmer for 1–1½ hours until the meat is tender. Mix the cornflour (cornstarch) with a little water and use to thicken the sauce, stirring constantly. Add the mushrooms, adjust the seasoning, and simmer for a further 5 minutes. Serve at once, sprinkled with herbs.
TOTAL CALORIES: 510
CALORIES PER SERVING: 255
SERVES 2

Three Bean Salad

Metric/Imperial
125 g/4 oz canned red kidney beans, drained
125 g/4 oz canned cannellini beans, drained
125 g/4 oz canned flageolet beans, drained
2 spring onions, finely chopped
125 g/4 oz tuna, drained of all oil
100 g/3½ oz cauliflower florets
100 g/3½ oz peeled prawns
few stoned black olives
dressing of your choice (page 115)
2 radicchio or chicory heads

American
¼ lb canned red kidney beans, drained
¼ lb canned cannellini beans, drained
¼ lb canned flageolet beans, drained
2 scallions, finely chopped
¼ lb tuna, drained of all oil
¾ cup cauliflower florets
½ cup shelled shrimp
few pitted black olives
dressing of your choice (page 115)
2 radicchio or endive

Wash the kidney beans in a colander and drain well. Mix the beans together in a bowl. Stir in the spring onions (scallions), tuna, cauliflower, prawns (shrimp) and olives. Spoon over the chosen dressing and mix well. Arrange the radicchio or chicory (endive) on a serving dish and pile the salad in the centre.
TOTAL CALORIES: 840 (without dressing)
CALORIES PER SERVING: 420 (without dressing)
SERVES 2
Note: Egg Dressing (page 115) is very good with this salad.

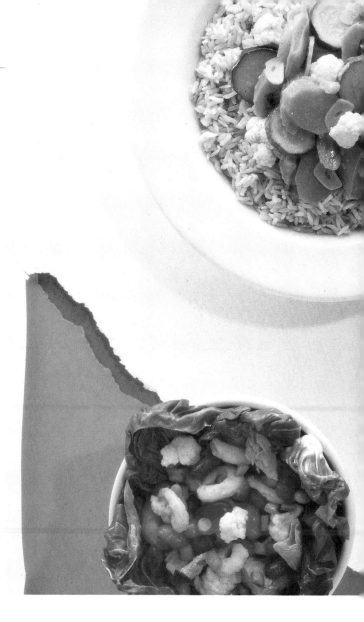

Thyme and Parsley Stuffing
This is sufficient for about 4 portions and will be enough for a small chicken.

Metric/Imperial
125 g/4 oz fresh wholewheat breadcrumbs
2 tbsp freshly chopped parsley
good pinch dried thyme
salt and freshly ground black pepper
grated rind of ½ lemon
2 tsp lemon juice
skimmed milk, to bind

American
2 cups soft fresh wholewheat bread crumbs
2 tbsp freshly chopped parsley
good pinch dried thyme
salt and freshly ground black pepper
grated rind of ½ lemon
2 tsp lemon juice
skimmed milk, to bind

Mix all the ingredients together well.
TOTAL CALORIES: 290
CALORIES PER SERVING: 75

Clockwise from the front: Three Bean Salad, Vegetable Curry, Swiss Steak

Trout with Almonds

Metric/Imperial
1 × 200 g/7 oz trout, cleaned
juice of ¼ lemon
15 g/½ oz flaked almonds
watercress and lemon wedges

American
1 × 7 oz trout, cleaned
juice of ¼ lemon
2 tbsp flaked almonds
watercress and lemon wedges

Sprinkle the trout with lemon juice and place under a preheated moderate grill (broiler) and cook gently for about 5–7 minutes each side or until tender. Meanwhile, place the almonds in a small frying pan (skillet) and heat gently until golden brown. Sprinkle over the trout and serve with sprigs of watercress and lemon wedges.
TOTAL CALORIES: 350
SERVES 1

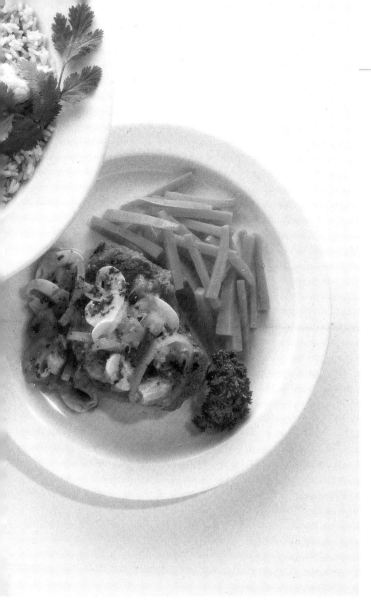

Vegetable Curry

Metric/Imperial

1 tbsp corn oil
2 tsp ground coriander
1½ tsp ground cumin
½ tsp turmeric
½ tsp ground ginger
2 large cloves garlic, thinly sliced
100 g/3½ oz carrots, sliced diagonally
4 spring onions, chopped
2 sticks celery, sliced diagonally
2 leeks, sliced
3 courgettes, sliced
1 small cauliflower, broken into florets
300 ml/½ pint stock, (homemade if possible)
150 ml/¼ pint plain yogurt
25 g/1 oz cashew nuts

American

1 tbsp corn oil
2 tsp ground coriander
1½ tsp ground cumin
½ tsp tumeric
½ tsp ground ginger
2 large cloves garlic, thinly sliced
⅔ cup sliced carrots
4 scallions, chopped
2 celery stalks, sliced diagonally
2 leeks, sliced
3 zucchini, sliced
1 small cauliflower, broken into florets
¼ cup stock (homemade if possible)
⅔ cup plain yogurt
¼ cup cashew nuts

Heat the oil in a saucepan, add the spices and cook for 5 minutes without browning. Add the garlic, carrots, spring onions (scallions) and celery. Cook for 2 minutes, then add the leeks, courgettes (zucchini) and cauliflower. Pour over the stock, bring to the boil, and simmer gently for 8–10 minutes. Stir in the yogurt and heat gently, without boiling. Sprinkle with cashew nuts and serve at once.
TOTAL CALORIES: 500
CALORIES PER SERVING: 125
SERVES 4

Vegetable Lasagne

Metric/Imperial

250 g/8 oz courgettes, sliced lengthwise
125 g/4 oz flat mushrooms, sliced
4 tomatoes, skinned and sliced
2 medium onions, sliced
1 tsp mixed dried herbs
600 ml/1 pint skimmed milk
3 eggs, beaten
125 g/4 oz mature Cheddar cheese, grated

American

½ lb zucchini, sliced lengthwise
1 cup sliced flat mushrooms
4 tomatoes, skinned and sliced
2 medium onions, sliced
1 tsp mixed dried herbs
2½ cups skimmed milk
3 eggs, beaten
1 cup grated sharp Cheddar cheese

Layer the courgettes (zucchini), mushrooms, tomatoes and onions, alternately in a dish, seasoning well and sprinkling with herbs. Mix the milk, eggs and cheese together and spoon over the vegetables. Cook in a preheated moderately hot oven, 190°C (375°F) or Gas Mark 5, for 25 minutes.
TOTAL CALORIES: 1040
CALORIES PER SERVING: 260
SERVES 4

Vegetable Terrine

Metric/Imperial

600 ml/1 pint aspic
2 tbsp dry sherry
1 tbsp freshly chopped parsley
1 tbsp freshly chopped basil
250 g/8 oz fresh asparagus, trimmed
175 g/6 oz carrots, thinly sliced
175 g/6 oz small turnips, thinly sliced
4–6 canned artichoke hearts, sliced
175 g/6 oz courgettes, thinly sliced
125 g/4 oz French beans, halved

American

2½ cups aspic
2 tbsp dry sherry
1 tbsp freshly chopped parsley
1 tbsp freshly chopped basil
½ lb fresh asparagus, trimmed
6 oz carrots, thinly sliced
6 oz small turnips, thinly sliced
4–6 canned artichoke hearts, sliced
6 oz zucchini, thinly sliced
¼ lb green beans, halved

Blanch and drain all the fresh vegetables. Mix the liquid aspic with the sherry and fresh herbs. Spoon a thin layer over the base of a 1 kg/2 lb loaf tin or terrine and chill until set. Dip each of the selection of vegetables in the aspic, then arrange in layers in the terrine, pouring a thin layer of aspic over each time. Set each layer in the refrigerator. Continue layering until all the vegetables and aspic are used, finishing with the aspic. Chill for 2 hours. To turn out quickly, dip the terrine in a bowl of boiling water, then invert onto a serving dish. Garnish with parsley and basil if desired.
TOTAL CALORIES: 280
CALORIES PER SERVING: 70
SERVES 4 as a starter or light meal

Veal Escalope with Ham

Metric/Imperial

150 g/5 oz veal escalope
1 slice lean ham
salt and freshly ground black pepper
1 tsp oil
1 tomato, sliced

American

5 oz veal scaloppini
1 slice lean ham
salt and freshly ground black pepper
1 tsp oil
1 tomato, sliced

Beat the veal between 2 sheets of greaseproof (waxed) paper until thin and flat. Place the ham on half the veal, season well and fold over, securing with string. Heat the oil in a frying pan (skillet) and cook the veal for 8–10 minutes on each side until tender. Drain well on kitchen paper towels, remove the string, and serve at once garnished with fresh tomato slices.
TOTAL CALORIES: 245
SERVES 1

Veal Florentine

Metric/Imperial

150 g/5 oz veal escalope
150 g/5 oz spinach
salt and freshly ground black pepper
2 tbsp marsala
25 g/1 oz mozarella cheese, sliced

American

5 oz veal scaloppini
5 oz spinach
salt and freshly ground black pepper
2 tbsp marsala
1 oz mozarella cheese, sliced

Place the veal under a preheated hot grill (broiler) and cook for 5–6 minutes each side. Meanwhile, cook the spinach in the water still clinging to the leaves after washing. When cooked, drain the spinach well and place in an ovenproof dish. Place the veal on top, season and pour over the marsala. Arrange the cheese over the veal and return to the grill (broiler) until the cheese has melted.
TOTAL CALORIES: 340
SERVES 1

Vegetable Salad

Metric/Imperial
3 tbsp tomato juice
1 shallot, finely chopped
1 tbsp dry white wine
dash of Tabasco
6 coriander seeds
1 bouquet garni
1 clove garlic, crushed (optional)
2 courgettes, sliced diagonally
2 sticks celery, chopped
few cauliflower florets
50 g/2 oz button mushrooms, sliced
1 carrot, grated coarsely
1 tbsp green peppercorns, drained

American
3 tbsp tomato juice
1 shallot, finely chopped
1 tbsp dry white wine
dash of hot pepper sauce
6 coriander seeds
1 bouquet garni
1 clove garlic, crushed (optional)
2 zucchini, sliced diagonally
2 celery stalks, chopped
few cauliflower florets
¼ cup sliced button mushrooms
1 carrot, grated coarsely
1 tbsp green peppercorns, drained

Place the tomato juice, shallot, wine, Tabasco (hot pepper sauce), coriander seeds, bouquet garni and garlic in a saucepan, bring to the boil and simmer for 5 minutes. Turn off the heat and leave until completely cold, then strain into a jug.

Place the vegetables and peppercorns in a bowl and pour over the dressing. Toss well to mix, then spoon into a serving dish.

TOTAL CALORIES: 90
CALORIES PER SERVING: 45
SERVES 2

Watercress Soup

Metric/Imperial
½ oz butter
1 bunch watercress, chopped
1 small onion, chopped
2 tsp flour
salt and freshly ground black pepper
450 ml/¾ pint skimmed milk

American
1 tbsp butter
1 bunch watercress, chopped
1 small onion, chopped
2 tsp flour
salt and freshly ground black pepper
2 cups skimmed milk

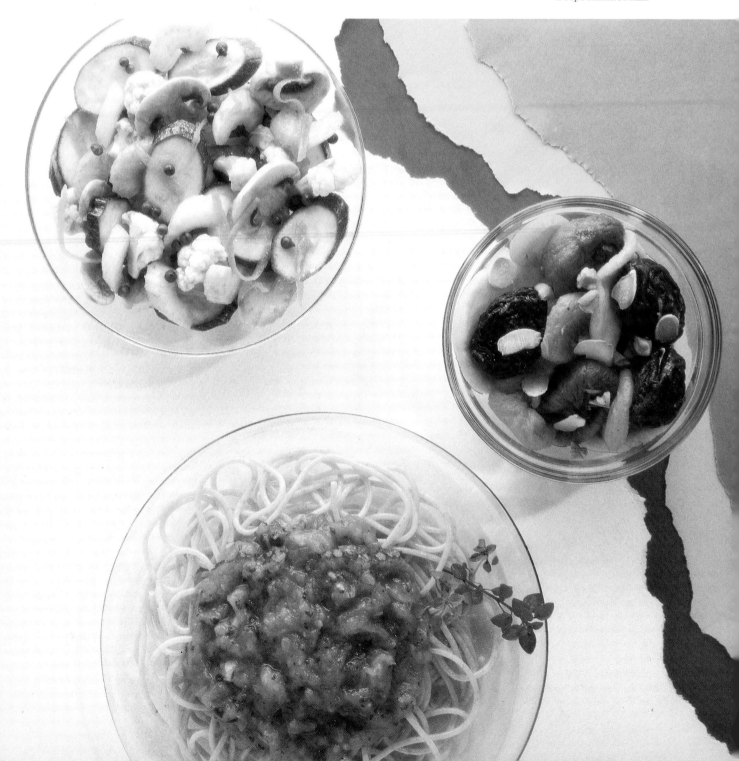

Melt the butter in a saucepan and add the watercress and onion. Cook gently for 5–7 minutes and then sprinkle over the flour and seasoning. Stir well and continue to cook for 1 minute. Gradually pour in the milk and bring to the boil. Simmer for about 10 minutes, then cool slightly and purée in a blender. Return to the clean pan and adjust the seasoning. Serve either hot or cold.

TOTAL CALORIES: 390
CALORIES PER SERVING: 195
SERVES 2

Whipped Cream Topping

Metric/Imperial
5 tbsp whipping cream
5 tbsp plain yogurt
1 egg white

American
1⅓ cups whipping cream
⅓ cup plain yogurt
1 egg white

Whip the cream until thick, then gradually beat in the yogurt. Beat the egg white until stiff, then fold into the cream and yogurt mixture.

TOTAL CALORIES: 340

White Sauce

Metric/Imperial
1½ tsp butter
25g/1 oz flour
300 ml/½ pint skimmed milk
salt and freshly ground black pepper

American
1½ tsp butter
¼ cup flour
1¼ cups skimmed milk
salt and freshly ground black pepper

Melt the butter in a saucepan and stir in the flour. Cook, stirring, for 1 minute and then gradually add the milk. Keep on stirring all the time to prevent lumps. Bring to the boil and simmer for 2 minutes, stirring until smooth, and season well.
    Makes 300 ml/½ pint (1¼ cups).
TOTAL CALORIES: 260

Wholewheat Macaroni with Cheese and Ham

Metric/Imperial
50g/2 oz Bel Paese cheese, diced
50g/2 oz low fat soft cheese with herbs and garlic
50g/2 oz Gruyère cheese, grated

Clockwise from the front:
Wholewheat Spaghetti with
Tomato and Basil Sauce, Vegetable
Salad, Winter Fruit Compote

1–2 cloves garlic, crushed
2 tsp freshly chopped thyme
2 tsp freshly chopped parsley
2 tsp freshly chopped chives
125g/4 oz very lean ham, diced
salt and freshly ground black pepper
175g/6 oz wholewheat macaroni

American
⅓ cup diced Bel Paese cheese
¼ cup low fat soft cheese with herbs and garlic
½ cup grated Gruyère cheese
1–2 cloves garlic, crushed
2 tsp freshly chopped thyme
2 tsp freshly chopped parsley
2 tsp freshly chopped chives
½ cup diced lean ham
salt and freshly ground black pepper
6 oz wholewheat macaroni

Put the cheeeses and garlic into a saucepan, add the herbs and heat through very slowly. Stir in the diced ham and season well with salt and pepper.
    Cook the macaroni in boiling salted water for 7–9 minutes or until 'al dente'.
    Drain the macaroni and add to the sauce. Mix well, turn onto a heated serving dish and serve at once.
TOTAL CALORIES: 1500
CALORIES PER SERVING: 375
SERVES 4

Wholewheat Pan Pizza

Metric/Imperial
125g/4 oz wholemeal bread mix
lukewarm water
Topping:
50g/2 oz tomato purée
100g/3½ oz tomatoes, skinned and sliced
1 clove garlic, sliced
¼ tsp dried basil
¼ tsp dried marjoram
1 × 350g/12 oz can asparagus, drained
100g/32 oz tiny button mushrooms
few stuffed olives
75g/3 oz Bel Paese cheese, thinly sliced
salt and freshly ground black pepper

American
¼ lb wholewheat bread mix
lukewarm water
Topping:
2 tbsp tomato paste
½ cup skinned and sliced tomatoes
1 clove garlic, sliced
¼ tsp dried basil
¼ tsp dried marjoram
1 can (12 oz) asparagus, drained
1 cup tiny button mushrooms
few stuffed olives
⅓ cup thinly sliced Bel Paese cheese
salt and freshly ground black pepper

Mix together the contents of the bread mix and measure the required amount. Place in a bowl and stir in sufficient lukewarm water to form a firm but elastic dough. Knead for 5 minutes, then cover and leave in a warm place for 50 minutes or until the dough has doubled in size. Lightly grease a non-stick heavy-based 18–20 cm (7–8 in) frying pan (skillet). Knead the dough again and roll out to the size of the pan. Place in the pan (skillet) and work a little dough up the sides.
    Spread the tomato purée (paste) over the bottom, then cover with the sliced tomatoes. Sprinkle with the garlic and herbs, and arrange the asparagus and mushrooms on top with the olives and cheese. Season well.
    Cook over a medium heat for 15–20 minutes, then place under a pre-heated grill (broiler) until the cheese is golden. Transfer to a heated serving dish and serve hot.
TOTAL CALORIES: 740
CALORIES PER SERVING: 185
SERVES 4

Wholewheat Spaghetti with Chicken Livers

Metric/Imperial
100g/3½ oz chicken livers
1 small onion, finely chopped
25g/1 oz button mushrooms, sliced
1 clove garlic, crushed
pinch of chilli powder
¼ tsp mixed dried herbs
1 tbsp dry sherry
salt and freshly ground black pepper
25g/1 oz wholewheat spaghetti
2 tbsp plain yogurt
freshly chopped thyme

American
½ cup chicken liver
1 small onion, minced
¼ cup sliced button mushrooms
1 clove garlic, crushed
pinch of chili powder
¼ tsp mixed dried herbs
1 tbsp dry sherry
salt and freshly ground black pepper
1 oz wholewheat spaghetti
2 tbsp plain yogurt
freshly chopped thyme

Place the chicken livers, onion and mushrooms in a non-stick frying pan (skillet). Cook for 5 minutes, stirring occasionally, until the chicken livers are browned. Add the garlic, chilli powder, herbs, sherry and seasoning. Cover and simmer, stirring occasionally, for 5 minutes.
    Cook the spaghetti in boiling salted water for 9 minutes or until 'al dente'. Drain well.

Pour the yogurt onto the chicken liver mixture; heat gently but do not boil. Add the spaghetti and mix well. Serve at once, sprinkled with thyme.
TOTAL CALORIES: 300
SERVES 1

Wholewheat Spaghetti with Tomato and Basil

Metric/Imperial
500g/1 lb tomatoes, skinned, seeded and chopped
100g/3½ oz onion, very finely chopped
2 tbsp freshly chopped basil
salt and freshly ground black pepper
dash of Worcestershire sauce
150g/5 oz wholewheat spaghetti
25g/1 oz freshly grated Parmesan cheese

American
2 cups skinned, seeded and chopped tomatoes
⅞ cup minced onion
2 tbsp freshly chopped basil
salt and freshly ground black pepper
dash of Worcestershire sauce
5 oz wholewheat spaghetti
¼ cup grated Parmesan cheese

Put the tomatoes, onion, basil and seasoning into a saucepan. Boil rapidly for 15–20 minutes, stirring, until the sauce has thickened. Add the Worcestershire sauce; season.
    Meanwhile, cook the spaghetti in boiling salted water for 6–8 minutes until it is 'al dente'. Drain, spoon over the sauce and sprinkle with cheese.
TOTAL CALORIES: 750
CALORIES PER SERVING: 375
SERVES 2

Winter Fruit Compote

Metric/Imperial
175g/6 oz dried apricots
125g/1 oz dried figs
50g/2 oz dried apples
300 ml/½ pint apple juice
grated rind and juice of 2 lemons

American
1 cup dried apricots
⅔ cup prunes
1 tbsp dried figs
½ cup dried apples
1¼ cups apple juice
grated rind and juice of 2 lemons

Place the dried fruit, apple juice, lemon rind and juice in a bowl and soak for 4 hours. Transfer to a saucepan, cover and slowly bring to the boil, then simmer for 20–30 minutes until tender. Chill before serving.
TOTAL CALORIES: 880
CALORIES PER SERVING: 220
SERVES 4

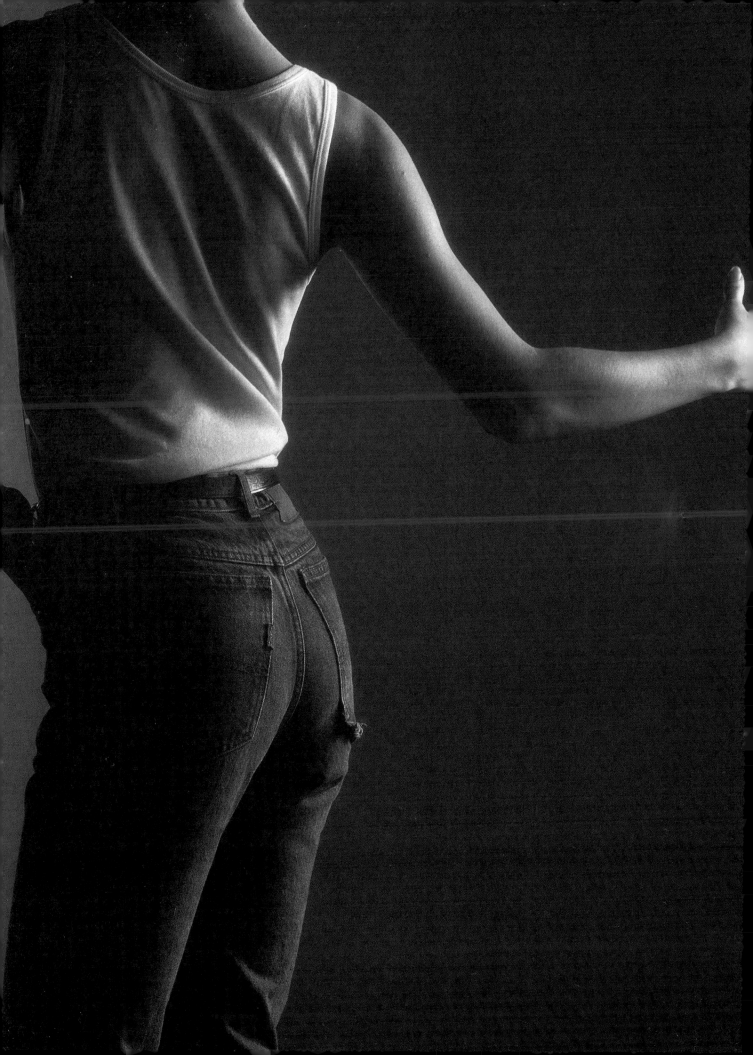

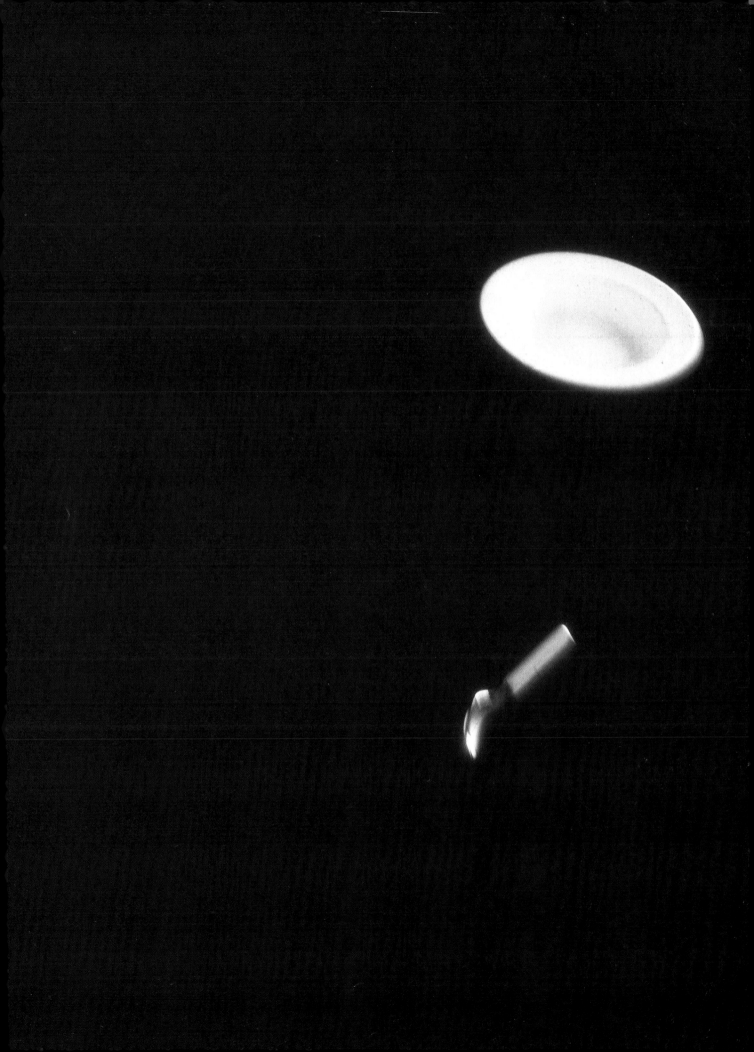

The exercise programme

Exercise mania has us in its grip. Suddenly everyone seems to be out there – running laps, working out, lifting weights, stretching hamstrings…Everyone except you, that is. You've heard that you will look and feel better for it physically – emotionally too – and you long for a strong, supple, healthy body. But it seems impossible to get started.

The sheer difficulty of knowing how and where to start can seem daunting enough. As awareness of fitness has increased, so ways of getting fit have multiplied. There are hundreds of different methods, each claiming to be better than the next. Who is right? What is best? Running or swimming? Swimming or yoga? Straightforward toning exercises or weights? Free weights or fixed weights? Fixed weights or Nautilus? Isometric or Isotonic? Dynamic or static? Conditioning or stretching? New York stretching or Californian stretching? The sheer confusion of choice alone can bring on a sense of overwhelming inertia…

What is needed is a programme which will integrate these methods because each has something to offer, but not everything. Combining them leads to a more complete form of fitness than following any one to the exclusion of the rest. This 24-week programme has been designed to promote all-round fitness and to get you into your best shape ever, by introducing each of these fitness basics – posture in week 1, stretch in week 3, aerobics in week 8, weights in week 9 and so on.

To guard against the possible risks of injury or of overdoing it, the programme is graduated, starting very gently and getting increasingly demanding as you get fitter. It takes a full 6 months to get into shape, to transform a flabby, out-of-condition body into a lean, fit one. Try to take short-cuts or treat exercise as a race and you are heading for trouble. The exercise boom may have focused some healthy, and much-needed, attention on our state of fitness, or lack of it, but it has also doubled the queues of people seeking the services of doctors, physiotherapists and osteopaths for sprained knees, bad backs, torn tendons and other sports-related aches and pains. The headlong rush to get fit is always self-defeating. You've got to be able to walk again before you can run again.

Avoid being an exercise drop-out by going at a reasonable pace and by remembering that healthy exercise has much more to do with beating the sluggish uninspired part of yourself than it does with beating anyone else. Twinges of pain are warnings to be careful, not challenges to be overcome.

Although you will find that the particular exercise focus changes each week, a general emphasis on self-awareness runs throughout the programme. As you become fitter, so you also become more aware of how your body feels as it moves and, gradually, more attuned to what your own unique fitness needs are. By week 24 you will not only be fit, strong and supple but also self-confident in the knowledge that you are well able to take good care of yourself and to continue exercising in the way that is right for you. And that's what being really fit and healthy is all about…

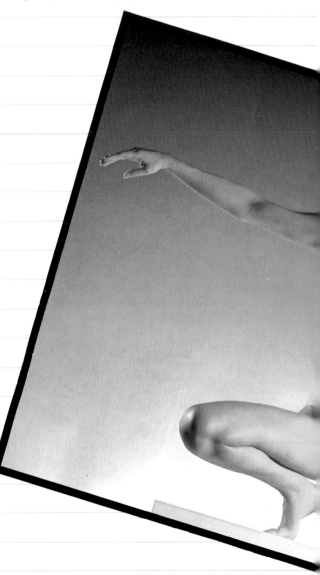

The 24-week plan

Follow the programme, starting today, from week one, repeating exercises as indicated on the lists at the beginning of each week. New exercises are underlined in black. Run through the programme every day if possible (and at least 3 times a week) at whatever time you like – but never directly after a heavy meal. Try to establish a regular exercise time because you will find it easier to stick to your programme if it becomes a normal part of your day. Wear clothes that are comfortable and which allow freedom of movement. Leotard, tracksuit, vest and pants, and loose baggy T-shirt over tights are all good. If knees are weak, leg warmers can be very useful.

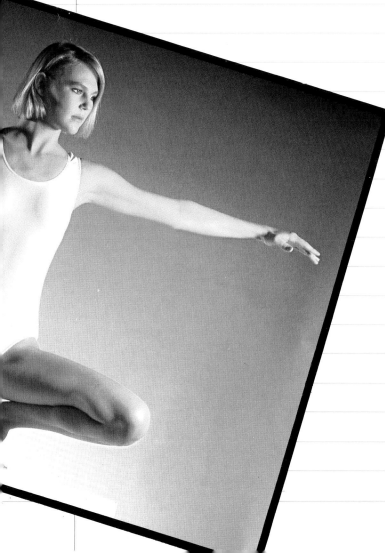

The colour of leotard in each illustration varies with the type of exercise according to the key below. When an exercise combines two or more elements, the leotard is striped.

stretch   co-ordination

loosener   relaxation

         aerobics

mobility

     balance

tester

     therapeutics

strengthener

WEEK 1: POSTURE

Good posture comes first for two reasons: it determines your shape and ensures you are working the right muscles and joints, so getting the most from your exercises...

If you have been told good posture means 'tummy in, chest out, shoulders back', you have been told wrong, for good posture starts from the back, not the front, and is achieved by a natural lengthening of the spine. The spine largely determines your shape because it communicates with every part of the body via skull, shoulders, ribcage and pelvic girdle. If its position is right, everything from top of head to toes automatically comes into line.

These Preliminaries will help realign your body by returning your spine to its correct position. Sense what happens to your body as you do them and repeat them often through the day – not just when you exercise. Feel what it is like to stand correctly with spine lengthened, shoulders down, pelvis centered and weight balanced and enjoy the feeling of lift that flows through you as you lengthen upwards.

This week's programme
Preliminaries
1 × 2
2 × 4 each way twice
3 × 8 each side
4 × several
5 × 16
6 × 1
7 × 5 each level
8 × 4 each side
9 × 1 each side
10 × 3
11 × up to 8 each side
12 × 8
13 × 2 each leg
14 × 4
15 × several
16 × several
17 × 7 each way
18 × 1

PRELIMINARIES

I HEAD AND NECK *Stand sideways to a mirror and let head drop down. Now lengthen at back of neck as you lift back of head. Feel yourself growing taller. Notice how lifting from back of head lengthens top of spine. But don't cheat by poking chin out as this will shorten top of spine by increasing curve at back of neck. Drop shoulders down away from ears to allow top of spine to lengthen upwards.*

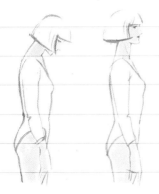

Maximum lengthening of the spine from coccyx to base of skull: good posture in a nutshell...

Posture is *the* instant shape-improver, much more effective than crash dieting. You can make your figure look 100 per cent better, *immediately*, by standing and moving correctly.

When posture is right, the bones and ligaments of the skeleton counteract the pull of gravity leaving muscles free for movement; when posture is wrong, muscles take over the work of the bones, producing unnecessary strains and tensions...

II PELVIS

Still standing sideways on to mirror, stick your bottom out and notice how this makes your tummy bulge too. See also how small of back has become more curved. Does this shortening of spine make the whole of your back feel tight? The correct position of spine is achieved by tilting pelvis into a central position. Place one hand on lower back, the other on tummy and gently push lower back forwards. Notice how small of back lengthens as pubic bone lifts a little and tummy is contained. This centering of pelvis is crucial to posture.

III WEIGHT BALANCE

Stand with legs slightly apart. How is your weight placed? Do you stand more on left side or right? Do you slightly bend one knee, placing all your weight on the other leg? Try doing this and notice what happens to your hips and shoulders. Now readjust posture so that hips and shoulders are level and you are standing with weight centrally balanced between heels and balls of feet.

Once you have done them, run through Preliminaries again. Now you are ready to start exercising.

1 **NECK** *Stand correctly, remembering to lift at back of neck, and slowly lower head forwards as far as you can. Return it to centre and then, keeping lift in back of neck, lower it slowly backwards. Don't let it drop. Return head to centre and tilt it to right until you feel a gentle stretch along left side of neck, then bring it back to centre and repeat to left. Turn head to right, looking round as far as you can, then return to centre and repeat to left. Now repeat the exercise.*

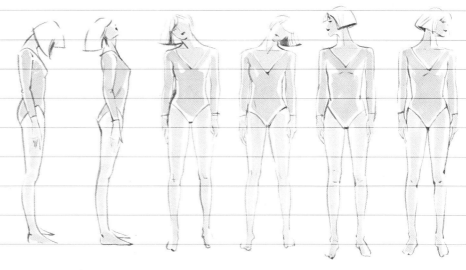

Ease into exercising with general stretches to lengthen muscles and prepare them for more strenuous work to come. Warmed extended muscles are more responsive to exercise, less susceptible to injury . . .

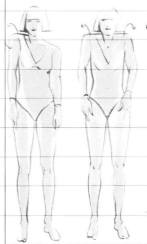

REMEMBER Drop shoulders and lengthen back of neck all the way through your exercise routine.

2 **SHOULDERS**
These loosen up the shoulder area, which is often stiff, and can be practised whenever you are aware of any tightness or tension there. Standing straight, take one shoulder forwards, lift it and then push it back and down. Repeat twice for each shoulder and then rotate them together 4 times, first forwards and then back. It is important to end on the backward movement as most people tend to let their shoulders come too far forwards.

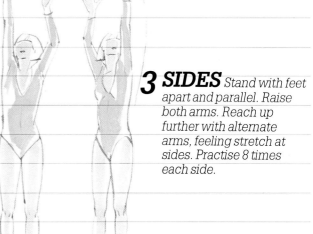

3 **SIDES** *Stand with feet apart and parallel. Raise both arms. Reach up further with alternate arms, feeling stretch at sides. Practise 8 times each side.*

4 **UPPER BACK**
Raise arms to shoulder level in front of you. Reach forwards with alternate arms and bring them back into place several times. Repeat with both arms together. Then try interlacing hands, turning palms away from you. Tuck buttocks underneath you and push away with hands, feeling stretch across back of shoulders.

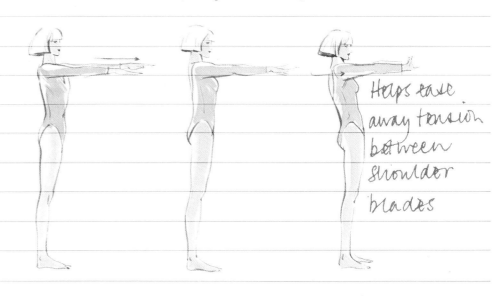

Helps ease away tension between shoulder blades

5 LEGS
Stand with feet slightly apart and parallel. Bend knees, keeping heels on floor. Straighten legs, lifting up onto balls of feet. Practise 16 times.

CAUTION When bending knees, make sure they are directly above toes and do not fall inwards.

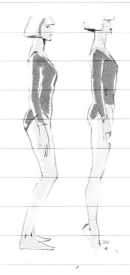

Strengthens legs and gets circulation going after standing still

The weight of the head (over 4.5 kg/10 lb), the habit of holding it stiffly and the everyday effects of stress make for tense tight muscles that can lead to pain and headaches. This movement sequence will help loosen the muscles around the neck and so relieve strain.

6 BACK
This is an excellent exercise for beginners provided you are supported, so lower back is protected. Think about your posture as you do it and feel how helpful it can be for lengthening the back. Bend knees and bend forwards from hips, folding arms and resting elbows on a counter at about hip height. Walk backwards with knees slightly bent until you are making a right angle between trunk and legs. Now lengthen back of neck as you bend knees a bit more. Feel how this helps back to lengthen. Gradually straighten knees keeping length in back so it remains as flat as possible. Repeat bending and straightening several times.

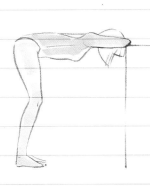

A strong stretch in the shoulders and arms may be felt at first as chest area expands.

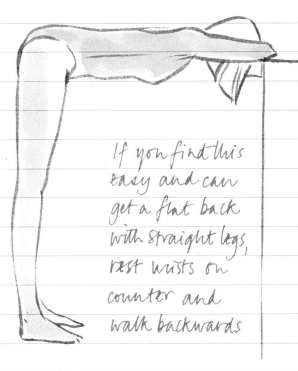

If you find this easy and can get a flat back with straight legs, rest wrists on counter and walk backwards

7 BUST
Clasp hands in front of you and clench them sharply together 5 times at waist, shoulder and eye level in order to work every part of the supporting muscles.

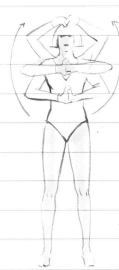

Strengthens muscles which help support the breasts

Muscle has just so much elasticity before it contracts back to its original shape. While slow easy stretching extends it according to these natural limits, quick bouncing movements do not. They should be avoided, or at least left till really fit, because they invoke the stretch reflex – which causes muscles to contract as a protective measure. Repetitive bouncing movements can cause damage to muscle and connective tissue because of the speed of the contraction, so keep stretches slow and controlled throughout the exercise programme.

8 WAIST

Stand with feet apart and slightly turned out. Lift ribs away from hips. Bend to side and hold for 3 counts, maintaining feeling of lift as you bend. Feel stretch along opposite side. Come back to centre and repeat to other side. Practise 4 times.

Good posture is essential to get the most from this, so check you are standing well throughout.

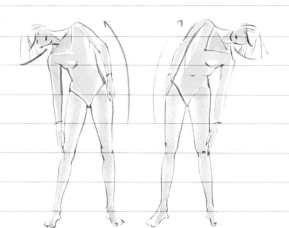

Imagine a pane of glass just behind and in front of you to prevent you tipping forwards or backwards

If your posture is perfect, your abdominal muscles will act like a belt to hold in your tummy. If you slouch, they will weaken and your tummy will stick out however slim you are.

Check posture by checking shoes. Where are the soles more worn down? If toes or heels, you are tipping too far forwards/ too far back when you walk; if outsides, you are rolling your feet outwards; if insides, weight is tipping inwards and knees are probably knocking together too.

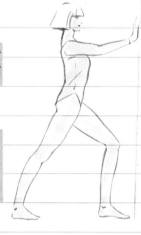

9 CALVES

Stand with one leg forwards and one back, heels firmly on floor, front knee bent and other straight with muscles at front of thigh contracted. Now lean forwards, using a wall for support if you find it helps, until you can feel a strong pull in calves. Maintain pull for 10 counts, and release.
Change legs and repeat.

10 BACKS OF THIGHS

Stand with feet a little apart and parallel. Bend knees as you bend forwards from hips, keeping back long. Slowly go down into a squat, so that front lower ribs are resting on about the middle of thighs. Allow heels to lift a little. Place hands on either side. Breathe in. As you breathe out, straighten legs as much as you can, but don't worry if you are unable to straighten knees. Feel stretch in backs of legs and continue to breathe out as you hold position for 4 counts. Breathe in as you squat down again. Practise 3 times.

If you feel stretch behind knees, fine; if any pain in lower back, however, this exercise is not for you. Try mobility sequences for spine on page 242 and return to this when back becomes more mobile.

THE AIM.... to keep ribs as close as possible to thighs as you straighten legs

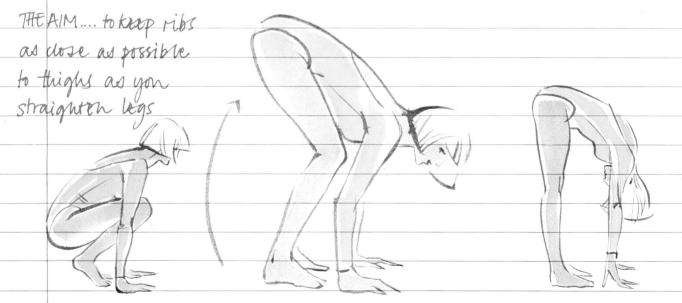

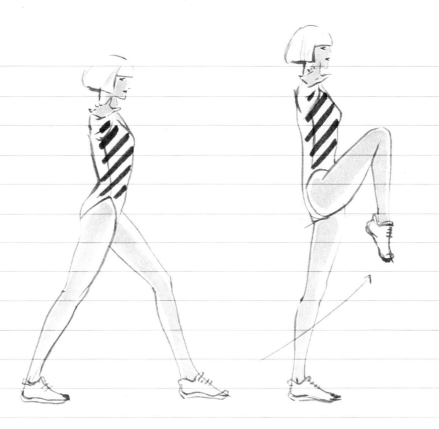

11 LUNGE *Stand well with feet together and arms out to side at shoulder level. Transfer weight from foot to foot, lifting heels and keeping toes on floor, several times. Then step from foot to foot, lifting feet about 20 cm (8 ins) from floor each time.*

When you feel well balanced, try this gentle aerobic exercise. Take one leg forwards, bending knee until it is directly over toes, and the other back so that you are now in a lunge position. Bend back knee and lift leg up in front of you. Replace it on floor behind. Practise up to 8 times and then change legs.

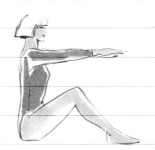

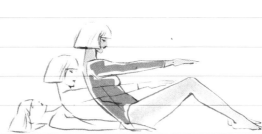

Feel tummy muscles working strongly

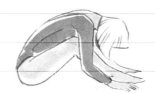

12 ABDOMEN *Sit on floor with knees bent, feet hip-width apart and arms straight out in front at shoulder level. Breathe in. As you breathe out, lean back tilting pelvis and lowering head. Press lower back into floor. Breathe in and come up. Breathe out and flop gently forwards. Breathe in and come up. Practise 8 times, in a good smooth rhythm.*

13 OUTER THIGHS *Lie on back with arms at shoulder level. Raise left knee into chest and extend leg upwards, flexing foot. Pass it over right thigh onto floor, aiming to get foot as close to right hand as possible. Feel stretch in left thigh and hold for 4 counts, breathing out and trying to keep shoulder blades flat on floor. Now lift leg again and, bending knee as before, lower to floor. Repeat with right leg. Then complete exercise again.*

Bonus: Gives a marvellous twist in the spine

If aware of any strain in back, leave this one out and practise Therapeutic exercises on page 242 instead. Return to it when back gets stronger.

14 BACK

Sit with bottom against a wall and soles of feet together and as close to you as possible. Place hands on ankles and lengthen spine upwards so that shoulder blades and back of crown of head are touching wall too. Pull thighs downwards*, maintaining length in spine and hold for 4 counts. Practise 4 times.

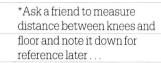

*Ask a friend to measure distance between knees and floor and note it down for reference later . . .

Used as a meditation pose for its excellent effects on posture and breathing. When spine is lengthened, ribs are lifted and chest opens, enabling you to breathe well.

CAUTION If you feel any pain in knees, bring feet away from you until comfortable.

(handwritten) BONUS stretches inner thighs and loosens hips.

15 BACK

Now come away from wall and see if you can lengthen back upwards unsupported in another position. At first do this side-view to a mirror to check back is straight. Sitting, take legs apart until you feel a slight stretch in inner thighs. Now lengthen spine upwards as much as you can*. Look in mirror. Is back lengthened or rounded? If unable to straighten up completely, use hands to help. Place them behind you and push them into floor. Now hold position for a few moments and then round back and bend knees. Repeat several times, gradually increasing holding time to a minute or more.

As stretch in inner thighs subsides and you feel you can take more, push on hands, lifting trunk off floor a little; then lower a little further forwards so legs go further apart.

*How far can you comfortably take legs apart while maintaining length in spine? Ask a friend to measure distance between feet and note it down for reference later . . .

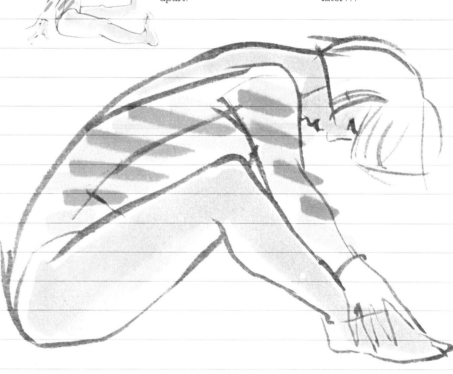

(handwritten) Releases tension in back and makes a good loosener after the strong posture exercises.

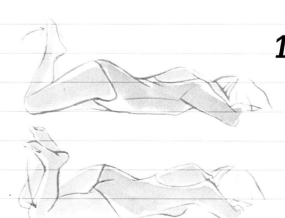

16 BACK

Lie on front, hands flat one on top of the other and forehead on hands. Bend knees and let feet sway to each side several times.

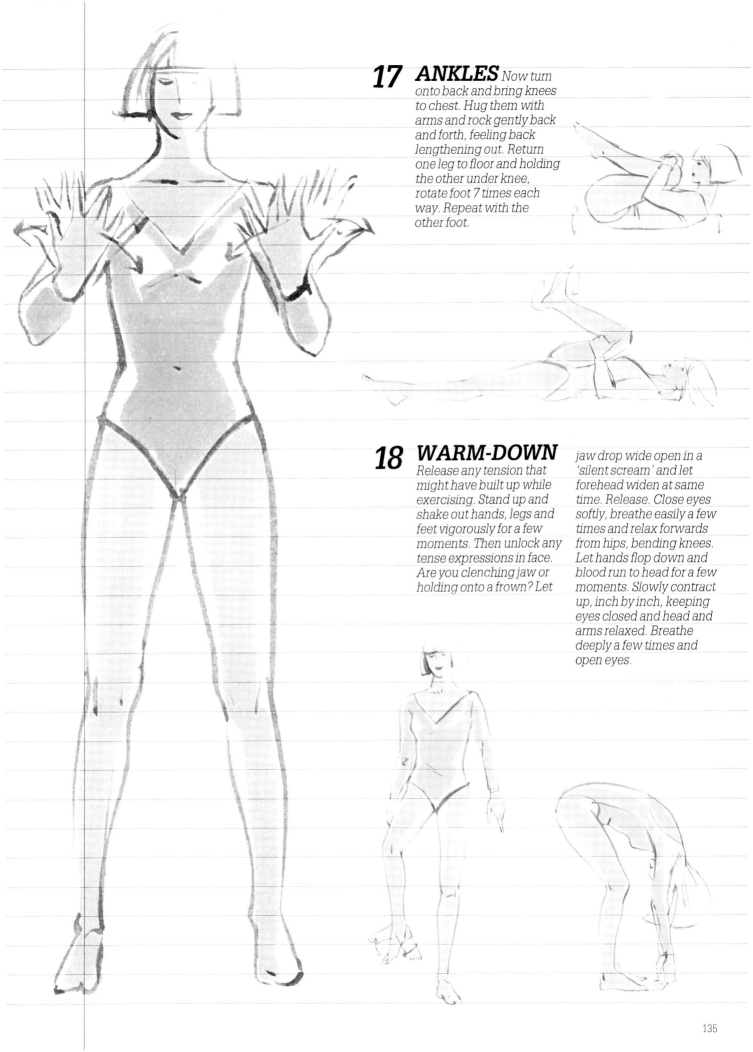

17 ANKLES *Now turn onto back and bring knees to chest. Hug them with arms and rock gently back and forth, feeling back lengthening out. Return one leg to floor and holding the other under knee, rotate foot 7 times each way. Repeat with the other foot.*

18 WARM-DOWN
Release any tension that might have built up while exercising. Stand up and shake out hands, legs and feet vigorously for a few moments. Then unlock any tense expressions in face. Are you clenching jaw or holding onto a frown? Let jaw drop wide open in a 'silent scream' and let forehead widen at same time. Release. Close eyes softly, breathe easily a few times and relax forwards from hips, bending knees. Let hands flop down and blood run to head for a few moments. Slowly contract up, inch by inch, keeping eyes closed and head and arms relaxed. Breathe deeply a few times and open eyes.

WEEK 2: BREATHING

Good breathing is the secret of successful exercising, enabling you to work to the best of your abilities and having considerable benefits for heart and health.

Although none of us needs to learn how to breathe any more than we need to learn how to make the heart beat, we do need to *relearn* how to use the whole of our breathing apparatus – namely the 12 pairs of ribs, and their intercostal muscles, that attach to either side of the spine and come round to form the sides and front of the chest.

To use your ribcage correctly, your posture must also be correct. If not, all the breathing exercises in the world will be to no avail for it is only when the spine is lengthened and chest lifted that the ribcage has the freedom it needs.

This week's programme
Preliminaries
14, see note, × 4
19 × 1
20 × several
6, with pelvic tilts
21 × several
22 × several
23 × 3 each side
24 × 1
25 × 8
26
27 × up to 12 each leg
12 × 8
13 × 2 each leg
28 × 4
15, progression **29** × 4
16 × several
30 × 7 each way
31

19 GOOD BREATHING

Now move away from wall and stand up, maintaining length in back and openness in chest. Place one hand on chest and the other on abdomen. Take a few slow deep breaths. Which hand moves first? If it is the upper one, you are breathing from the top of your chest, hardly using ribcage at all. Now continue breathing slowly and evenly, but concentrate on taking each breath down to bottom of ribs. Can you feel abdomen moving gently out as chest fills with air and the diaphragm, an involuntary muscle, moves downwards? Continue breathing in this way several times and then place hands across middle of back. Notice ribs are working there too. Breathing uses whole of the chest area, not just the front.

N.B. Back strengthener (**14**) will be familiar. Notice that your spine is not flattened against the wall but curves slightly in at the small of your back – just enough to get your hand through. This natural curve is good, if not too exaggerated, because it helps your chest to open and your ribs to work freely.

Now slump your shoulders forwards and notice what happens to your ribcage. See what happens, too, when you stiffen up and flatten your chest.

Returning to the correct position, become aware of your breathing. See how easy it is when you give yourself enough room.

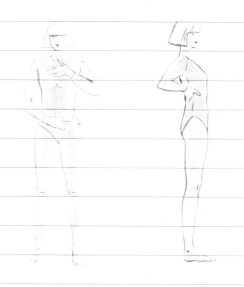

Few of us realize the extent of the breathing space available to us. We never think of our lungs expanding at the back as well as the front, for example.

20 NECK

Here is a progression of the exercise practised last week. Breathe in as you turn head to side. Breathing out, lower head slowly forwards and then breathe in again as you lift it to other side. Practise several times.

Close eyes so you can attend fully to movement of ribs as you breathe

Breathe in through the nose as you prepare for the exercise, out through nose or mouth as you do it, and in again through the nose as you release. Instructions are given to help you. Don't worry if you feel like breathing in when the instructions say out. This often happens to begin with, particularly if you usually hold your breath when you exercise. Help counteract it by reminding yourself to BREATHE OUT. The out-breath is always the important one; the in-breath will look after itself.

21 BACK

Here is a progression on last week's flat back exercise (6). Start as before and go into flat back, resting elbows on counter for support. Now do a few pelvic tilts as you stand with knees straightened and back supported. Breathe in. As you breathe out, tilt pelvis, contracting tummy muscles and allowing back to round. Breathe in as you flatten back again. Practise several times.

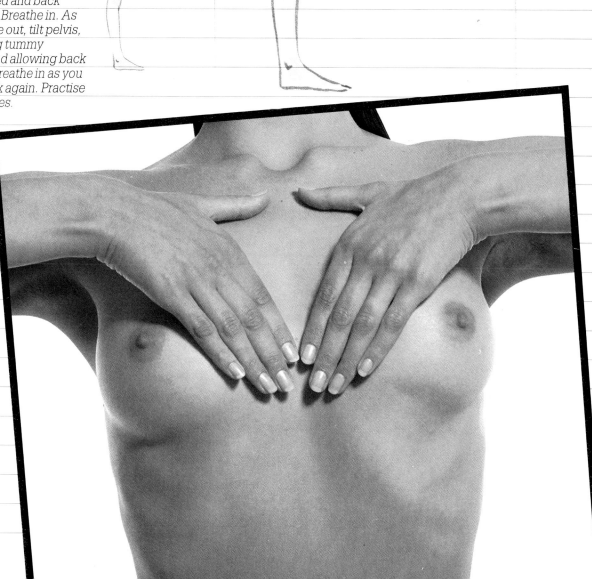

22 LOOSENER

LOOSENER Start by standing well, feet hip-width apart. Breathe in. As you breathe out, contract in and curl forwards, bending knees and allowing arms to flop forwards. Breathe in as you straighten knees. Enjoy it several times, moving easily and freely.

Notice you breathe out as front of body contracts, in as it expands: this is the principle behind all breathing when exercising.

Remember your good posture throughout

It is vital to breathe out properly. 70 per cent of all the body's waste is expelled on the breath. Compare with defecation (3 per cent), urination (7 per cent) and sweating (20 per cent) and you will see that in order to eliminate waste, and keep body tissues healthy and uncongested, it behoves us to breathe fully and freely. Vigorous sustained aerobic exercise will help to do this by giving lungs a good workout.

23 WAIST

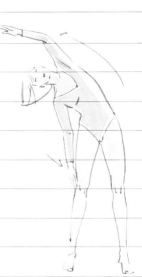

WAIST This is a progression from last week's stretch (8). Stand with feet apart and parallel. Breathe in as you lift left arm (keeping shoulder pulled down). Breathe out as you bend to right, stretching as far as you can. Breathe in as you come up a little, allowing arm to bend. Breathe out as you stretch again to side. Repeat twice and then change arms.

Use your breathing to help you when you exercise – a long exhale can help you stretch a bit further or contract your muscles more strongly...

24 CHEST AND BACKS OF THIGHS

CHEST AND BACKS OF THIGHS Stand with feet apart. Breathe in and take hands behind, clasping them together. As you breathe out, lift hands up as far as possible and bend forwards from hips. Breathe normally as you hold stretch for 4 counts, then hold it for a further 4 taking good deep breaths and feeling reaction in abdomen. Shake head gently to make sure neck muscles feel free. Breathe in and straighten.

Excellent for posture

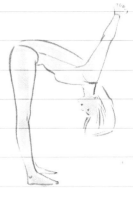

If you can't yet bend from hips with flat back, bend knees as you go forwards.

25 LEGS

LEGS A progression on last week's strengthener (5). This time, take legs wider apart and point feet out so that legs turn out from hip joint and knees are aligned over toes. Place hands on hips to help keep pelvis centered. Breathe in as you straighten legs and lift heels. Practise 8 times.

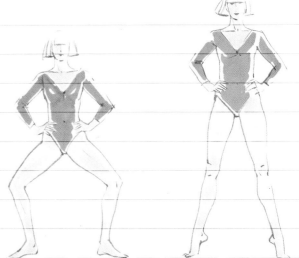

26 UPPER BODY

This excellent exercise encourages good breathing, strengthens chest, bust and arms and gives a stretch along backs of legs. Stand arm's length away from a wall with feet together and arms at shoulder level. Place palms flat on wall in front. Breathe in. As you breathe out, bend arms and lean forwards, keeping spine in a long straight line. Breathe in as you return to starting position. Practise 4 press-ups, rest a moment, and repeat.

As exercise gets easier, step back further

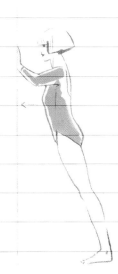

27 KICK

Try this progression of last week's aerobic exercise (11), keeping lunge position but instead of bending knee and lifting leg, kick it out in front. Practise up to 12 kicks each leg.

Place your hands on your chest after doing the leg kicks. If not actually panting, you will certainly be breathing rapidly and from the top of your chest. Next time you feel tense or anxious, examine your breathing again. Are you breathing too fast and too high? Take slower, deeper breaths and feel yourself relax...

28 ABDOMEN

Lie flat on back with body in a long straight line, shoulders down and arms at sides. Bend knees, so that feet are flat on floor, hip-width apart. Breathe in. As you breathe out, lift head and shoulders off floor. Hold for 3 counts if you can. Breathe in as you lower to floor. Practise 4 times* and then roll head from side to side to release front neck muscles (they have to work strongly in this exercise). Take a good deep breath to release any tension in chest too.

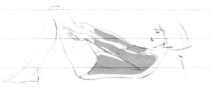

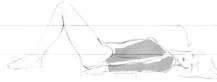

If you feel strain in neck, place one or two cushions under head.

*Next time you try this, see how many you can do comfortably, *without straining*. It may be no more than 4 or 5. Note it down for reference later...

It is important to get your breathing right on the strong abdominal exercises (12 and 28) because the chest on the in-breath is like a full balloon: the intake of air builds up pressure, pushing the tummy out. It is physiologically impossible, therefore, to contract it at the same time. It is by breathing out that you work these muscles...

29 BACK *Try this active progression of last week's back strengthener (15). Starting as before, sitting on floor with legs well apart and spine lifted, hold for as long as you can breathing normally. Then breathe in, lifting spine a little more. Now interlace fingers, take palms away from you and, as you breathe out, do a pelvic tilt allowing back to round and knees to bend, pushing forwards with hands. Breathe in straightening legs strongly and lifting back. Coordinating movements with breathing should produce a nice steady rhythm. Practise 4 times. Bring legs together and shake them out to release any tension after this strong exercise.*

BONUS Gives a good stretch across back

Do you feel like yawning when you exercise? If so, it is a good sign because it is the body's natural way of getting more air and means you are working muscles well, increasing their demand for oxygen.

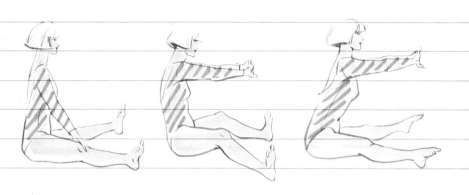

Your breathing not only reflects every physical effort but every emotional disturbance too. When angry, your breathing becomes shallow and quick; when excited, you take longer out-breaths, breathe in more quickly; when depressed, you continue to take air in and let hardly any out. When very strongly moved or surprised, you (momentarily) stop breathing altogether...

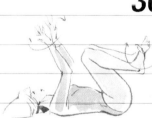

30 ANKLES AND WRISTS *Now turn onto back and press knees into chest. Hold arms loosely in air, as shown, and then rotate feet and hands together, 7 times each way.*

31 RELAXATION *Still lying on back, slide feet down along floor. Bring them together and flex feet as you lift head to look between them. Now lower head and allow legs to rotate easily outwards. Turn palms of hands upwards so arms rotate outwards too. Take 3 or 4 good deep breaths thinking about using ribcage to its maximum so that it lifts up and out on in-breath and sinks back on out-breath. It may help to imagine you are lying by the sea: with each in-breath waves wash over you and with each out-breath they race back to the ocean. Stay there for a while, with eyes closed. Notice how breathing becomes shallower and more even as body quietens and needs less and less oxygen to keep it going.*

Looking down midline of body helps you to check that you are lying in a straight line

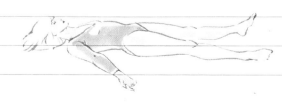

WEEK 3: STRETCH

Good breathing can be applied very successfully to long, slow stretching – the essential preliminary to any activity whether it is jogging, yoga, aerobics, weight training or simply getting out of bed in the morning...

    The gentle stretches you have been doing will have helped lengthen your muscles in preparation for this week's stronger ones. As you do them, you may find strong resistance in parts of your body. This is an uncomfortable sensation – not pain (*see note, over*) – and it will make your body want to tighten up to protect itself. Help prevent this natural tendency by breathing OUT as you work through the stretch and you will find that the sensation subsides, enabling you to stretch still further.

This week's programme
Preliminaries
32 × several
3 × several
33 × 6 backwards
34 × 8 each side
35 × 8 each leg
27 × 8 each side
36 × 8 each side
6, progression **37** × 4
25 × 8
26, taking feet further from wall × 8
24, trying to straighten legs × 1
12 × 4
28, taking head, shoulders and ribs off floor × 4
13 × 3 each leg
30 × 7 each way
29 × 4
38 × 1 each leg
39 × 1
31

Listen to your body and be aware of its needs. If stiff or tense at the start of your session, spend longer than usual on the stretches until you feel really loosened up. Swinging straight into a demanding routine will otherwise merely be adding to tensions that are already there...

32 **WARM-UP** *Stand well, with feet hip-width apart and parallel. Breathe in and stretch up as you lift arms. Breathe out as you bend knees and swing down. Straighten knees a little before bending them to help you swing up again on an in-breath. Enjoy this warm-up several times and then continue with small upwards stretches as though climbing a rope-ladder to ceiling.*

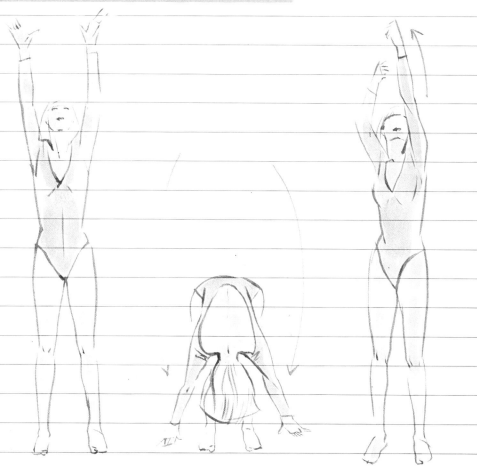

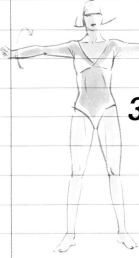

33 SHOULDERS

Lower arms sideways to shoulder level, turning feet out a little so that legs rotate from hips. Now make 6 small backward circles with arms, feeling a good stretch across front of chest each time.

Stretching, and particularly regular stretching, brings all sorts of benefits: greater flexibility, more freedom from tension, less likelihood of stiffness or physical injury, a strong sense of mental and physical well-being. Hold each stretch for count of 8, then, if comfortable, for a further 8 for extra lengthening – breathing well throughout.

IMPORTANT Learn to distinguish between the good stretch feeling of the well-used muscle and pain, which is more acute and actually *hurts*. Exercise should never hurt. If pain is felt, stop at once and consult your doctor.

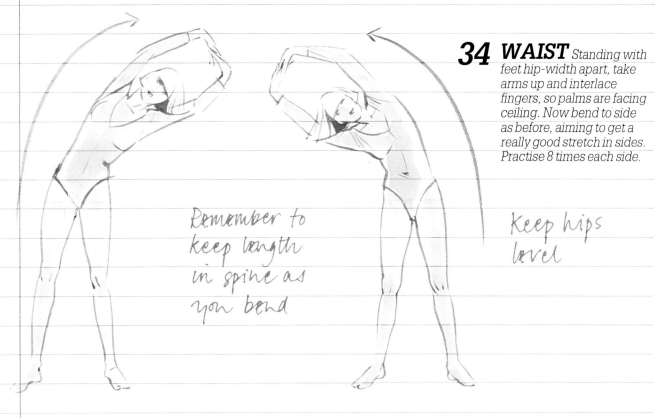

34 WAIST

Standing with feet hip-width apart, take arms up and interlace fingers, so palms are facing ceiling. Now bend to side as before, aiming to get a really good stretch in sides. Practise 8 times each side.

Remember to keep length in spine as you bend

Keep hips level

If you find that you can stretch further on one side than the other, give the stiffer side a chance to catch up by working it a little more and adding a few more repetitions.

Aim for same looseness in hips when walking

35 HIPS

Stand well with spine lifted, holding onto wall or back of chair for support. Now raise outside arm to shoulder level and swing leg forwards and back loosely from hip joint 8 times. Change legs and repeat.

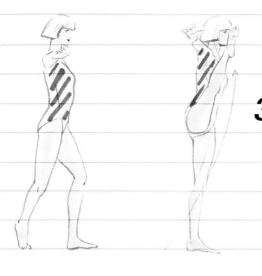

Stiffness not only restricts movement, it restricts pleasure too. Stretching can help bring more joy and spontaneity to your lovemaking by making you more supple, more sensuous, more confident in and about your body...

36 KICK *Stand with arms out sideways at shoulder level. Take one leg behind you and across, so that you are standing with weight on forward foot and toes of other foot resting on floor behind. Now breathe in and bend supporting leg a little. Breathe out as you kick to side with toes pointed. Practise 8 times, then change legs and repeat.*

37 BACK *Take legs wide apart and stand with feet parallel. Breathe in, raise arms to ceiling and stretch upwards. As you breathe out, go forwards from hips into flat back position. Continue on down till hands reach floor and stay there, breathing well, as you allow stretch to subside. Breathe in and lift. Breathe out and lower hands to floor again. Repeat 3 times to the rhythm of your breathing.*

If not much stretch is felt, walk hands backwards towards feet.

38 BACK AND LEGS *Sit on floor with back well lengthened. Breathe in and lengthen back a little more. As you breathe out, bend forwards from hips and hold flexed foot first with inside hand and then with both hands together. Breathe in and lift. As you breathe out, lower over extended leg. Hold for a few moments and, if stretch subsides, lengthen body down a little further. Repeat exercise with other leg, breathing well throughout. If you cannot reach feet with hands, use towel or belt round foot as illustrated on next exercise.*

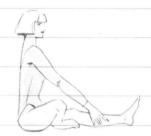

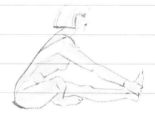

Eventually this becomes relaxing, particularly when you are loose enough at hips to rest head on legs. If you haven't yet found this, relax by stretching out as last week.

39 BACK AND LEGS *Now try forward bend with both legs straight and feet flexed. Use a towel or belt round feet at first, as shown here. Holding onto towel, breathe in and lift up. Maintaining length in your back, breathe out and bend forwards from hips. Creep hands further down towel and go as far as you can, keeping back quite straight*. Don't let it round. With practice you will soon hold outsides of feet.*

The body's response to stress is to stiffen up – shoulders tense, fists clench, expression freezes as blood races to the large muscle groups and the body armours itself for 'fight, flight or fright'. This primitive survival response can produce deeply-ingrained tensions that interfere with our zest and enjoyment of life. Using stretching and breathing to overcome internal tensions may help you manage external ones better...

*Now try this without a towel, looking in a mirror. How far can you go maintaining your flat back? Mark it with a dotted line on the diagram for progress reference later on...

A very
important
stretch that
lengthens
hole of
rick of
body + legs

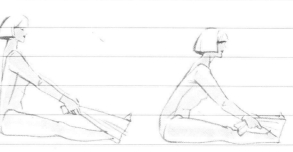

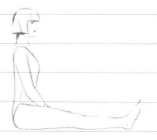

WEEK 4: AWARENESS

Exercising can increase awareness as long as each movement is sensed fully and not just repeated a set number of times. That is the message of Moshe Feldenkrais, Israeli physicist, teacher and philosopher, whose work has done so much to show how movement can be a path both to greater self-awareness and to unlocking hidden potential. 'Know what you are doing,' he says, 'and you can do what you want.'

This week's exercises 40-45 are based on his work. They are not 'exercises' in the traditional sense – not being designed to lose inches or strengthen muscles – but to increase awareness by freeing you from habit, and guiding you towards new ways of moving. New ways of moving can ultimately become new ways of being, because freeing the body enables the mind to develop freely too. Do the exercises slowly, concentrating on every stage, to help sharpen awareness.

This week's programme

Preliminaries
40 × several
41 × several
42 × several
43 × several
44 × 40 each side
45 × several
39, or with one leg bent if difficult **38**, × 1
13 × 4 each leg
34 × 8 each side
46 × 8 each leg
27 × 8 each leg
36 × 8 each leg
47 until comfortably out of breath

Active recovery cool-down, see page 161
37 × 6
26 until muscles being to tire
12 × 4
28 until muscles begin to tire
18 × 1
41 × several
31

---

40 **HABITS** *Interlace fingers together several times. Notice which thumb is on top and which little finger on the bottom. Is it always the same? Now repeat movement, but this time interlace fingers in non-habitual way so other thumb is on top. Does it feel strange and 'wrong'? Try it several times. Now do the same thing with your arms and then legs – crossing them first in the way that feels most natural and then doing the opposite. These movements are all habits and, though apparently unimportant, indicative of other habits that restrict and limit us.*

Until muscles begin to tire means stopping the exercise at the point where the muscles feel well-used, even capable of more, but where you feel no longer fresh enough to continue to do the exercise correctly. Too few repetitions are better than too many...

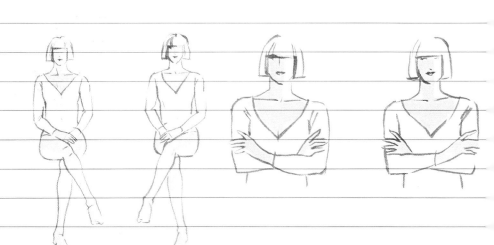

144

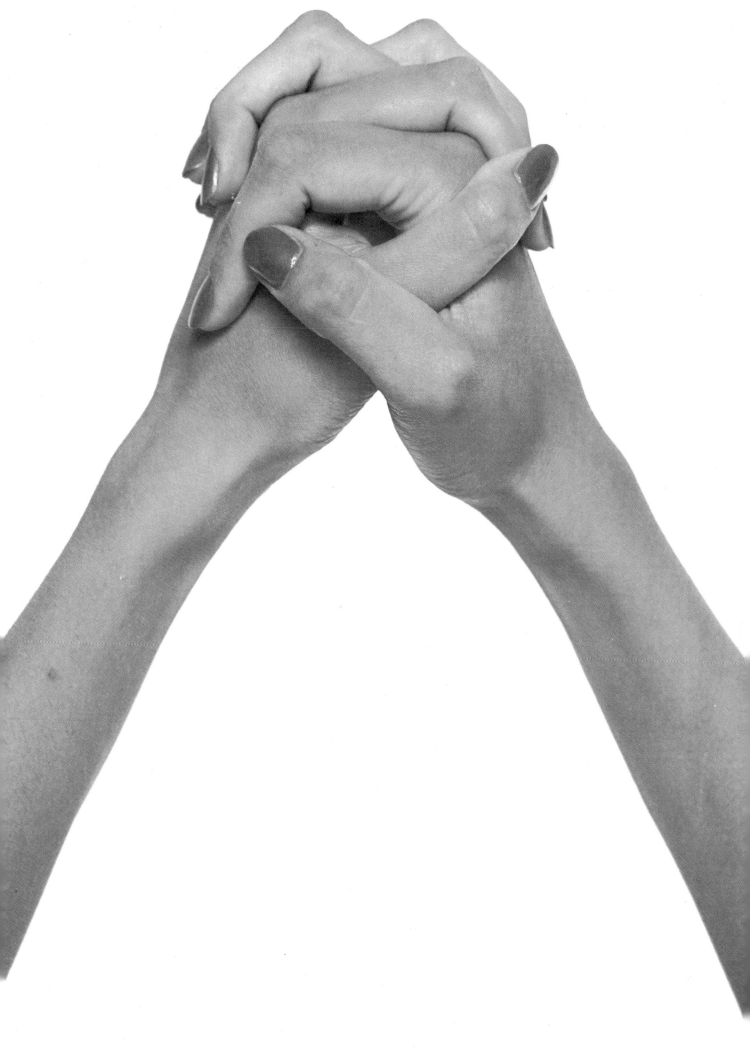

41 SPINE, HIPS, SHOULDERS

Lie on back with knees bent and feet flat on floor, about 15 to 20 cm (6 to 8 ins) apart. Arms, head, knees and shoulders should all be soft and relaxed. Notice what happens to your breathing as you try these movement combinations. Start by lifting one shoulder off floor several times and setting it back down. Repeat with other shoulder. Then with one hip and again with the other. Slide knees to floor and take a rest. Raise knees again and try lifting one shoulder and its opposite hip several times. Repeat with other shoulder and hip. Now lift both shoulders together several times and follow with both hips. Slide knees to floor and rest a moment. Raise knees again and lift one shoulder and hip on the same side together several times. Repeat with other shoulder and hip. Slide knees down and rest a moment and then try all the combinations again. Do they feel any easier?

'There is an essential difference between consciousness and awareness, although the borders are not clear in our use of language. I can walk up the stairs of my house, fully conscious of what I am doing, and yet not know how many steps I have climbed. In order to know how many there are I must climb them a second time, pay attention, listen to myself, and count them. Awareness is consciousness together with a realization of what is happening within it or of what is going on within ourselves while we are conscious.' Moshe Feldenkrais

Vary your way of moving each time, sensing the differences for yourself. Start very slowly, seeing how long you can take to make a movement, and then try it more quickly; practise making very large exaggerated movements then tiny ones – the smallest you can make.

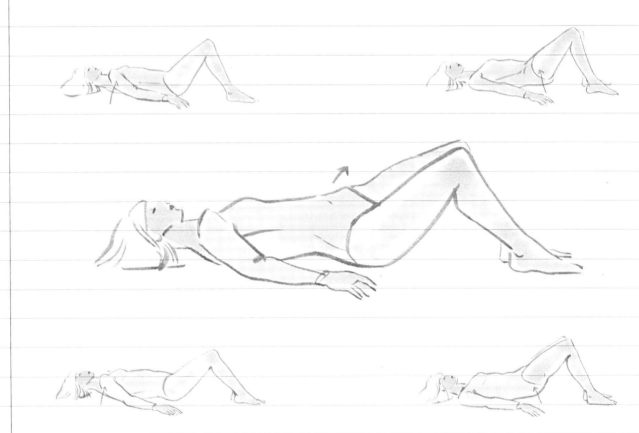

Do the sequences slowly and gently, and you will find your body gains quickly in agility as you gain in awareness. Differences can often be felt after just a few minutes. In addition bear the following in mind:

1. DON'T PUSH THROUGH PAIN. Each movement should be easy and fluid.

2. SLOW IS BETTER THAN FAST. Swift movements and mindless repetition reinforce habit; slow movements let you find new ways of moving. If aware of any stiffness or pain, slow down even more, so you can learn how to move without pain.

3. THE MEANS IS MORE IMPORTANT THAN THE END. Having a goal in mind limits you from the start because you shut off alternative possibilities. Keep an open mind, attend simply to each movement as you do it, pausing at each stage, and you will soon become aware of all the choices open to you and so will be able to pick the one that works best...

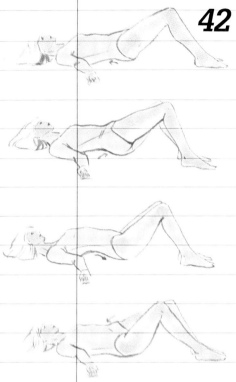

42 PELVIS

Lie on back and raise knees with legs in line with pelvis, hands by side and feet resting flat on floor. Imagine there is a clock face on the back of your pelvis, with 6 o'clock beneath coccyx and 12 o'clock just below navel. Move pelvis to 12 o'clock and notice that lower back lies flat on floor. Move between 6 and 12 o'clock slowly a number of times, being aware of how you organize this simple movement in your pelvic region.

Now imagine 3 o'clock beneath left hip and 9 o'clock beneath right hip. Rock slowly from side to side 20 times feeling both points. Rest a moment. Now move from 1 to 7 back and forth across face of pelvic clock; from 10 to 4; from 2 to 8; from 5 to 11 all several times.

Try this sequence: 12 to 1; 1 to 12; 12 to 11; 11 to 12 to 1; 1 to 12 to 11 to 10; 10 to 11 to 12 to 1 to 2; 2 to 1 to 12; 12 to 1 to 2 to 3; 3 to 2 to 1 to 12 to 11; 11 to 12 to 1 to 2 to 3; 3 to 2 to 1 to 12 to 11; 11 to 12 to 1 to 2 to 3; 3 to 2 to 1 to 12 to 11 to 10; 10 to 11 to 12 to 1 to 2; 2 to 1 to 12 to 11 to 10 to 9; 9 to 10 to 11 to 12. Stop and rest. Was there any area, say from 9 to 11, which was difficult or painful? Return to that area and move back and forth through it until movement becomes easier. Rest again. Now return to 6 to 12 movement. Is it any easier? Are you beginning to reclaim awareness of your pelvis? Rest a moment.

Now move to the 6 position. Move from 6 to 7; 7 to 6 to 5; 5 to 6 to 7; 7 to 6 to 5 to 4; 4 to 5 to 6 to 7; 7 to 6 to 5 to 4 to 3; 3 to 4 to 5 to 6 to 7 to 8; 8 to 7 to 6 to 5; 5 to 6 to 7 to 8 to 9; 9 to 8 to 7 to 6; 6 to 7 to 8 to 9 to 10 to 11 to 12. Stop and rest a moment. Then return to the 12 position and continue around face of clock in a clockwise direction, slowly taking 30 seconds to a minute for one rotation. Imagine you are the second hand making a sweep of the clock face. Repeat it several times. Stop and rest. Then make anti-clockwise circuits equally slowly. Stop and rest.

Your pelvis is your centre of gravity, sexuality and energy ... You have probably not moved it fully in years. Enjoy the pelvic clock movements, letting your energy flow freely. Isn't your pelvis more responsive, more supple than you imagined it could be? What other areas have you ceased to be aware of in this way?

*BONUS
Gives the spine a good twist*

43 UPPER BACK

Lie on back with feet flat on floor, 30 to 45 cm (12 to 18 ins) from buttocks, and knees bent vertically above them. Now raise both arms towards ceiling and place palms of hands together, so that armpits and wrists make angles of a triangle. Let arms fall to one side several times, keeping elbows straight and palms together. Don't let triangle collapse or you lose benefit of exercise. Feel opposite shoulder pushing arms over and notice how neck tends to lift from floor as arms move downwards. Repeat movement until you begin to notice arms tiring. Stop and rest. Then repeat again several times. Rest. Repeat.

44 LOWER BACK

Lying as before, but with arms by side, place right leg over left. Let both knees fall to right, keeping shoulder blades on floor. Both legs should now be supported by left foot only. Feel weight of right leg pulling left one down to floor and notice that when knees move down to floor neck tends to move away from floor. Return knees to centre and notice that neck returns to floor. Practise 20 times breathing out as you move knees downwards, in as you return them to central position. Stop and rest a moment and then repeat 20 times again. This time become aware of twist in spine and lengthening of muscles at side of vertebrae. Now stop and rest again and then reverse position, so that left leg is crossed over right. Let your knees fall to left 20 times, being aware of your body again, then rest a moment and repeat. Which side is more supple?

CAUTION Gives powerful twist in lower back. If you have back problems do it very gently, stop if you feel any pain and try Feldenkrais mobility sequences in Therapeutics section instead.

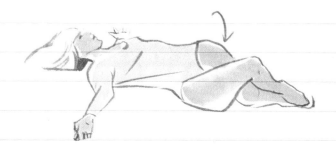

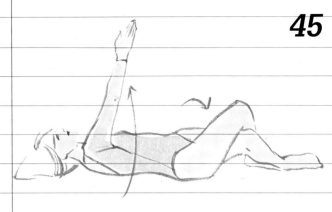

45 BACK *Now combine the last 2 exercises, letting hands and knees fall to opposite sides. Do this very gently and slowly, being aware of strong twist in spine. Do not force movement. Repeat several times. Then change way legs are crossed, let your knees fall to other side and take your arms over in opposite direction.*

Remember to keep elbows straight

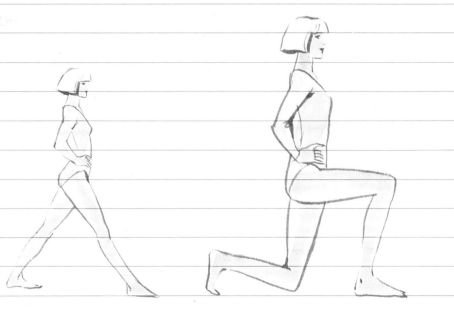

46 LEGS *Stand well with feet together. Take a large stride forwards with one foot, so that hips and feet are facing straight ahead. Do a small pelvic tilt and maintain it throughout. Breathe in. As you breathe out, bend front leg and lower back knee until it is touching (not resting on) floor. Return to starting position and repeat 7 times. Then repeat exercise with other foot in front.*

Good warm-up before running

Comfortably out of breath means stopping the exercise at a point well *before* breathlessness. You should be able to speak or to count yourself through the exercise while maintaining good technique for it to continue to have aerobic benefits. Once you start panting and gasping for air, the exercise has ceased to be aerobic and is no longer beneficial.

47 RUN *Running on the spot can be an excellent aerobic exercise but it needs a gradual build-up. Start simply by transferring weight from foot to foot, lifting heels only. Continue by lifting and stretching each foot. Then start to jump lightly from foot to foot so you are 'jogging' with feet about 10 cm (4 ins) off floor. Make sure you use whole of foot as you run – not just the balls. Gradually lift legs higher and continue until comfortably out of breath. Work down in same way afterwards to allow heart rate to slow.*

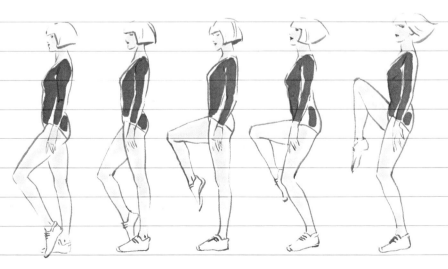

See also notes on running, page 218

WEEK 5: TWISTS

Maintaining mobility in the spine is your key to a strong healthy back. The stiffness that leads to back problems in later life is often caused by loss of mobility: 'If you don't move it,' the saying goes, 'you lose it'.

Vertebrae are actually designed to move and it's through rotating and twisting exercises that move the spine laterally, as well as forwards and back, that they are kept supple. But twists must be done correctly for best benefit. Remembering your good posture, always lengthen well first so that each vertebra has room to move and is not compressed on top of the other.

To begin with, you may find that you don't feel much of a twist at all – the vertebrae may feel locked and the whole spine stiff. But persevere and you will find that you can go round a little further each time. Your spine will soon become more supple with practice.

This week's programme
Preliminaries
32 × several
STRETCHES (fill in exercises on lines provided)
....
....
48 × 3
49 × several
46 × 8 each leg
AEROBICS until comfortably out of breath
....
ABDOMEN STRENGTHENERS until muscles begin to tire
....
....
51 × 1 each side
BACK STRENGTHENER
....
43, 44, 45 × several
39, or with one leg bent **38**, × 1
52 × several
WARM-DOWN/ RELAXATION

Sense which ways of moving work best for you and make the most of this information by creating your own exercise routine. This week's basic structure ensures you work out in a sensible order (*see note*); the rest is up to you. Fill in with exercises from previous week that you found helpful, changing the routine each time.

NB When exercising it's not just what you do that's important, it's the order in which you do it. Warm up first with general stretches; follow with twists and looseners; aerobics to get heart and lungs going; then strengtheners and more advanced stretches, finishing with at least 10 minutes relaxation...

48 CHEST *Stand well with pelvis centered, feet hip-width apart. Take a light broom or broomstick and hold it so your hands are about 1.2 m (4 ft) apart. Breathe in. As you breathe out, lift stick up, back and down as far behind you as you can. Breathe in. Breathe out and reverse process. If you find this very easy, bring hands further in until you can feel a good stretch across front and a contraction, or squeezing, in upper back. If it's very hard, take hands a little further out. Practise 3 times.*

mark off where hands are on stick and bring them in as shoulders become more supple

149

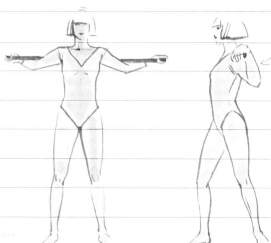
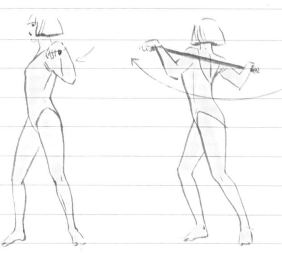

49 WAIST AND BACK

Place stick across shoulders as shown. Stand with legs hip-width apart, feet parallel and knees bent over toes. Check pelvis is centered. Breathe in. As you breathe out, twist to one side turning head and eyes too. Breathe in as you return to centre. Breathe out as you twist to other side. Repeat several times in a good slow rhythm, spotting something behind you each time to prevent dizziness.

keep hips facing forward as much as possible for maximum twist in back

BONUS Stick helps you twist further because when shoulders are kept still, ribs are lifted and back is lengthened.

How many repetitions are right for you? Bear in mind it's not just practice, but *perfect* practice, that makes perfect. Once you get tired or sloppy, you start practising your own mistakes – so reinforcing them. Stop at the point where you *begin* to feel too tired to do the exercise correctly.

Did you find last week's way of working beneficial? Has it helped with your stretches, made you feel looser, more 'at home' in your body? If so, always include some Feldenkrais work when you exercise...

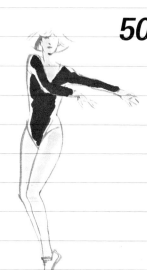

50 JUMPS

Prepare for this by standing with feet hip-width apart. Bend knees as you take arms over to one side, then straighten legs and lift heels from floor as you raise arms up to ceiling. Bend knees again and take arms to opposite side. Repeat 8 times, then start jumping lightly with both feet together, twisting body from side to side. Let arms swing freely in opposite direction. Continue until comfortably out of breath.

51 WAIST

Sitting cross-legged on floor, feel two 'sitting' bones beneath you as you lengthen spine upwards and drop shoulders down. Place one hand across body onto opposite knee and take free hand onto floor behind. Breathe in and push down onto hand to lengthen spine a little more. Breathe out as you twist, pulling gently further round as you are able. Repeat to other side. Cross legs other (non-habitual) way and repeat.

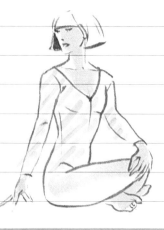

52 BACK

Lie on back with legs bent up, arms out at shoulder level and palms flat on the floor. Keeping knees together, take legs to one side and head to other. Keep shoulder blades on floor throughout. Repeat several times in an easy rhythm.

BONUS Excellent tension releaser

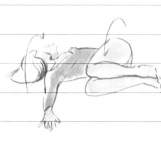

Are you becoming aware of some of the benefits of regular exercise? Do you feel stronger, supple, more self-aware and in tune with your body? Are you beginning to understand its needs?

Although you should feel well-used after exercising, you should not feel exhausted – rather alert, refreshed and ready for more. If you are not yet finding this, a good massage can often help because it gives that sensation of feeling calm yet energized at the same time...

WEEK 6: RELAXATION

It may seem odd to include a week on relaxation in a programme about movement, but the ability to relax is one of the most important elements of fitness. It is no use being strong and agile if you cannot relax because it is the balance between the two that produces real health.

Tension is tiring and wasteful – the inner result of outer pressures and problems that are often beyond your control. Help must therefore be sought from within. Finding inner resources that you can use to release muscular tension and to calm the mind is what learning to relax is about. For, although we all have these resources, we need to be taught how to apply them.

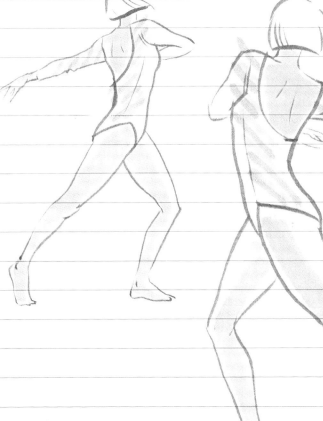
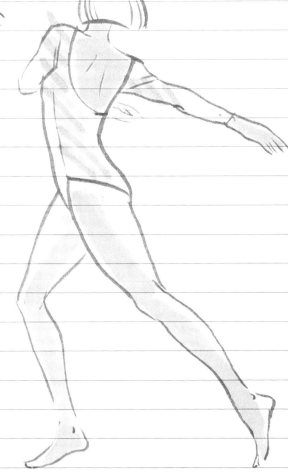

This week's programme
Preliminaries
32 × several
3 × several
53 × several
34 × 8 each side
46 × 8 each leg
47 until comfortably out of breath
54 until comfortably out of breath
Active recovery cool-down see page 161
37 × 6
26 until muscles begin to tire
24 × 1
28 until muscles begin to tire
52 × several
55 × several
44 × 40 each side
39, or with one leg bent **38**, × 1
56 × 1
57 × 3 mins each foot
56 × 1
58

53 WARM-UP A
progression on last week's exercise with the broomstick. Stand with arms at shoulder level and swing around bending knee and lifting heel as you go. Focus on something on a wall behind to help prevent dizziness. Repeat to other side and continue twisting from side to side in a good easy rhythm until you feel really warmed up.

Tension exhausts mind as well as body. A brain buzzing with problems and preoccupations soon loses its creativity – its ability to find new solutions and to come up with fresh ideas. Freedom from anxiety requires a greater mental freedom and that can only happen when the mind is calm.

There are many different routes to relaxation and they don't all require you to be still. In fact, activity can be one of the best. Slow progressive stretching helps release tense contracted muscles while a more vigorous work-out can promote tremendous physical and mental calm.

54 JUMP KICK

Standing with both feet together, hop onto one leg as you bring other up towards chest. Now jump both feet together again and extend same leg forwards in a kick. Repeat, alternating legs, until comfortably out of breath.

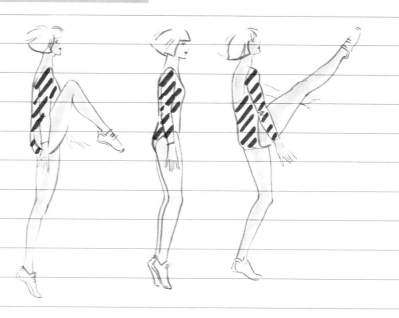

55 ABDOMEN *Lying on back with knees bent and feet flat on floor, breathe in. As you breathe out, push back of waist firmly into floor so pubic bone rises upwards. Pull tummy in at same time. Breathe in and release. Repeat several times.*

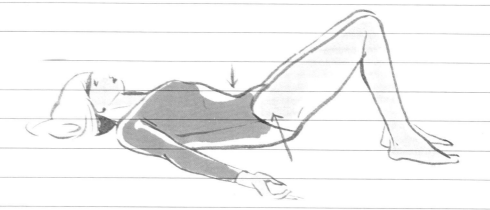

56 ROLL *Stand with feet hip-width apart and weight of body evenly distributed between them. Centre pelvis. Now lower head very slowly, tucking chin in. Continue lowering head towards floor and let shoulders drop forwards too, so arms are hanging heavily down. Bend knees as you go on curling VERY SLOWLY towards floor. Breathe well several times, then curl up again, equally slowly, keeping knees bent. Feel pelvis centering itself as you return equally slowly to upright position and straighten legs.*

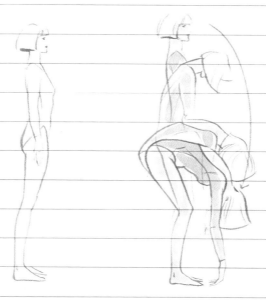

As you go down note tension points - places that feel difficult or stiff and interrupt flow of movement

57 FEET

Take a small firm ball – a squash ball is ideal – and place it beneath right foot. Roll it gently around in small circles, putting weight on foot. Imagine ball is covered with ink and you want to cover entire underside of foot – heel, sole, inner and outer edges, underneath toes. Continue for at least 3 minutes, closing eyes and enjoying massage.

Now look at yourself carefully in a mirror. Is there a difference between the two sides of your body? Does right side feel more relaxed? Is right shoulder lower than left? If so, it is because massage has eased muscles on right side of body. Repeat massage with other foot and see if, afterwards, both shoulders are level. Then repeat previous exercise and see if those areas of tightness have disappeared...

Feet must be bare for this one

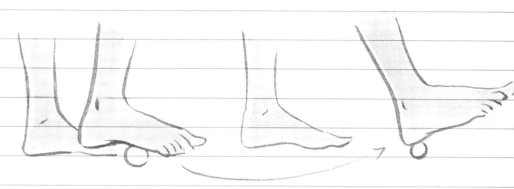

58 RELAXATION

Lie flat on back on floor. Press on elbows and back of head to raise chest a little, then pull shoulders away from ears. Lower chest again, spreading shoulder blades outwards and dropping chin slightly, so that back of neck is lengthened. Place one hand lightly on chest and other on abdomen and let them rest there. Rotate thighs outwards and wiggle knees until comfortable. This is your starting position.

Now roll head from side to side to make sure any tension in neck is released. Press head down into floor and stop. Pull shoulders down away from body once more and stop. Tilt pelvis, pressing back of waist into floor, and stop. Push heels away from you, lengthening backs of legs, and stop. Take a good deep breath, feeling lower hand rise as air is drawn deep into lungs. As you breathe out, release into floor and feel lower hand falling as air leaves lungs, but don't let your chest collapse. Run through your body checking for areas of tension. Are your jaws clenched? Are you frowning? Have shoulders crept up again? Is breathing still easy? Be aware of your body as you do this, then let go of everything, close eyes and relax, feeling breathing becoming shallower and shallower as you enter a state of deep relaxation.

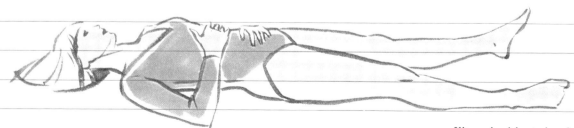

Ask someone to read this through as you do it

If lower back hurts, bend knees so feet are flat on floor, press lower back into floor until pain subsides, then slowly slide legs down again.

WEEK 7: STRENGTH

Building up strength may sound strenuous and difficult, but as soon as you begin you will discover that strength is about finding things easy. You will not feel so stiff after exercise; you will not get out of breath so soon; you will be able to manage everyday stresses and strains better and your posture and general shape will improve as your muscles become firmer and more toned. You should feel better too because while you are building up strength you will be giving your heart and lungs the boost they probably need.

As you work through your programme this week, be aware of what strengthening is all about. Sense your muscles tightening and contracting strongly as you exercise. Feel the warm tension and work them to the point where they begin to tire, but never continue until it becomes painful.

59 | **CALVES** *Start on all-fours, with legs fully extended and heels on ground. Now flex one knee and take weight onto other leg, pressing heel down into floor. Can you feel the stretch? Alternate from leg to leg in a nice steady rhythm 16 times.*

Excellent warm up for running as it stretches whole of back of leg

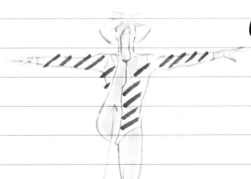

60 | **KICKS** *Start jumping up and down lightly on both feet for 4 counts. Now bend one leg slightly as you kick other out to front, then down, then to side, then down, then to front again, then down, then to side again (8 counts). Go back to jumping lightly with both feet together for 4 counts and repeat with other leg. Continue until comfortably out of breath.*

Aerobic exercises are strengtheners because they work the heart which is a muscle too and needs exercise just like any other muscle in the body ...

This week's programme

Preliminaries
32 × several
3 × several
53 × several
34 × 8 each side
59 × 16
47 until comfortably out of breath
Active recovery cool down, see page 161
54 × several
60 until comfortably out of breath
Active recovery cool-down, see page 161
37 × 6
61 until muscles begin to tire
24 × 1
62 × 3
28, trying to bring head and shoulders off floor until muscles begin to tire
52 × several
63 × 4 each side
64 × several
65 × several
66 × up to 6 each leg
44 × several
67 × up to 5
68 × 1
58

61 UPPER BODY

A progression on the wall press-ups... Using a table makes exercise stronger because you lift more of body up against gravity. Do 4 press-ups, keeping back long and straight. Rest a moment, and repeat. How do you feel? Stop now if muscles feel well used; continue if you feel you can take more and stop when muscles begin to tire*.

*Note down how many sets of 4 you can do comfortably, without straining or dipping in back, for reference later...

make sure table is firm and will not slip

A folded blanket beneath the heels gives them something to press against — makes for more of a stretch

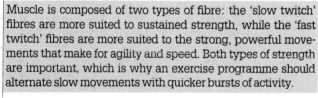

Muscle is composed of two types of fibre: the 'slow twitch' fibres are more suited to sustained strength, while the 'fast twitch' fibres are more suited to the strong, powerful movements that make for agility and speed. Both types of strength are important, which is why an exercise programme should alternate slow movements with quicker bursts of activity.

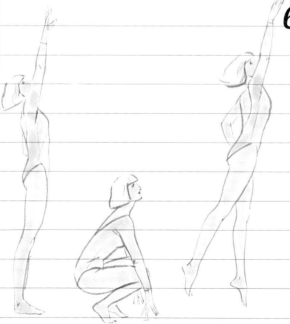

62 SQUAT JUMP

Stand by a wall, reach up with one hand and mark where you touch. Now crouch down and spring up to touch as high as possible above. Ask a friend to mark the spot. Try it 3 times, then take the best and measure distance between it and original mark.

The ability to push body weight up against gravity in one burst of energy is determined by fast-twitch muscle fibre.

Although height and weight should be taken into account for strictest accuracy, a measurement over 40 cm (16 ins) indicates you are likely to have a higher proportion of fast-twitch fibre...

The ratio of slow to fast-twitch muscle fibre does not change though it varies from individual to individual, determining which types of sport people are most suited. More slow-twitch fibres makes the endurance athlete, such as the marathon runner, while more fast-twitch fibres makes the more powerful shorter-distance athlete, such as the sprinter or the hurdler.

Find out which you are closest to with the squat jump test (exercise 62).

63 ABDOMEN *Lie on back with legs bent and feet flat on floor, arms about 30 cm (12 ins) away from body at sides. Breathe in. As you breathe out, take one hand across body to meet the other. Return to starting position and repeat to other side. Practise 4 times.*

Excellent for tightening tummy

For extra strength, try making a noise as you breathe out. Some exercise physiologists maintain that this makes you 5 to 10 per cent stronger than staying silent...

Most of these strengtheners work on the front of the torso and not on the back because back muscles are almost invariably too tight and abdominal muscles too loose – penalties of poor posture and sedentary living. Concentrating on strengthening the front will tighten the tummy and help you gain greater length in the back, so improving your posture.

64 INNER THIGHS *Lie as before, with large cushion or pillow between knees. Breathe in. As you breathe out, do a pelvic tilt and press knees firmly together. Breathe in and release. Breathe out and repeat. Continue several times and finish by holding pelvic tilt, breathing normally and squeezing legs together several times quickly.*

'The more feeble the body is, the more it commands; the stronger it is, the more it obeys...' Jean-Jacques Rousseau

65 OUTER THIGHS *Lie on side with legs stretched out, making sure body and legs are perfectly in line. Raise leg, keeping foot flexed and knee facing forwards. Do not aim for great height as this will mean turning leg out from hips and will defeat object of exercise. Lower leg half-way down and raise again. Continue until muscles begin to tire. Then lower leg and lift both legs off floor with feet together*. Take them as high as you can (at first this might only be an inch or two) and release. Turn over and repeat whole exercise with other leg.*

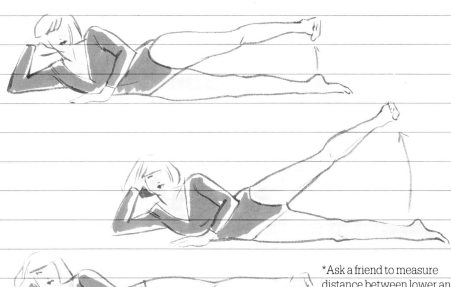

BONUS
tightens side of abdomen as well as outer thigh

*Ask a friend to measure distance between lower ankle and floor on each side and note it down for reference later...

66 BACKS OF THIGHS AND BUTTOCKS

Lie on front with pelvis supported by a cushion and forehead resting on hands in front of you. Take legs hip-width apart and bend them. Slowly lift them alternately up to 6 times each.

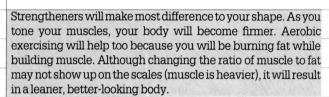

Strengtheners will make most difference to your shape. As you tone your muscles, your body will become firmer. Aerobic exercising will help too because you will be burning fat while building muscle. Although changing the ratio of muscle to fat may not show up on the scales (muscle is heavier), it will result in a leaner, better-looking body.

The most effective strengtheners ask muscles to shorten against gravity because they then have to work hard to support the weight of the body. Good examples: curl-ups, press-ups and this week's new front of thighs exercise (67).

67 FRONT OF THIGHS

Kneel with legs hip-width apart and arms out straight in front at shoulder level. Breathe in. As you breathe out, do a pelvic tilt and lean back until you can feel thighs working strongly to maintain position. Breathe in and come up. Practise up to 8 times

Muscles become sore and stiff through a build-up of metabolites – by-products of muscle contraction. These are carried away from the muscle by tiny blood capillaries. If a muscle is contracted for a long time, the capillaries are constricted, the blood cannot move freely and metabolites build up. After a while, the muscle will not be able to contract properly and the whole body may feel weak and stiff. Help prevent this by holding each position no longer than is comfortable and by warming down well after exercise…

Excellent strengthener as entire weight of body is supported by muscles working at front of thigh.

68 THIGHS

Still kneeling, bring knees together and take feet apart. Sit down between feet, if you can, and place one hand under each foot. Do a pelvic tilt and go back onto elbows, one at a time. Slowly lower head back. If you feel you can go further, slide arms out sideways and lower body onto floor, still maintaining pelvic tilt. You should feel no pain or squeezing in your lower back as you do this. Eventually this position becomes very relaxing.

If it's painful to sit between feet, sit on a cushion and let stretch come in that position; don't continue any further and relax as last week.

WEEK 8: AEROBICS

It is the mixture that makes exercise effective – activity with stillness, strength with suppleness, effort with easy movement...

Aerobics, a craze which has already collected more than its fair share of casualties, can defeat rather than enhance total fitness if carried out to the exclusion of everything else. As a part (an important part) but not the all, aerobics is great for working heart and lungs and enjoyable with it, provided that you build up gradually, as here.

All aerobic movements learned so far are now combined to make one continuous 4-minute sequence. Extending overall aerobic exercising time is important because it is the steady, sustained type of activity that produces the best benefits for heart and health.

This week's programme

Preliminaries
32 × several
69 × several
53 × several
34 × 8 each side
59 × 16
70
71
Active recovery
   cool-down, see page 161
37 × 6
61 until muscles begin to
   tire
28 until muscles begin to
   tire
52 × several
63 × several
64 × several
65 × several
66 × up to 6 each leg
44 × several
39, or with one leg bent
   38, × 1
30 × several
58

Aerobics literally means 'with air'. If you cannot sustain an activity for more than a minute or so – sprinting, swimming flat out and running upstairs are all good examples – the exercise is anaerobic because the demand outstrips the supply and builds up an 'oxygen debt' which leaves you breathless and gasping for air.

While aerobic exercise is steadier than anaerobic exercise and can be sustained comfortably for a reasonable time, it must also be vigorous enough to raise heart beat sufficiently to give a training effect. To begin with very gentle levels of activity, such as brisk walking, may do this but, as you get fitter, you will need to step up the pace.

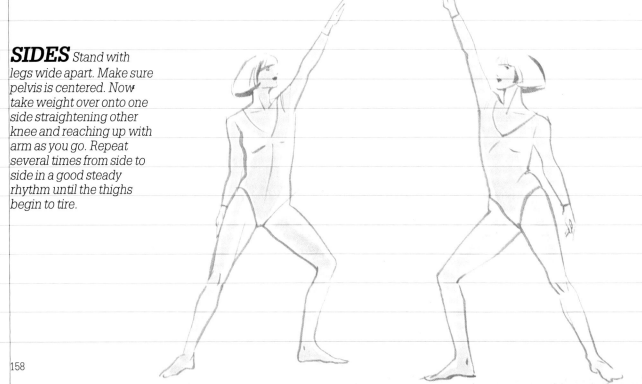

69 **SIDES** *Stand with legs wide apart. Make sure pelvis is centered. Now take weight over onto one side straightening other knee and reaching up with arm as you go. Repeat several times from side to side in a good steady rhythm until the thighs begin to tire.*

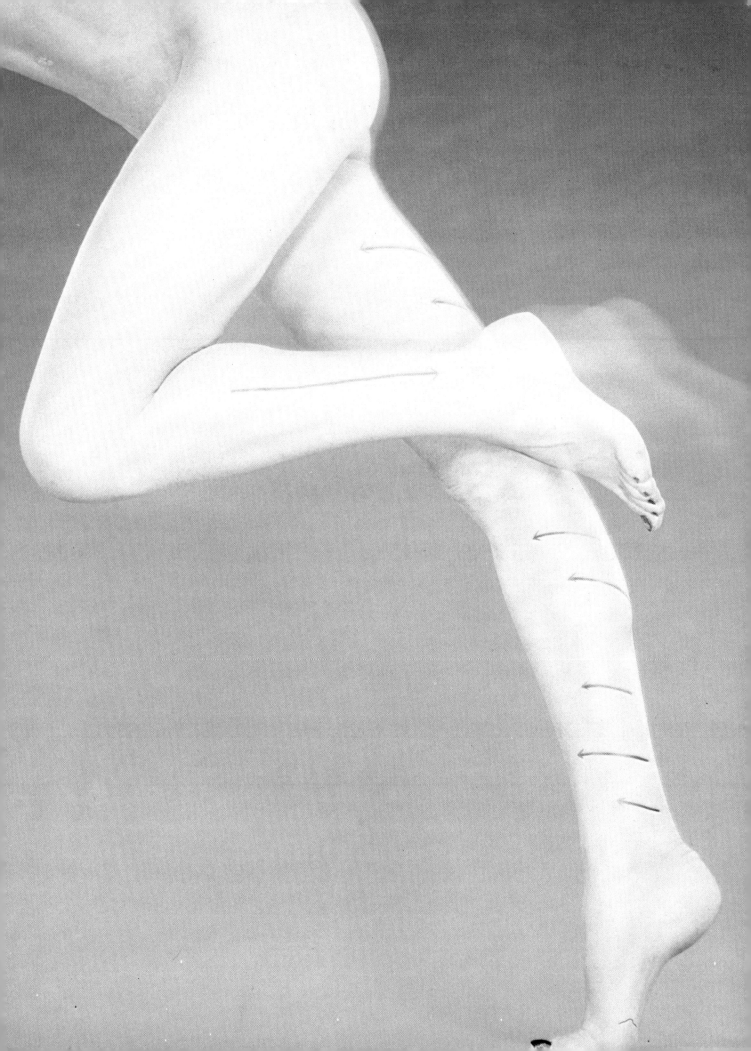

70 PULSE *Set aside one day each week and take pulse 3 times: before you start exercising, at the height of activity (just before you start cooling down) and again 10 minutes later.*

To take your pulse: locate it on the thumb side at the base of your left wrist. Curl your fingers – not your thumb – on the pulse and, using a stop watch or second hand on an ordinary watch, count for 20 seconds. Multiply by 3 for a minute's count.

Determine your maximum heart rate by taking your age from 220 (heart beats per minute). Aim to increase your fitness by sending your pulse rate up to between 70 and 85 per cent of maximum.

When you exercise aerobically, the lungs take in more air and the heart beats faster to send more oxygenated blood to the muscles for energy. With regular aerobic exercise, the heart actually becomes more efficient and sends more blood with each beat, so it does not need to beat as fast. This training effect can be monitored very easily by taking your pulse regularly, as indicated *left*.

See how much fitter you are getting by noticing a drop in your resting pulse rate (it may be as much as 10 beats or even more); by finding how much harder you have to work to get your exercise pulse up to target (your body's way of telling you your heart muscle is getting stronger and your cardiovascular endurance is improving); and by noticing how much closer your third reading (exercise 70) is to normal each time.

Gauge how much exercise is right for you by taking your pulse

If you take longer than 10 minutes to reduce pulse to normal, you have exercised too hard . . .

71 SEQUENCE *Start by running on the spot, padding from foot to foot and gradually getting higher (1 minute). Then reverse movement, so you are bringing feet back instead of forwards (30 seconds). Now combine them, running forwards for 8 steps and back for 8; repeat 4 times (1 minute). Regain your breath a bit* with side lunges (30 seconds) and then go into side kicks (15 seconds), jump kicks with straight leg (15 seconds), star jumps (15 seconds) and twist jumps (15 seconds). If at any stage you feel out of breath, slow down and return to the quiet padding before you start building up the intensity again.

Good quality training shoes are useful because they provide good support, help prevent jarring. They should be well cushioned with at least 1.5 cm (¾ in) under the heel and 1 cm (½ in) under the sole. Once feet and legs get stronger, you may find you don't need them – but you must have a good sprung surface if working barefoot.

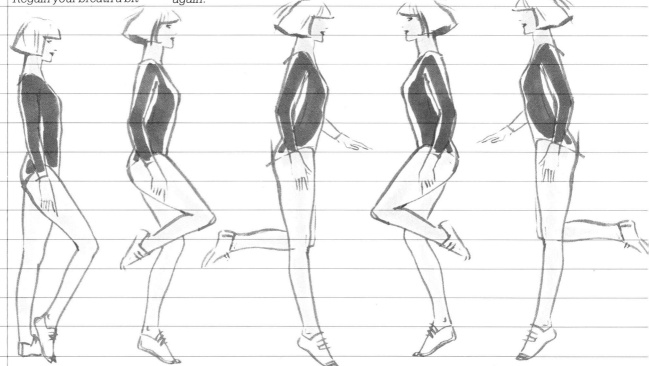

If breasts feel uncomfortable, wear a good supporting bra to help prevent ligaments from stretching and breasts from sagging. If you have any problems with breast lumps, check with your doctor before starting.

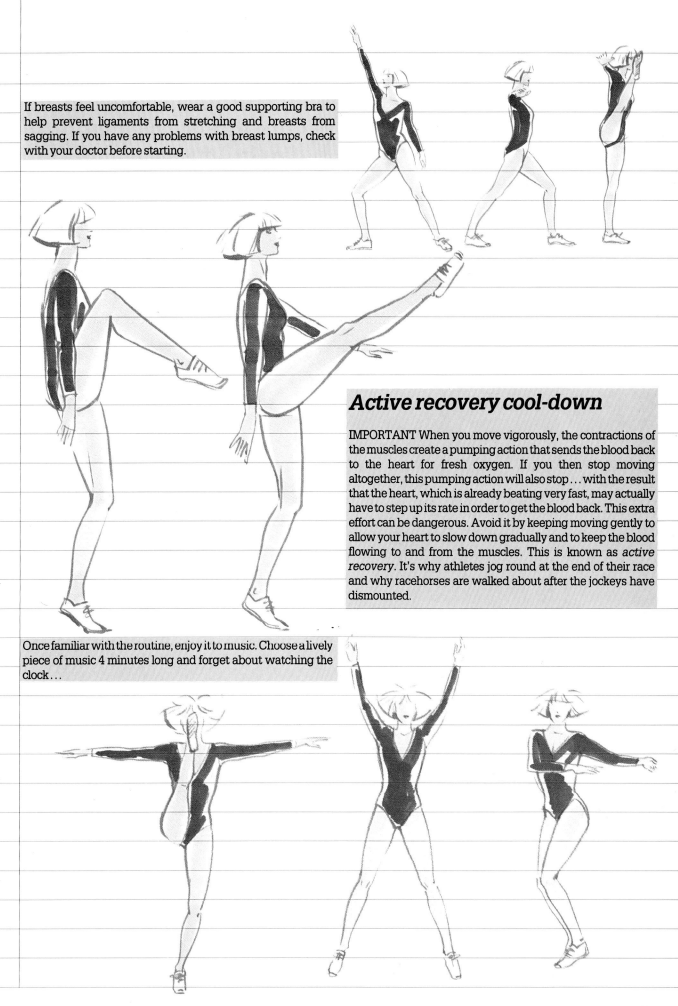

Active recovery cool-down

IMPORTANT When you move vigorously, the contractions of the muscles create a pumping action that sends the blood back to the heart for fresh oxygen. If you then stop moving altogether, this pumping action will also stop ... with the result that the heart, which is already beating very fast, may actually have to step up its rate in order to get the blood back. This extra effort can be dangerous. Avoid it by keeping moving gently to allow your heart to slow down gradually and to keep the blood flowing to and from the muscles. This is known as *active recovery*. It's why athletes jog round at the end of their race and why racehorses are walked about after the jockeys have dismounted.

Once familiar with the routine, enjoy it to music. Choose a lively piece of music 4 minutes long and forget about watching the clock ...

WEEK 9: WEIGHTS

Working with weights demands more from muscles, multiplies benefits, accelerates results…but make sure you can work with your own body weight first. Try these exercises on their own and add weights only if and when they become comfortable.

All strengthening exercises work on an *overloading* principle; to exercise a muscle effectively you must overload it by working it harder than usual. While straightforward strengtheners are fine to begin with, benefits decrease once muscles become stronger. So overload again, this time with weights.

This week's programme
Preliminaries
32 × several
69 × several
53 × several
34, bouncing a little further for 3 counts to each side, × 4 each side
72 × 6 rotations
59 × 16
71
Active recovery cool-down, see page 161
37, gently bouncing 3 times as you lower × 4
28, with arms folded in front until muscles begin to tire
52 × several
63, lifting shoulders off floor until muscles begin to tire
73 × 6 at each level
74 × 8 each leg
65, adding weights until muscles begin to tire
75 × up to 8
66, with weights and legs straight up to 8 each leg
16, leaving weights on for more swing × several
39, or with one leg bent **38**, × 1
30 × several
58

72 SHOULDERS
Strap a 0.5 kg (1 lb) weight to each wrist or improvise with food cans of an equivalent weight held in the hand. Stand with arms outstretched at chin level and rotate arms backwards 6 times.

Strap-on weights attach to wrists and ankles and can be bought from any sports shop and many department stores. Or improvise with food cans held in the hand and an old sock filled with sand tied loosely around the ankle. Start with weights of 0.5 kg (1 lb) each and work up to 1.5 kg (3 lb). That's your maximum: after that add repetitions, not weight…

73 CHEST
Lie on back with knees bent and weights strapped to wrists or held in the hand. Extend arms sideways at shoulder level. Breathe in. Breathe out as you bring weights up and cross arms over in front. Breathe in as you lower them. Practise 6 times and then repeat whole exercise at eye and waist levels in order to work every part of pectoral muscles.

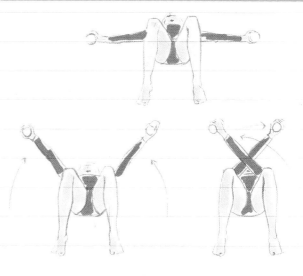

Weights can be used to build muscle strength or endurance. *Strength*, achieved by using heavy weights and few repetitions, strengthens muscle in a few specific areas and builds bulk – the type of training weightlifters do. *Endurance*, achieved by using light weights and many repetitions, tones and tightens the entire muscle and does not add bulk.

Attaching weights to wrists and ankles increases the toning effect of the exercise because greater resistance must be overcome as the arm or leg is lifted against gravity.

74 FRONT OF THIGHS

Sit on a table so that thighs are well supported up to knee, with a 0.5 kg (1 lb) weight strapped round each ankle. Breathe in. As you breathe out, slowly lift one leg up until it is completely straight. Breathe in and lower. Practise, alternating legs, 16 times.

Can be excellent for strengthening knees, particularly if weak, but consult your doctor first if you do have a problem.

If you can't extend leg fully, try exercise without weights.

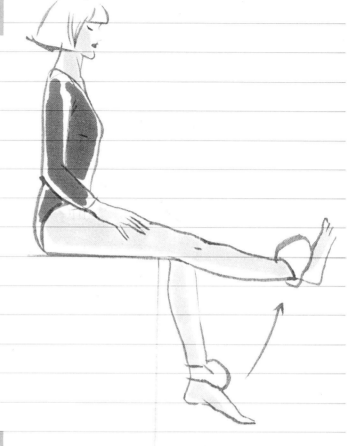

Curl-ups are one of the best tummy tighteners because the muscles have to contract from a position of maximum length as you bring your body up against gravity. Doing them this week with your arms folded in front will make the exercise stronger, as you cannot use arms to help pull you up.

Rember to use your breathing to help as you exercise

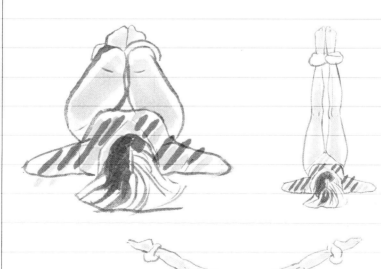

75 INNER THIGHS

Lie on back with arms outstretched and a 0.5 kg (1 lb) weight attached to each ankle. Slip hands beneath pelvis to ensure that lower back remains pressed into floor. Raise legs by bending them first into chest and then straightening them up. Take them slowly apart as wide as you can and then bring them together again equally slowly. Practise up to 6 times.

If back hurts, work at Feldenkrais mobility sequence for spine, page 242, and skip this for the moment.

WEEK 10: BALANCE

Balance, the keynote of an effective exercise programme, is also an important aspect of fitness in its own right. Do you know how good yours is?

Don't be disheartened if, having completed the tests, the answer is not very good. No-one need be stuck with a poor sense of balance. It can be improved by more attention to posture, and by relaxation techniques or meditation to help calm the mind. Practice can be helpful too. But don't confuse practice with effort. Effort, can interfere with balance by overriding subliminal messages coming from the brain and central nervous system. Stop trying so hard and you may do better.

This week's programme

Preliminaries
57 × 3 mins each foot
56 × 1
76 × several
77 × 1 each leg
69 × several
53 × several
72 × 6 rotations
24 × 1
78 × 3
59 × 16
79

Active recovery
cool-down, see page 161
37 × 4
28 until muscles begin to tire
52 × several
63 until muscles begin to tire
80 × several at each stage
73 × 6 at each level
65 × several
75 × several
39, or with one leg bent
  38, × 1
58
77 × 1 each leg

76 **BALANCE** *Stand with feet hip-width apart and shift weight from foot to foot to help you assess which side of your body is carrying most weight. Now imagine you are on a tightrope. Stand well with spine lengthened and both feet together. Lift one heel. Imagine someone is pulling that knee forwards with an invisible piece of string. Then take that foot and place it in front of the other. Transfer weight onto forward foot and immediately lift back foot and place that in front,* *again imagining someone is pulling knee forwards. Practise taking several steps along your tightrope. Note breathing and position of head. Now try walking backwards, maintaining length in back and not turning head round to see where you are going. Take several steps backwards, then stand with feet together again. Does balance feel different?*

Notice that when walking you maintain balance by having all your weight on one foot at a time. How straight is your tightrope? Try exercise again with eyes shut. Mark where you start and take same number of steps forwards and backwards. Where do you finish?

As you need to be calm and unflustered to balance well, it can be a very good barometer of your state of mind. It is sure to be affected if overtired or agitated and is often less good before a period; increased clumsiness and liability to accidents are now recognized symptoms of pre-menstrual tension. So don't be surprised if it seems easier some days than others.

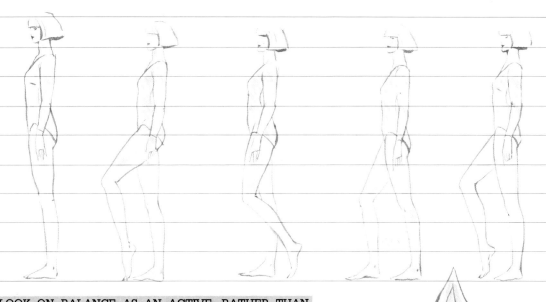

LOOK ON BALANCE AS AN ACTIVE, RATHER THAN
PASSIVE, QUALITY... However still and balanced a body
seems, it is never static. A dynamic distribution of energy in the
nerves and muscle of the body will be taking place all the time
to keep it upright, prevent it toppling over. The slightest shift in
posture and thousands of tiny adjustments will be made...

77 **BALANCE** *Stand
on one leg and lift other
foot onto inner thigh, using
hands to help you. Place it
as high as you can. Now lift
arms to ceiling and remain
in this position for as long
as you can. Can you close eyes and still keep
balance? Change sides
and repeat.*

This 'tree pose' may be easier
on one side than the other; if
so, practise weaker side more
often.

78 **LEGS** *Stand well with
feet together and arms by
side. Bring arms up to
shoulder level and then lift
heels. Slowly go down into
squat position. Can you go
right the way down, so that
bottom is resting on heels,
and up again, without
losing balance? You must
go all the way up with
heels lifted, only returning
them to ground when
completely upright. Try 3
times keeping smooth
rhythm.*

CAUTION Don't go all the way
down if knees are weak.

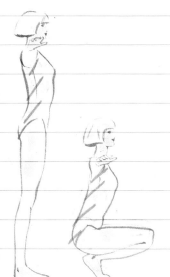

*If you can
remain in pose
with eyes closed
for 1 minute,
your balance
is good*

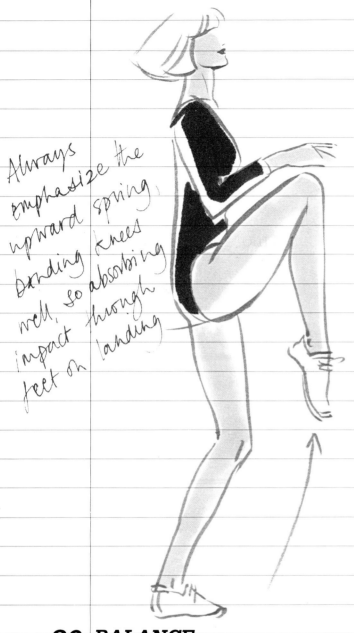

Always emphasize the upward spring, bending knees well, so absorbing impact through feet on landing

79 AEROBIC *Now try lifting knees really high as you spring from foot to foot when running on the spot. Ensure you are getting a good height by placing arms out in front, as shown, and bringing thighs up to touch. Resist temptation to bring hands down to meet them! Continue until comfortably out of breath and then wind down a little with some easy jogging and padding before continuing aerobic sequence. Extend more energetic parts of sequence by a few seconds to bring total up to 5 minutes.*

REMEMBER Balance improves with physical confidence and physical confidence improves with fitness.

80 BALANCE *Sit with knees bent and feet flat. Rock from side to side and then round in a circle so that you can feel your two 'sitting' bones. When weight is evenly balanced on both, you will know pelvis is centered. Place hands under heels and lift both legs up, with knees still bent. When you feel stable, rock gently back and forth several times.*

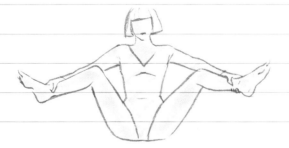

Then try this balancing trick. Breathe in and do a pelvic tilt. As you breathe out, lift arms and legs into air to make a wide V-shape. Can you maintain your balance in this position?

Practice and patience will help if you can't achieve this right away; take time on each stage so you learn to balance steadily before straightening legs.

Does balance improve after activity? Try the 'tree pose' before and after the programme and see. If balance improves, exercise is having exactly the right benefits for you, helping you to feel revitalized and calm at the same time. If balance does not improve, ask yourself whether you are rushing into the exercises – and, if so, take them more slowly.

WEEK 11: COORDINATION

Coordination, like balance, is an aspect of fitness we can all improve on. A lucky few may be blessed with exceptional coordination, but the rest of us have to learn to move our bodies well. From the infant guiding spoon to mouth to the tennis player returning a ball, the lesson is the same: coordination, like any other skill, is to be mastered with practice.

The key to doing these exercises well – and most sports too – lies as much in the mind as in the body. Keep a relaxed, non-judging attitude. Worrying about your performance will cause muscles to tense up and shorten, leading to awkward jerky movements which will interfere with your coordination and may even inhibit movement altogether. Let your body find its own rhythm and you will feel the movements becoming smoother and easier.

This week's programme

Preliminaries
77 × 1 each leg
56 × 1
42 × 1
81 × 1
69, changing rhythm every 4 lunges to bend opposite knee to outstretched arm × several
53 × several
72 × 6 rotations
24 × 1
61 until muscles begin to tire
82 × several
59 × 16
83

Active recovery cool-down, see page 161
84 × several
28 until muscles begin to tire
52 × several
85 until muscles begin to tire
86
87
65 × several
75 × up to 6
88 × 4
58

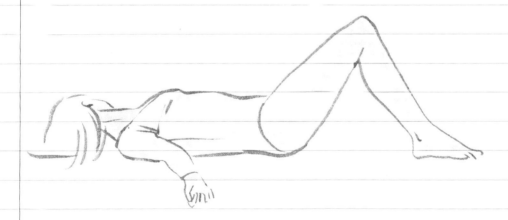

81 **HEAD AND PELVIS** *Lie on back with knees bent and feet flat on floor, as for pelvic clock. Visualize a clock on the back of your head with 12 o'clock at top, 6 o'clock where spine joins skull, 3 o'clock under left ear and 9 o'clock under right ear.*
a. *Now read instructions for pelvis on page 147 and perform them with head.*

Take time, do them thoroughly and rest often.
b. *Do you notice that your pelvis moves in conjunction with your head? Move them both together from 6 to 12 and back again several times. Now move pelvis to 6 and head to 12; pelvis to 12 and head to 6. Repeat several times and rest.*

c. *Move pelvis and head to 12 and make a complete clockwise circle with both, travelling slowly and gently around clock. Rest. Travel in an anti-clockwise direction equally slowly. Rest.*
d. *Finally, for a gentle but challenging lesson in coordination, move pelvis and head to 12 and let pelvis travel in an*

anti-clockwise direction while head travels in a clockwise direction. Do this slowly and gently. Stop and rest when you get confused and then start again. Repeat several times and then reverse the direction. Rest. Stand up and walk around. How does your pelvis feel? Your head? Your neck? Your back?

167

82 COORDINATION

Stand with arms outstretched at shoulder level and lift foot about 5 cm (2 ins) off floor. Now rotate foot as you move it out towards back in an anti-clockwise direction. Bring it in again, this time rotating it in a clockwise direction. Try it several times with each foot. Then try bringing arms forwards, rotating hands in an anti-clockwise direction, and backwards, rotating hands smoothly in a clockwise direction. Practise several times. Then put both together. Repeat several times or until you get it right.

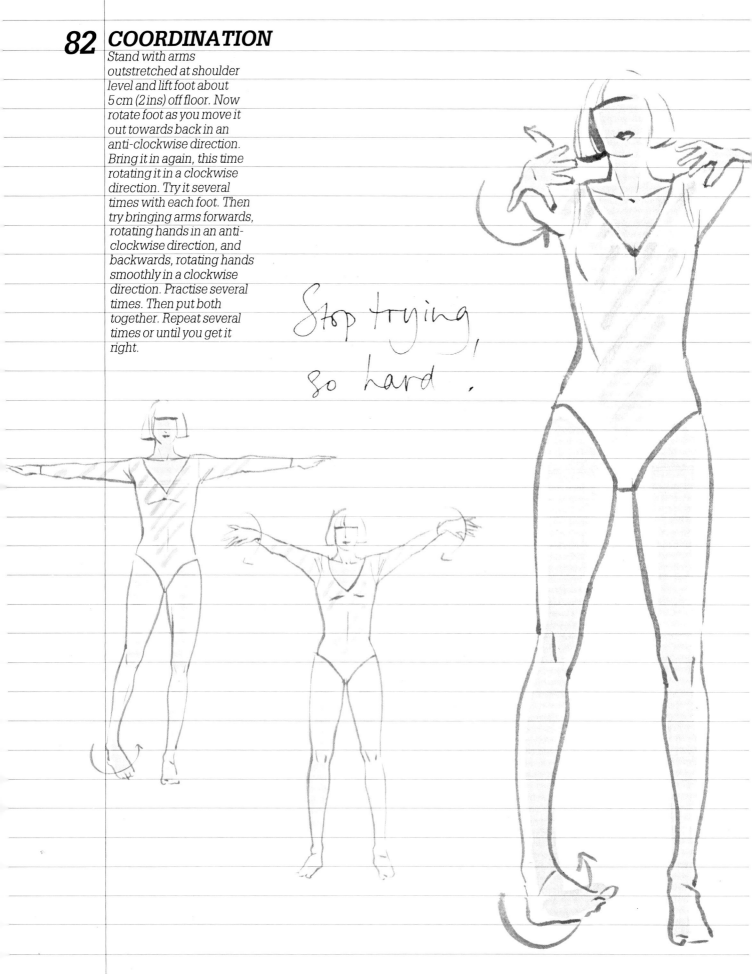

Stop trying, so hard.

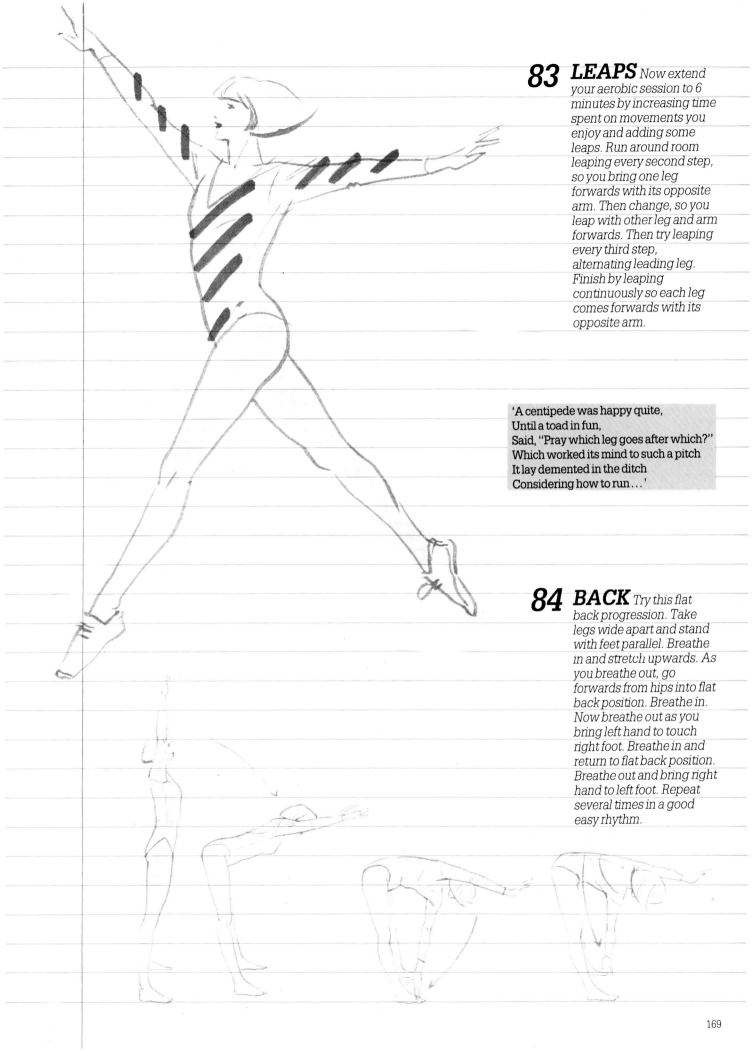

83 LEAPS Now extend your aerobic session to 6 minutes by increasing time spent on movements you enjoy and adding some leaps. Run around room leaping every second step, so you bring one leg forwards with its opposite arm. Then change, so you leap with other leg and arm forwards. Then try leaping every third step, alternating leading leg. Finish by leaping continuously so each leg comes forwards with its opposite arm.

'A centipede was happy quite,
Until a toad in fun,
Said, "Pray which leg goes after which?"
Which worked its mind to such a pitch
It lay demented in the ditch
Considering how to run...'

84 BACK Try this flat back progression. Take legs wide apart and stand with feet parallel. Breathe in and stretch upwards. As you breathe out, go forwards from hips into flat back position. Breathe in. Now breathe out as you bring left hand to touch right foot. Breathe in and return to flat back position. Breathe out and bring right hand to left foot. Repeat several times in a good easy rhythm.

169

85 ABDOMEN
Lie on back with legs bent and feet flat on floor. Clasp hands behind head. Breathe in. As you breathe out bring right knee towards left elbow, letting other leg come off floor as comfortable. Breathe in and release. Breathe out and bring left knee towards right elbow. Continue in a good rhythm until muscles feel well used.

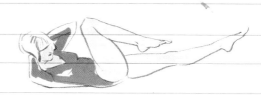

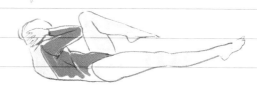

Exercise becomes harder as you take straight leg lower

86 LEGS
Lie on back. Bend one knee so foot is flat on floor. Stretch other out and raise it about 10 cm (4 ins) off floor. Beat it vigorously in air for 16 counts. Repeat with other leg.

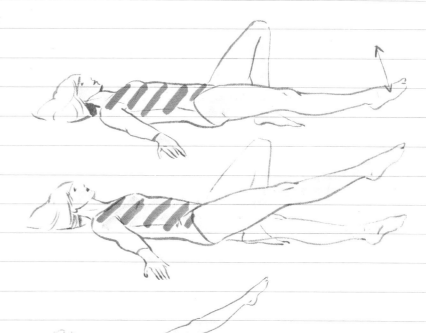

87 LEGS
Now try previous exercise again, but this time as you beat one leg bend and straighten other every 4 counts. Change legs and repeat.

88 BACK AND BUTTOCKS
Lie on front with pelvis resting on a cushion, and forehead resting on hands in front. Raise both legs bending knees and bring them out to sides, rotating feet inwards as you go. Return them to centre, rotating feet outwards. Repeat twice and then try rotating feet in opposite directions as you bring legs out and in again.

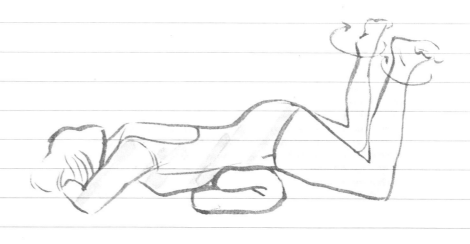

Because coordination is a function of brain as well as body, mental relaxation techniques can often help. If you find these exercises difficult, try them again after the relaxation and see if you improve...

WEEK 12: HALF-TERM EXAMS

Half-way through, and time to see how well you are doing. Although competition plays no part in getting fit, a sense of progress and achievement does. So run through these tests to see how much you have improved and to gain fresh incentive for the next 12 weeks.

Some benefits should be clear already. How do you feel compared to when you started? If the answer is stronger and fitter, more energetic and less tired, more in tune with your body and its needs – then you pass with honours because that is what exercising is all about.

These tests assess the specific aspects of fitness that add up to true health – posture, flexibility, strength, balance, stamina, the ability to relax…Excelling in just some of them is not enough, you must be up to scratch on every one before you can consider yourself in really good shape.

This week's programme
Preliminaries
32 × several
69 × several
53 × several
34 × 8 each side
89 × 1 each side
59 × 16
83, with pulse test (70, see note)
Active recovery cool-down, see page 161
84 × several
90 × 1
91
92
52 × several
85 until muscles begin to tire
65, with progress test **93**, × several
75 × up to 6
94 × 1
95 × 1
96 × 1
97 × 1
44 × several
58
98 × 1 min

Examine yourself on one day only this week and use the others to run through the basic programme, concentrating on weak areas…

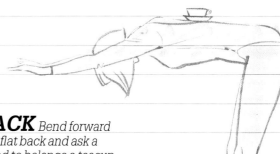

89 SIDES *Put palm of hand against a wall at shoulder level and, standing sideways, try to stretch other hand over head to touch, without twisting at waist. Repeat to other side.*

You should find this easy; if not, practise until you do.

90 BACK *Bend forward into flat back and ask a friend to balance a teacup and saucer there. The teacup should be full and you should be able to hold it absolutely still without slopping…*

Jon should find this easy – if not practise until you do

These exams differ from the academic type in 3 ways. First you are the only person taking part; second there is no examiner – you should *know* if you have made the grade; and, third, there are no prizes – simply greater confidence and well-being.

91 UPPER BODY

Do table press-ups in sets of 4, with a small rest in between, and continue until muscles begin to tire. How many sets of 4 can you do maintaining perfect technique – i.e. without straining or dipping in the back? Turn back to week 7 (exercise 61) and check your progress.

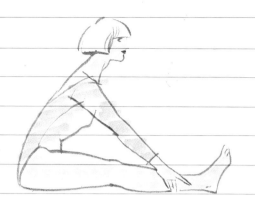

92 ABDOMEN

How many curl-ups can you do comfortably with arms folded in front? Turn back to week 2 (exercise 28) and check progress by seeing how well you did on the preliminary stage of this exercise. If you can do as many or more of this more demanding progression, you are doing very well.

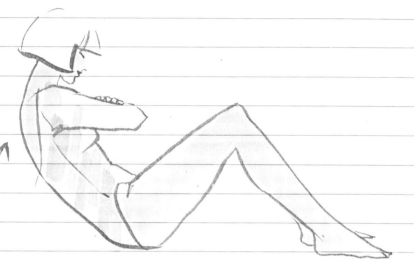

93 OUTER THIGHS

Lie on side, supported by elbow, and take both legs up in air as high as you can. When you feel quite stable, ask a friend to measure the distance between lower ankle and floor on both sides and then turn back to week 7 (exercise 65) and check your progress.

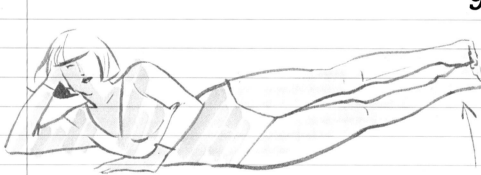

94 BALANCE

Can you now manage to do the V-trick with both legs fully extended? If not, practise until you can.

CAUTION Not for weak backs

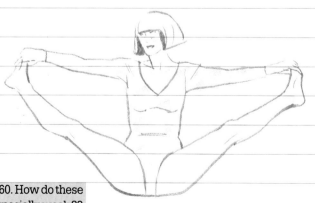

Take your pulse 3 times as directed on page 160. How do these readings differ from the previous 4 weeks – especially week 8? If both resting and post-exercise pulse have dropped by several beats, you are doing well . . .

95 **BACK** *Sit with bottom against a wall and soles of feet together as close to you as possible. Place hands on ankles and lengthen spine upwards as much as possible. Pull thighs downwards and ask a friend to measure distance between knees and floor. Now turn back to week 1 (exercise 14) and see how you have progressed. Come away from wall and repeat test with back unsupported and take another measurement. If this is less than your original, and your back is quite straight, you are doing very well indeed . . .*

If you can't get knees below waist level, practise hip loosening exercises in Therapeutics section, page 243 until you can.

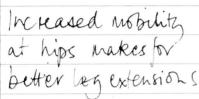

Increased mobility at hips makes for better leg extensions

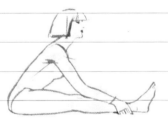

96 **BACK** *Sitting on floor, take legs apart until you feel a good stretch in inner thighs. Lengthen back well and, if you cannot maintain position with spine lengthened, bring legs in until you can. Ask a friend to measure distance between feet and then turn back to week 1 (exercise 15) to check your progress.*

Exercises 95, 96, 97 test for mobility in the hips as much as for strength, and length, in the back: lengthening the spine allows the hip joint to rotate outwards more easily (95), giving better leg extensions (96) and enabling the back to bend further from the hips (97).

97 **BACK** *Turn back to week 3 (exercise 39) and look at the dotted line you made on the diagram. Now sit sideways on to a mirror with feet out in front as before. Lengthen well up spine as you breathe in and, as you breathe out, bend forwards from hips keeping back quite straight. Can you go further than before?*

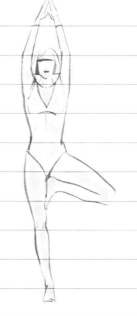

98 **BALANCE** *Has your balance improved over the last 2 weeks? Try the 'tree pose' (exercise 77) with eyes closed and ask a friend to time you. If you can maintain position without wobbling or opening eyes for a full minute you are doing very well.*

WEEK 13: SHAPERS I

If you know what your weak points are, and why you have them, you are already half-way towards a more evenly proportioned body. The next two weeks' exercises can take you the other half of the way by showing how you can help overcome them.

The length and basic shape of the legs, the width of the shoulders, waist and hips and the size of the breasts are all genetically determined. Although these basic proportions cannot be changed, you can do a tremendous amount to make your body the firmest and best-looking possible of its type.

It is not just any old exercise that firms and tightens, *it is the right type*. Flab, the bit that dieting leaves behind, can spoil the line of the slimmest body. Because it collects in areas of the body that are not frequently used, such as the underside of the upper arm and innerside of the thigh, you will need some well-chosen exercises *in addition* to a balanced diet and an active lifestyle in order to keep in shape. Now to work...

This week's programme
Preliminaries
32 × several
69 × several
53 × several
34 × 8 each side
99 × several
100 × 8
59 × 16
83
Active recovery cool-down, see page 161
84 × several
101 × up to 8
102 × 4
51 × 1 each side
103 × 4
52 × several
85 until muscles begin to tire
73 × 6 at each level
64 × several
66 × up to 8 each leg
39 × 1
68 × 1

Place thumbs just below base of skull to feel neck muscles tighten

This week, start with some healthy self-appraisal. Areas that can be improved upon will determine where you need to get to work. Do the relevant exercises 3 to 5 times a week throughout the rest of the programme, and you will soon see an improvement. Expect to notice real differences after 12 weeks...

99 | **CHIN** *Clasp hands at back of head, as shown, and press head back while pulling forwards with hands at same time. Repeat several times.*

Think back to front for double chins: jawline is kept trim by muscles at the back, not the front, of the neck.

100 UPPER ARMS

Stand in flat back position, with feet hip-width apart and knees bent. Bend arms forwards so that upper arms are parallel to floor and elbow is at a right angle. Breathe in. As you breathe out, straighten arms backwards fully extending elbows. Breathe in and return to starting position. Practise 8 times, keeping movement controlled – don't just fling arms back.

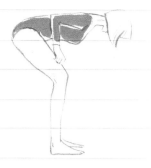 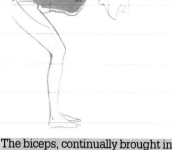

When exercise is comfortable use weights and gradually build repetitions.

The biceps, continually brought into action by any movement that brings hands towards shoulders, such as lifting, are always firm; but the triceps which lie on the underside of the upper arm are often a problem, being brought into action only when the arm extends backwards. This movement can become an effective tightening exercise when weights are used (100). Other helpful exercises: 73 and 91.

101 UPPER BODY

Kneel on all-fours and walk hands forwards until your back makes a nice straight line all the way from back of knees to back of head. Breathe in. As you breathe out, bend elbows and lower body to floor, keeping back straight. (It is useful to do this sideways on to a mirror to begin with to check back is flat and not sagging in middle.) Breathe in and raise up again. Practise up to 8 times in a good steady rhythm.

Firms arms, chest and upper back – areas most women don't exercise enough.

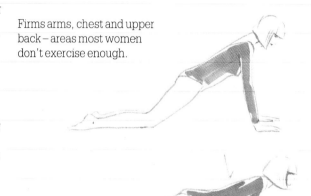

Do not rest body on floor between press-ups

Chest exercises won't increase breast size or firm up breasts that have already sagged because the breast is not a muscle; but they can do much to keep breasts firm and lifted by working the underlying supporting muscles. Helpful exercises: 7, 73, 101, 102.

102 SIDES

This excellent exercise works the latissimus dorsi muscles at side and helps counteract flabbiness around bra strap area – a very common problem. You will need a strong partner and a broom handle. Kneel on floor and hold broom handle with hands well apart and arms fully extended above head. Ask partner to stand behind you with his hands on centre of handle. Breathe in. As you breathe out, gradually pull handle down as he resists. The whole movement should take about 10 seconds and handle should be pulled down until it touches back of neck. Practise 4 times.

Experiment a little to establish how much resistance partner should apply.

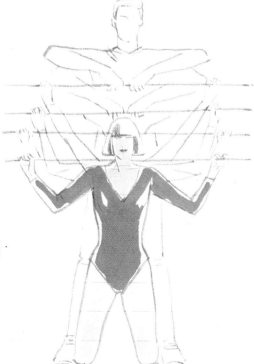

103 ABDOMEN

Lie on back with legs bent and arms at sides. Breathe in. As you breathe out, lift head off floor, pulling forwards with hands. Breathe in and return to floor. Breathe out and lift head and shoulders off floor. Breathe in and return. Breathe out and lift head, shoulders and ribcage off floor. Breathe in and return. Breathe out and come all the way up to a sitting position. Now curl all the way down to floor again, in stages as before, breathing out as you curl down, in as you come up . . . Practise 4 times, remembering your breathing.

Thick waists are slimmed by bending and twisting movements. Helpful exercises: 34 and 51. Do several each time you exercise.

Weight training machines, such as those used by the Nautilus system*, can be great for conditioning under-used areas because they isolate specific muscle groups. If there is a Nautilus gym in your area, twice-weekly workouts would make an excellent supplement to these exercises.
*Now widely available in gyms in the UK and US.

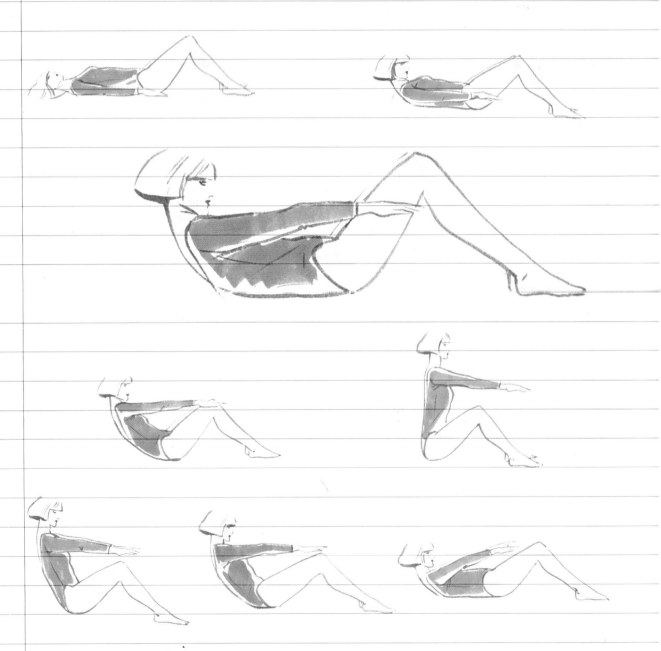

Work towards doing
this with arms
folded in front

The abdomen is wrapped in muscles which run vertically, horizontally and diagonally like the lines on the Union Jack. These soon become slack and weak through lack of use. Make the most of this natural built-in girdle by working each set of muscles (exercises 103, 65 and 85 respectively).

WEEK 14: SHAPERS II

The shaping-up theme continues. Attention, this week, on buttocks, hips and thighs. Remember to incorporate the relevant shapers from last week too...

This week's programme
Preliminaries
32 × several
69 × several
53 × several
34 × 8 each side
104 × 12 each leg
59 × 16
83
Active recovery cool-down, see page 161
84 × several
101 until muscles begin to tire
103 × 4
52 × several
85 until muscles begin to tire
105 × several
106 × 16 with each ball
107 × 8 each side
108 × several
39 × 1
58

104 BUTTOCKS AND HIPS

Attach a light 0.5 kg (1 lb) weight to each ankle. Holding onto back of chair for support, transfer weight onto inside leg; now take leg out to side as far as possible, keeping foot flexed. Return to floor and rotate foot outwards to angle of about 45° and then extend leg backwards in a straight line as far as comfortable, keeping back vertical and not arching or leaning forwards. Return leg to starting position. Practise 12 times, then change legs and repeat.

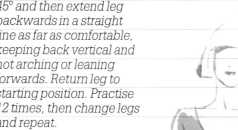

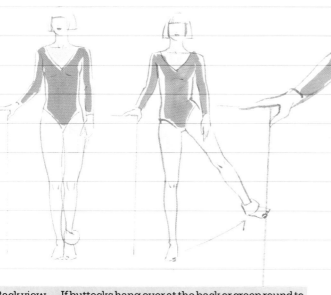

Back view... If buttocks hang over at the back or creep round to the sides, contributing to a bulge at the hips, they need firming. Helpful exercises: 104, if you cannot see a definite dent at the sides beneath the hips; 66 and 105 if your shape at the back is not firm and well defined.

Firms slack buttock muscles at side, reduces bulge at hips

105 BUTTOCKS

Lie on back with legs falling gently outwards. Do a pelvic tilt and squeeze buttocks together several times. Then repeat, but this time hold each contraction for 6 counts before releasing. Practise several times.

Buttock muscles soon respond to exercise

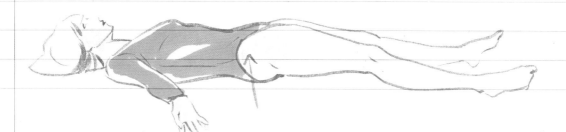

106 INNER THIGHS

Lie on back with knees bent, feet flat on floor. Place a football-sized ball between knees and squeeze quickly together 8 times. Then try 8 slower contractions, continuing to squeeze for 6 counts. Now place a smaller tennis-sized ball between knees and repeat exercise.

Using different sized balls works entire range of muscles

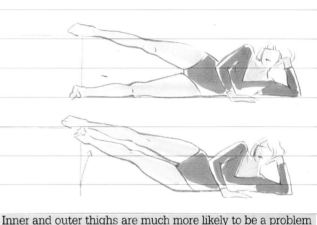

107 INNER THIGHS

When comfortable add weight to lower ankle

Lie on side, as shown, with body in a straight line and knees facing forwards. Place upper foot on chair seat and point toes. Now flex lower foot and bring it up to meet the other. Hold for 3 counts and release. Practise 8 times, then turn over and change legs.

Inner and outer thighs are much more likely to be a problem than front or back because they are used for lateral movements and rotation only. The muscles at the front of thigh, which are used for forward motion, usually remain firm and toned even in the overweight. Helpful exercises for inner thighs: 64, 75, 106, 107…alternate for variety. Helpful exercises for outer thighs ('saddlebags'): 65 and 108.

108 OUTER THIGHS

Lie on side, supported by one elbow, with lower leg bent back at knee. Flex foot of upper leg and raise until it is parallel to floor. Hold for 6 slow counts and slowly lower. Repeat until muscles begin to tire, and then turn over and repeat with other leg.

When exercise is comfortable add weights to ankle

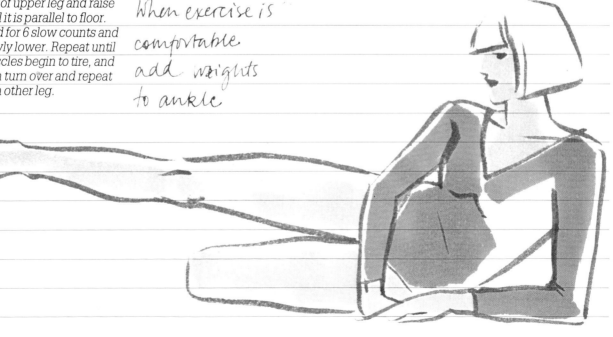

WEEK 15: MOBILITY

The freedom to move easily is one of our most basic freedoms and, very often, the one we think least about. But we should treasure it. Keeping mobile by being mobile can prevent any amount of stiffness later on.

Keeping mobile means taking each joint through its full range of movement every day (knees are the exception, see over), *not* contorting your body into strange shapes. It doesn't matter a bit whether you can do the splits or get your foot around your neck. These are gimmicks. But it does matter tremendously if you cannot move as and how you wish. There is nothing more demoralizing than a stiff, awkward body that protests every time you ask it to move.

As you work through the exercises this week, sense yourself becoming more supple. Results should be rewardingly swift. As your range of movement develops you may find yourself capable of more in other directions too: freedom from physical stiffness can lead to greater mental and emotional freedom...

This week's programme
Preliminaries
32 × several
69 × several
53 × several
24 × 3
109 × several
110 × 8 each direction
111 × 8 each leg
46 × 8 each leg
83
Active recovery
  cool-down, see page 41
74 × 4 each leg
103 × 4
52 × several
85 until muscles begin to tire
112
Active recovery
  cool-down, see page 161
113 until ankles and calves begin to tire
42 × 1
43, 44, 45 × several
114 × 3 each way
68 × 1
N.B. Remember to include Shapers from last two weeks where appropriate...

---

109 **ELBOWS** *Stand with feet about hip-width apart and a book, or flat object, in the palm of each hand. Now bring hands in towards you as you bend elbows out and stretch arms out again. Repeat smoothly several times.*

Don't clutch onto books – they should simply balance on the flat of your hand.

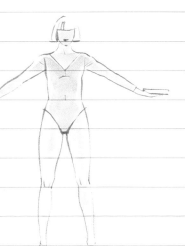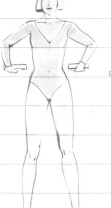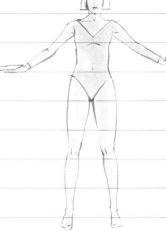

Thumbs should face back in both positions

You should do mobility work before aerobics and the stronger stretches and strengtheners because it helps you both to work more effectively and to guard against injury – particularly important in cold climates where joints tend to be stiff and need to be warmed up well before attempting anything more demanding.

110 SHOULDERS

Stand with feet about 60 cm (2 ft) apart. Hold a broom handle in front of you and lift it up to shoulder level. Raise one arm up above head, letting the other drop to waist. Now use both arms to take stick backwards as far as it will go. Then bring it down behind you so that shoulder blades are squeezed together. Continue round back to the front again, raising opposite arm to the one before. Practise 8 times in each direction. This exercise is much used by javelin throwers.

BONUS Improves coordination. As you get better change direction every 4 times, then every 2 . . .

Bring hands in as shoulders become more supple

111 **HIPS** *Stand holding onto back of chair for support. Bend outside leg so thigh is parallel to floor and toes are pointed. Now make a wide circle with leg, keeping back vertical and feeling stretch on inside of hip as you bring leg right round to back. Return to starting position. Practise 8 times with each leg.*

Sense hip moving deep within socket as you bring leg backwards and forwards.

The straighter your back, the more hips must work.

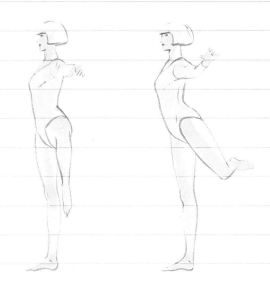

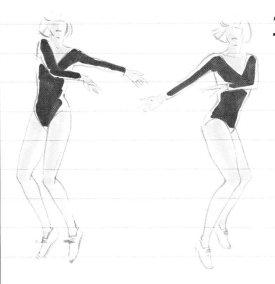

112 **AEROBIC SEQUENCE** *Add another, improvised, aerobic sequence to your routine. Pick a lively piece of music 4 minutes long, start and finish with gentle padding (see note) and then choose from aerobic movements you have already learned, adding new ones given here.*

a. Progress the twist jump so you are jumping with about one walking step between feet.

b. Try some scissor jumps, first straight forwards and then to diagonal, back to centre and then to other diagonal. Feet should be one walking pace apart.
c. Stand well with heels about 10cm (4ins) apart and spring up, landing with alternate feet forwards. Make sure that knees bend directly over toes and don't lean forwards: tuck pelvis under and jump up and down looking straight ahead.

What intensity of aerobic exercise is right for you? As you get fitter make it more demanding. Move faster and jump higher, always emphasizing the upward spring. If you begin to tire, slow down and go back to some gentle padding before increasing the pace again.

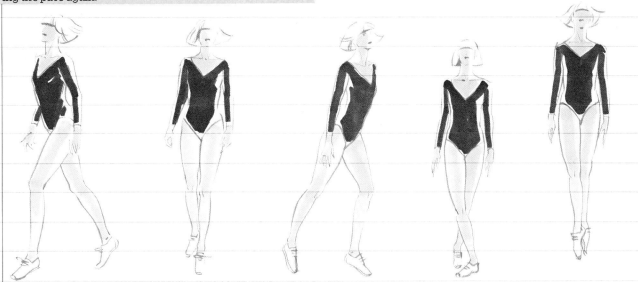

You will find that no mobility exercises are given for the knee because the knee is designed to work safely on one plane only (see page 243). This vulnerable joint is kept stable by the muscles at the front of the thigh. Strengthen these and you will help keep the knee trouble-free. Most effective strengthener: exercise 74. Try it this week holding the fully extended position for 4 counts before slowly lowering.

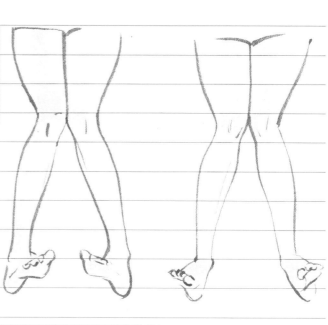

113 ANKLES *Sit on a chair with knees together and heels apart. Bring big toes together, trying to lift them up as much as possible. Then brush outwards along floor, pulling little toes up and pressing big toes down. Repeat until ankles and calves begin to tire.*

TEST Can you raise big toes at least 15 cm (5 ins) when heels are on floor? If not, practise until you can. You will be able to lift toes higher as ankles become more mobile.

Weak feet and ankles are easily injured. Strong, springy ones make you feel agile and lively and improve your balance. Exercises that increase mobility at ankles will help strengthen them and improve posture too . . .

114 SPINE *Sit with legs crossed and take right leg back, so that left foot is by right knee. You should be well balanced and able to feel both 'sitting' bones beneath you. Stretch left hand behind you, resting on fingers. Raise right arm and twist to left, bending from hips. Try to keep hips level and facing front as you reach forwards to diagonal and sweep round to right, changing position of arms as you go through centre. If you can, drop back onto elbow and look behind you. Then sweep back again, going forwards as far as possible and round to opposite side. Practise 3 times, then reverse legs and repeat.*

This is borrowed from contemporary dance, and stabilizes hips to give good twist in spine.

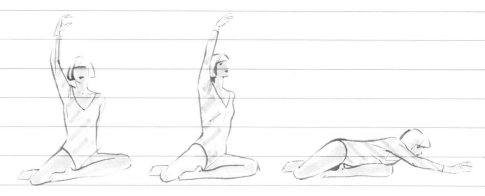

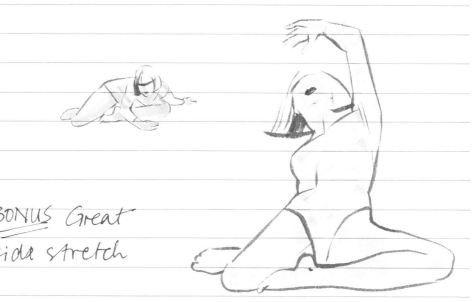

BONUS Great
side stretch

WEEK 16: DŌ-IN

The new-wave holistic approach to medicine underlines the interaction of body, mind and spirit and calls for a concept of health that embraces the whole in place of the parts, the individual instead of the illness. These ideas have always been central to the philosophies and exercise systems of the East and the Orient – yoga, T'ai Chi, acupuncture and many of the martial arts and Dō-in (pronounced 'doe-in'), an ancient and enlivening body massage.

Common to all these philosophies is a belief in a life force, known as Ki-energy, which is made up of the opposing forces of Yin (negative, female, spiritual) and Yang (positive, male, material). This energy, which has even been photographed (*see note*), is constantly ebbing and flowing. It is when it is well balanced that our physical and spiritual well-being is greatest.

The oriental therapies use different methods to regulate this flow of energy and so restore equilibrium. Dō-in is one of the simplest. It takes just a few minutes to learn and can be practised effectively at home by anyone.

This week's programme

Preliminaries
98 × 1 each leg
115 × 1
98 × 1 each leg
69 × several
34 × 8 each side
110 × 8 each direction
113 until ankles and calves begin to tire
101 3 × 4
59 × 16
83

Active recovery
  cool-down, see page 161
84 × several
103, hands clasped behind head × 3
52 × several
85 until muscles begin to tire
39 × 1
112

Active recovery
  cool-down, see page 161
43, 44, 45 × several
114 × 3 each way
68 × 1

Visual proof of an energy field, or 'aura', emanating from a living body has been given by Kirlian, a Russian scientist. He photographed it by passing an electric current beneath a photographic plate on which the body, or part of the body, is resting. The result was an eerie photograph in which the energy could be seen as a luminous halo. If ailing, the halo is dimmer, though photographs taken before and after spiritual healing sessions have shown increased brightness around the tips of the fingers as the new-found health emanates from the body...

115 DŌ-IN

Rub hands vigorously together at eye level. Shake them out, clap them together, squeeze and pull each finger out away from you, breathing out strongly. Continue until hands feel warm and fingers tingle. Put hands a little way from each other. Do you feel you are holding an invisible ball of energy? Now you are ready to start.

a. *Lightly rap top of head and brow with knuckles. Rub cheeks and nose, pinch and squeeze eyebrows, rotate eyes, blink vigorously and tap chin with tips of fingers. Now rub ears and pull lobes by letting elbows drop downwards.*

b. *Interlace fingers and squeeze along sides of neck with heels of hands. Work from base of neck up, breathing out as you press in, in as you release.*

c. *Cup elbow in hand and make a loose fist with other hand. Pound top of shoulders, working from neck outwards. Start lightly, then rap more vigorously.*

d. *Breathe in deeply and stretch up. Clench fists loosely and, as you breathe out, thump chest, opening mouth wide and making loud noises.*

e. *Rap from top of inside arm, to wrist and then up outside of arm . . .*

f. *Go into flat back, bending from hips. Rap each side of spine, working from head to buttocks.*

g. *Drop forwards from hips and rap buttocks.*

h. *Still standing, rap each leg in turn, from top of inner thigh to ankle. Return up outer side.*

i. *Rub feet vigorously all over, rap along sole of foot from heel to toes, press Achilles tendon and massage area above ankle. Finally massage toes individually, wiggling and rotating each in turn.*

Rapping yourself with fists and knuckles may look painful, but it's not at all. The key is to keep hands soft, fists loosely clenched and wrists flexible.

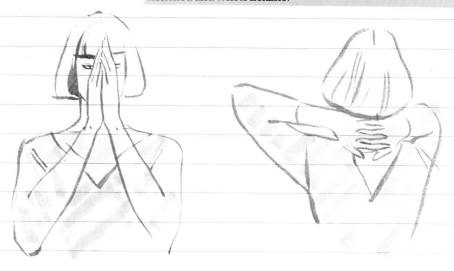
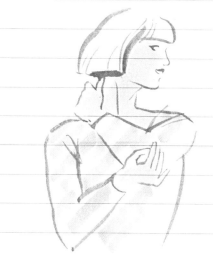
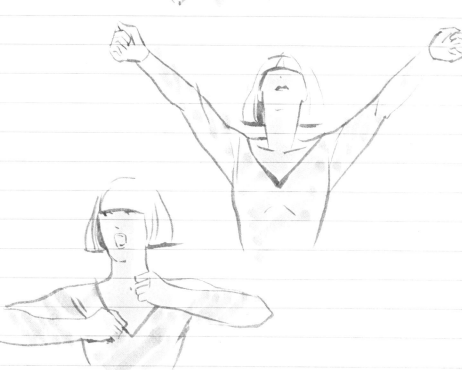

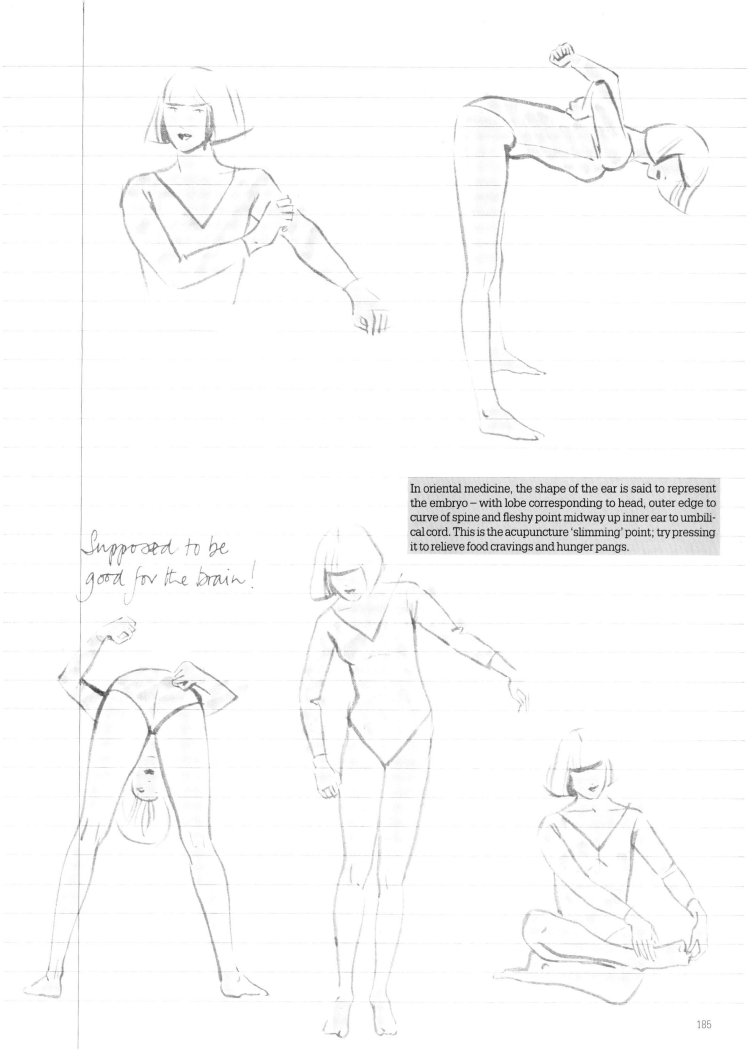

Supposed to be
good for the brain!

In oriental medicine, the shape of the ear is said to represent the embryo – with lobe corresponding to head, outer edge to curve of spine and fleshy point midway up inner ear to umbilical cord. This is the acupuncture 'slimming' point; try pressing it to relieve food cravings and hunger pangs.

WEEK 17: YOGA SUN SALUTATION

Yoga is not so much a form of exercise as a complete philosophy which aims to bring body and mind into close harmony through the practice of postures (*asanas*) and breathing control (*pranayama*). This communion of mind and body takes a lifetime to achieve and is obviously beyond the scope of any book.

Although advanced yoga postures and breathing techniques should be taught by a qualified teacher, the simpler postures, such as those given here, can be practised quite safely by anyone. They will free tension, improve flexibility and give you more joy and confidence in your body

You don't have to put yourself into bizarre positions or tie yourself into a pretzel to do yoga. Greater freedom and ease of movement is the aim and this comes with practice. If a position feels strained or painful, you are either not doing it properly or are not yet ready to do it. The challenge is to move your body just a little more freely and easily each time.

This week's programme
Preliminaries
116 × 3
34 × 8 each side
110 × 8 each direction
101 3 × 4
59 × 16
83
Active recovery
   cool-down, see page 161
84 × several
103, hands clasped
   behind head × 4
52 × several
85 × 1
39 until muscles begin to
   tire
112
Active recovery
   cool-down, see page 161
66, with weights and
   straight legs × 8 each
   leg
43, 44, 45 × several
114 × 3 each way
58

116 SUN SALUTATION

a. Stand with feet together and palms of hands joined in prayer position. Lengthen up spine and drop shoulders away from ears. Breathe easily in and out several times. Imagine the sun's energy pouring in, filling you with strength and vitality.
b. Breathe in deeply as you reach up with arms. Enjoy feeling of lift and maintain it as you continue to stretch backwards.
c. As you breathe out, bend forwards from hips going smoothly through flat back position until

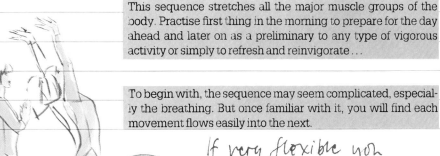

This sequence stretches all the major muscle groups of the body. Practise first thing in the morning to prepare for the day ahead and later on as a preliminary to any type of vigorous activity or simply to refresh and reinvigorate...

To begin with, the sequence may seem complicated, especially the breathing. But once familiar with it, you will find each movement flows easily into the next.

If very flexible you may be able to rest head on shins

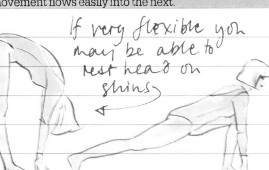

hands are flat beside feet, or at least touching floor. Keep legs straight.

d. Breathe in and extend right leg back so that it is fully extended with heel pointing towards back of room. Keep head up and look straight ahead. Your body should now make a straight line from heel of back foot to shoulders.

e. Breathe normally as you take left foot back and place it beside right. You are now in full press-up position (good preparation for week 24). Your back should be flat with no arching or sagging and pelvis tucked under.

f. Breathe in. As you breathe out, lower body so that toes, knees, chest, palms and forehead are all resting on floor. Pelvis should be raised off floor and hands should be as before, with elbows bent and arms by sides.

g. Breathe in. As you breathe out, release position and lie extended on floor with hands by head.

h. Bring hands up to shoulder level and breathe in as you raise head and chest, keeping pelvis flat on floor. Arch head back as you straighten arms.

i. Breathe out and raise hips to form an inverted V, with feet flat on floor and legs straight. Look at toes.

j. Breathe normally as you bring right foot forwards. Keep left foot back and fully extended, resting on toes.

k. Breathe in. As you breathe out, bring left leg up. Place feet together and straighten legs.

l. Breathe in as you straighten up from hips. Bring arms up, lengthening up spine, and then stretch backwards.

m. Breathe out and straighten. Bring hands back to prayer position. Practise whole exercise 3 times in a good rhythm.

This position, *astanga*, has 8 points of contact with floor.

Check position in mirror – all the same rules of posture apply when horizontal as when vertical . . .

Are hands any flatter than before?

Make the sequence more demanding by stretching further in each position, using out-breaths to help you. For a greater challenge still, take up Iyengar yoga. Iyengar, one of the great yoga masters, has developed a series of strong sustained stretches to overcome stiffness, help free the body.

187

WEEK 18: SEXUALITY

Sexuality is a quality we can all develop by becoming more aware, more confident, and by using our bodies more fully.

It was the psychologist Wilhelm Reich (1897-1977) who first suggested that mind and body can influence each other in such a way as to interfere with, or to enhance, sexual pleasure. Emotional disturbances, he said, lead to muscular 'blocks' that dam up biological energy and interfere with our capacity for giving and receiving pleasure. Reich called these blocks 'dead zones' because they are the opposite of the sexual impulse which is about being alive in its fullest, most enjoyable sense.

Most of us have dead zones in our bodies – and sometimes in our minds too. Help awaken them with long, slow stretching, specific strengtheners that call on underused muscles and some Feldenkrais work that will enhance awareness by focusing attention on your body.

This week's programme
Preliminaries
116 × 1 slowly, breathing well
43, 44, 45 × several
42 × 1
117 × 1
56 × 1
118 × several
34 × 8 each side
110 × 8 each direction
101 3 × 4
59 × 16
83
Active recovery
   cool-down, see page 161
84 × several
103, hands clasped behind head × 4
52 × several
85, until muscles begin to tire
64 × several
106 × 16 with each ball
112
Active recovery
   cool-down, see page 161
114 × 3 each way
58
N.B. Also this week, pelvic floor exercises **119**, see note

'Sexuality and anxiety are functions of the living organism operating in opposite directions: pleasurable expansion and anxious contraction…'
Wilhelm Reich *The Function of the Orgasm*

The pelvis can be a major dead zone. The Feldenkrais clock sequence should have helped you gain awareness and mobility there but if you still find it stiff and unresponsive, use your breathing to help you. Lying down, breathe out slowly and deeply and see how your pelvis starts to roll naturally forwards in a continuous forward curve. Reich maintained that this undulatory movement is the position of 'surrender' in which blocked energy is released and that it is the only position in which orgasm can take place.

117 AWARENESS

Lie on back with knees bent and feet flat on floor. Visualize your anus, picturing it as a circle, and squeeze it several times. Now visualize your bladder, picturing it as a tube, and squeeze that several times. Can you differentiate between them? Practise squeezing anus, then bladder, quite hard several times and then go back to squeezing anus softly. Do you notice a difference? Visualizing both anus and bladder together, squeeze them simultaneously. Rest a moment, then squeeze them separately several times. Are you finding it easier to move them independently? If not, continue practising a few times each day until you do…

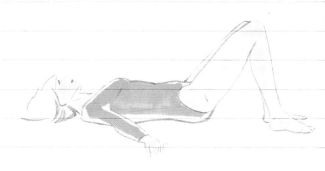

118 PELVIS *Standing with feet apart, hands on hips and knees slightly bent, rock pelvis back and forth several times. Then rock it from side to side. Finish with some complete rotations, clockwise and anti-clockwise, making sure that movement is coming from pelvis and not from thighs.*

Are you very stiff? You will get much more supple with practice . . .

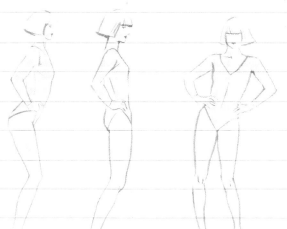

VARIATION . . . Try a figure-of-eight: circle right hip clockwise in a complete rotation; coming through centre, circle left hip anti-clockwise in a complete rotation. Do several then change direction.

The more you use and move your pelvis, the more you will become aware of it as your centre of gravity and balance.

119 PELVIC FLOOR *Locate pelvic floor muscles (see note) by trying to stop the flow of urine when you go to the lavatory. Once you have got the feeling, practise contracting and releasing them. Then try contracting them in stages: up one level; pause; up a little more; pause; all the way up; hold and release. Repeat 10 times slowly, then more quickly, several times a day.*

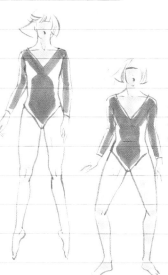

The muscles of the pelvic floor lie like the interconnecting circles of a figure-of-eight around the vagina and urethra (which leads to the bladder) and the anus. Although fundamental to pleasure and sensitivity when making love, few of us even realize where they are much less think of exercising them to keep them firm and strong. This week's exercises not only test their strength but your ability to differentiate between them . . .

Your partner will be able to tell whether you are doing this correctly if he can feel muscles tightening when you make love . . .

Finish with a test: can you jump up and down, legs wide apart as shown, coughing out as you do so without letting urine escape from the bladder? If so, your pelvic floor muscles are in good shape.

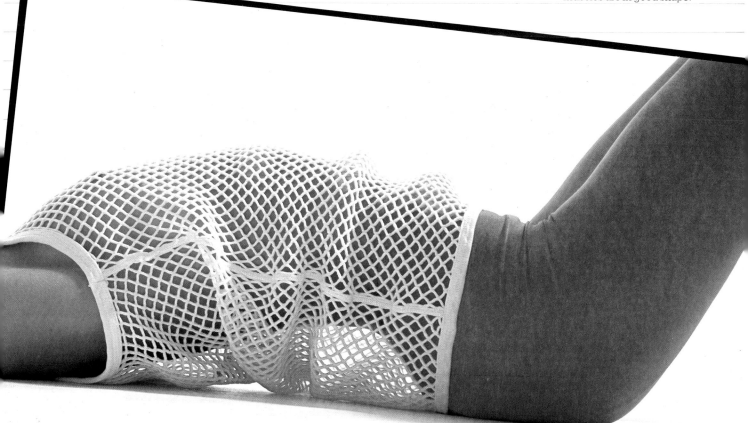

WEEK 19: ROCK AND ROLL

Free-moving, fun, fast and extremely energetic, rock and roll may look easy and carefree but it demands perfect-timing, good coordination, considerable strength, stamina and mobility (particularly in the ankles, hence exercise 121), and a lot of practice to get the footwork right. Start rehearsing today with the specially choreographed rock and roll sequences on page 208. Learn a new section, step by step, each day and you will have mastered the complete sequence by the end of the week...

This week's programme
Preliminaries
32 × several
69 × several
53 × several
120 × 8 each side
121 × 16 each position
113 until ankles and calves begin to tire
101 4 × 4
59 × 16
122
Active recovery
cool-down, see page 16
84 × several
103, hands clasped behind head × 5
52 × several
85 until muscles begin to tire
Rock and roll practice (see page 208)
112
Active recovery
cool-down, see page 16
123 × 4
114 × 3 each way
68 × 1

120 WAIST
Stand with feet well apart and parallel, hands on chest as shown. Turn torso to right, to back and to centre again rocking body 3 times as you go. Repeat to other side. Practise 8 times each side.

Rock and roll, the phenomenon of the 50s, seemed to arrive out of nowhere...but in fact it can be traced back as far as West African tribal dancing and, more directly, to the many dance crazes that swept the USA in the 20s and 30s when big bands and glittering ballrooms made dancing available to everyone. Rock and roll borrowed heavily from these crazes before adding some uptempo steps of its own...

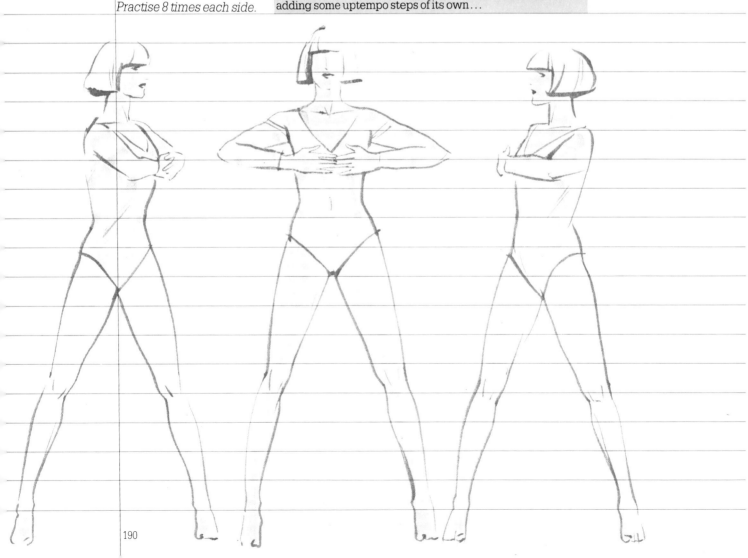

121 LEGS AND ANKLES

Stand well with feet together. Bend knees and lift up onto balls of feet. Straighten legs and return to starting position. Repeat 16 times; then try the same exercise with legs apart; with right leg in front of left; with left leg in front of right.

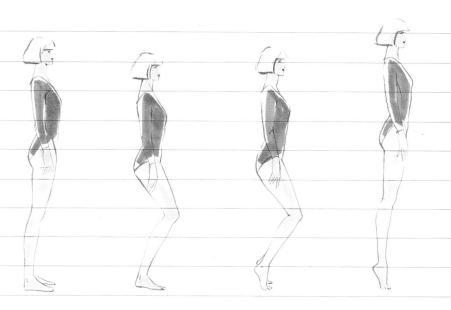

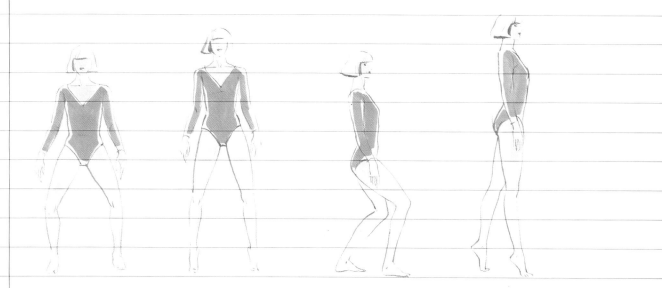

In the mood . . . Try doing the new exercises, and the aerobic sequence, to one of the rock and roll music suggestions on page 208.

122 LEGS

Stretch one leg back, the other forwards, and place hands on floor. Bounce hips towards floor for 7 counts. Then bring back leg in and bounce knees together for 3 counts. Change legs and repeat. Alternate in this way twice and then stretch one leg back, place its opposite elbow on floor and bounce hips down towards floor as before. Change legs and repeat. Practise twice.

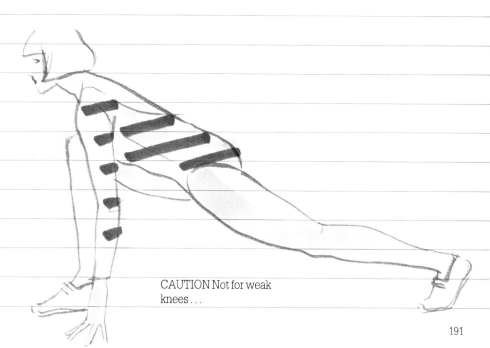

CAUTION Not for weak knees . . .

123 WAIST AND INNER THIGHS *Sit with legs apart, arms outstretched at shoulder level. Lift one arm up over head and stretch over towards opposite foot, maintaining length in spine. Return to centre, change arms and repeat to other side. Then reach forwards from hips feeling strong stretch in thighs as you go. Keep back straight. Repeat 3 times.*

VARIATION Try flexing feet

WEEK 20: MEDITATION

Meditation seems strange to many western minds, but the ability to put all activity aside and to find one's centre again is more important than ever in the rush and tumble of the western lifestyle where time to contemplate, to be passive and to *let* rather than *make* things happen is hardly ever on the schedule.

You don't need a guru or collection of Sanskrit words in order to meditate, just a mind that is open, receptive, willing to see what happens. Don't you owe it to yourself to find out why so many people become calmer and happier once they start meditating regularly? Follow the simple directions *below*.

'... that serene and blessed mood,
In which the affections gently lead us on –
Until, the breath of this corporeal frame
And even the motion of our human blood,
Almost suspended, we are laid asleep
In body, and become a living soul:
While with an eye made quiet by the power
Of harmony, and the deep power of joy,
We see into the life of things ... '
William Wordsworth. *Lines composed a few miles above Tintern Abbey*

This week's programme
Preliminaries
**20-minute meditation
   practice**
124 or **125**
56 × 1
57 × 3 minutes each foot
116 × 1, breathing well
110 × 8 each direction
120 × 8 each side
59 × 16
122
**Active recovery
   cool-down,** see page 161
103, hands clasped behind
   head × 5
52 × several
85 until muscles begin to
   tire
123 × 4
112
**Active recovery
   cool-down,** see page 161
42 × 1
81 × 1
117 × 1
58
124 or **125**

Three requirements for meditation:
1. No distractions. Meditate in a quiet place. Take a watch to check on time occasionally but not an alarm.
2. Comfort. Don't lie down – it's too easy to go to sleep; sit instead with spine straight and supported by cushions if necessary.
3. No judgements. Don't expect too much right away. Instead of being preoccupied with how well you are doing, adopt a calm, passive, non-judging attitude and simply enjoy the peace of quiet contemplation.

124 MEDITATION I

Sit with spine straight and legs out in front of you. Now bend one knee and place foot high on opposite thigh, then either lift second leg over first or tuck it beneath in half lotus or sit in simple cross-legs if neither position is comfortable. Place hands on knees, close eyes, relax body, soften face and turn attention inwards. You now need something to meditate on. Here are two alternatives. Practise both and continue with the one that you find works best.

Breathing. The important thing for this is to be aware only of the breath as it comes and goes. If other thoughts drift in, do not let them intervene; allow them to pass on. Starting on an out-breath, count each breath until you reach 10. If random thoughts rush in, go back to the beginning and start all over again. With practice, your concentration will improve.

The lotus position *padmasana*, the position of enlightenment symbolizes our own spiritual nature with our roots in the mud our stem rising through the water in search of light and our head blossoming in the clarity of self-realization...

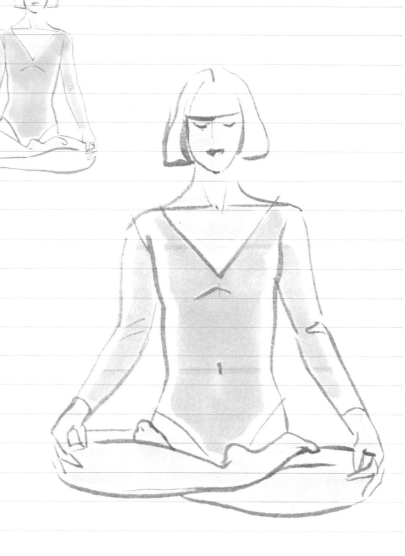

125 MEDITATION II

Sitting as above, and being lightly aware of your breathing, repeat a single syllable word on each out-breath, silently or out loud. You might like to choose a word yourself, or use a Sanskrit 'mantra' such as the Siddha 'OM' (pronounced 'Oh-m'). Or try the word 'ONE' recommended by Herbert Benson in The Relaxation Response. *Whichever you choose, allow your mind to dwell on it maintaining an attitude of passive, relaxed concentration.*

When the eyes are active, the brain is active too. If thoughts rush in while meditating, soften your eyes and you will find your mind becomes still again.

Breathing is a useful path to meditation because it is a bridge between the voluntary and the involuntary, the conscious and the unconscious. 'The mind rides the breath' is how the eastern gurus put it.

Breathing out is the breath of surrender, of letting go. When we expire, we die and release our hold on life; when we give birth the exhalation expels the baby; when we have an orgasm, we gasp; when we breathe out in meditation we surrender the self to greater consciousness. The Mahayama Buddhists in Tibet, in an extension of this practice, breathe in the suffering of others in the form of visualized black smoke and breathe out love and compassion in the form of a white light to heal and to bless.

WEEK 21: BASIC BALLET

The exacting standards of classical ballet are such that to be good you have to start young – not just because of the years of training required but also because its strict disciplines shape the body in a certain way. Happily, though, there is still much to be gained from ballet, such as improved strength and an enjoyable feeling of grace and renewed control over your body, without having to reach the great technical heights demanded of the classical dancer.

Many basic ballet movements make useful general exercises. They demand good control, correct technique and suppleness at certain joints – in particular the hips where the 'turn out' (rotation of the hip in the joint) is considered paramount. Strength, too, is important. The slight willowy shape of the classical dancer belies tremendous power, particularly in the legs and feet...

This week's programme
Preliminaries
116 × 2
126 × 4 each side
127 × 8 each side
128 × 4 each side
129 × 8
130 × 8 each side
131 × 8 each side
132 × 8 each side
110 × 8 each side
123 × 4
101 4 × 4
59 × 16
112
Active recovery
   cool-down, see page 161
103, hands clasped
   behind head × 5
52 × several
85, add 0.5 kg (1 lb)
   weight to each ankle
   until muscles begin to
   tire
114 × 3 each way
133
Active recovery
   cool-down, see page 161
43, 44, 45 × several
58

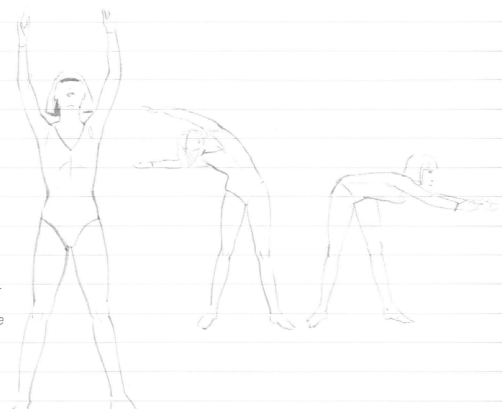

126 ***WARM-UP*** *Stand in second position (feet apart and turned out) with arms raised to ceiling. Bend over to right, bringing arms and head over too. Then twist into diagonal forward stretch, with flat back, and move round to opposite corner keeping hips level throughout. Now twist again so you stretch to left. Return to centre and lower arms to shoulder level. Repeat 3 times to each side in a nice easy rhythm.*

127 TENDU

Stand well in first position (heels together, toes out, arms and hands as shown), with pelvis tucked under and spine lengthened. Extend leg to side, brushing foot along floor until toes are fully pointed. Keep body centered and both legs straight. Practise 8 times; then change legs and repeat to other side.

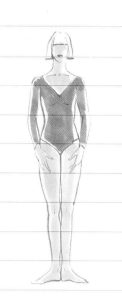
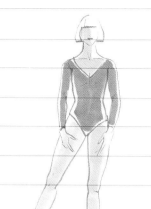
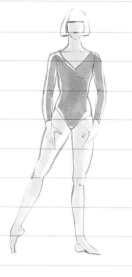

Leg turns out from hip in first position – one of the most basic ballet stances.

Preliminary to *battement* leg-raising exercises . . .

BONUS Good for balance.

128 PETITS BATTEMENTS

Stand well with feet together. Brush one foot forwards along floor and up, pointing toes, to height shown here. Repeat to side, back and to side again. Make sure you keep body centered, hips level and back vertical throughout. Practise 4 times with each foot and then repeat whole exercise, but this time flex and point foot 4 times each time you lift it.

BONUS Good for balance.

129 DEVELOPPÉ

Stand well with feet together, arms at shoulder level. Lift one leg so thigh is parallel to floor and hips are level. Extend leg forwards, pointing toe, in one slow controlled movement. Your whole leg should now be parallel to floor. Lower to tendu and bring feet together. Practise 8 times; then change legs and repeat exercise.

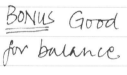

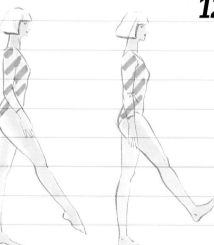

The more you lift knee the higher leg will go

Keep supporting leg straight throughout

Ballet is not a complete form of exercise: upper body loses out to lower body and suppleness to strength. So, if you want to use it as a means of keeping fit, complement with some good general stretches, plenty of flexibility work on shoulders and spine (the twists in particular) and strengtheners for the upper body.

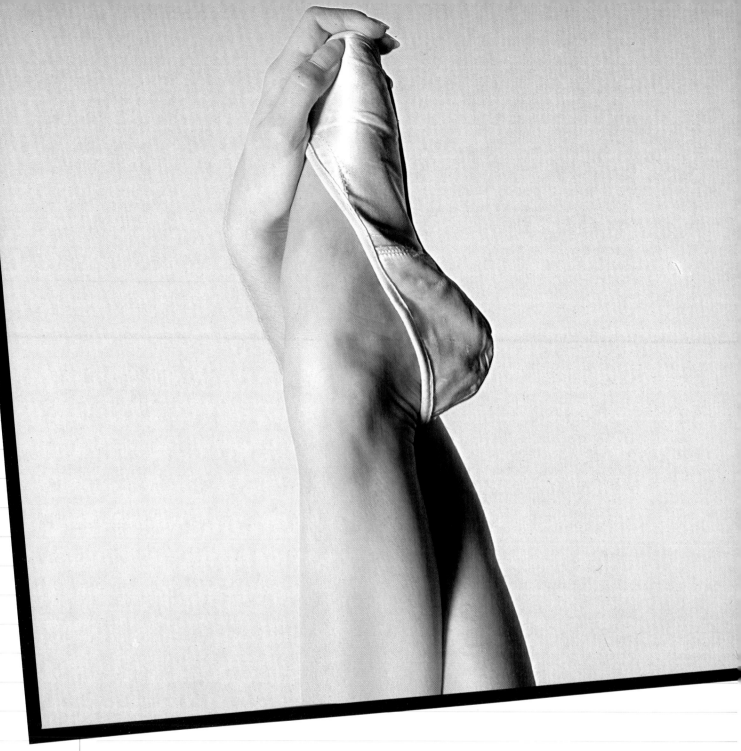

130 DEVELOPPÉ À LA SECONDE

Stand well in first position with arms at shoulder level. Lift one leg so toes are by inside of other knee and extend out to side. Practise 8 times, in a slow controlled manner; then change legs and repeat. Now try it again, but this time extend leg forwards instead of sideways keeping heel to the side to practise turn out.

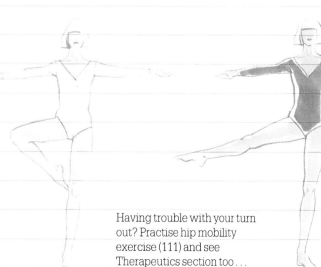

Having trouble with your turn out? Practise hip mobility exercise (111) and see Therapeutics section too . . .

Great strengthener & good for balance too . . . .

131 EPAULEMENTS

Stand in second position with arms at shoulder level. Press one shoulder forwards and down. Then repeat to other side, feeling connection between shoulders as you do so. Practise 8 times each side and then repeat exercise walking forwards, one step at a time, bringing each shoulder forwards with its opposite leg.

132 RETIRÉ *Stand in first position with arms at shoulder level. Lift one leg up until thigh is parallel to floor and place foot up inside of supporting leg so toes touch knee. Return to starting position. Practise 8 times each side.*

keep supporting leg straight throughout

133 JUMPS *Extend your freestyle sequence by 1 minute, adding any movements you enjoy and these ballet jumps. Stand in first position with arms as shown, bend knees in demi plié and spring up into air, pointing toes. Land lightly, bending knees in demi plié again, and spring up again, feeling leg muscles tighten. Be sure to keep pelvis tucked under and back vertical.*

CAUTION Failing to bend knees may jar spine.

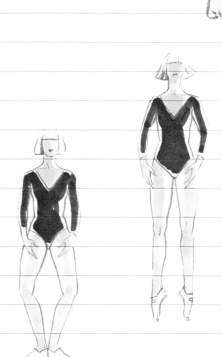

Helps you to think 'up' as well as 'forward' when you move

WEEK 22: BARRE WORK

Here are a few more basic ballet movements using a barre to help you balance. Look on it as an aid, not a leaning post, and hold onto it lightly with the tips of the fingers. If you place too much weight on it, the line of your body will be wrong and the exercise less effective. If you do not have a barre, use the back of a chair – a good substitute because you will know you are not using it properly if it starts tipping or lifting.

Thigh muscles work hard to maintain stability when doing pliés. If you find them difficult, or your knee hurts, only go as far as comfortable and if pain is felt, STOP.

This week's programme
Preliminaries
116 × 2
134 × 4
135 × 4
136 × 4
137 × 4
128, progression **138** × 4 each side
132 on demi-pointe, hand resting lightly on barre × 8 each side
139 × 8
110 × 8 each direction in sets of 2 each time
101 4 × 5
59 × 16
122
Active recovery cool-down, see page 161
103, hands clasped behind head × 5
52 × several
85, with weight until muscles begin to tire
140 × 4 each side
5-minute freestyle aerobic sequence
Active recovery cool-down, see page 161
39 × 1
43, 44, 45 × several
58

134 DEMI PLIÉ
Stand in first position, holding barre as shown, with spine lengthened and pelvis centered. Maintaining upright posture, bend knees so that they go directly over feet. Bend them as far as you can without lifting heels off floor for 2 counts. Return to starting position, fully extending legs, for 2 counts. Repeat 3 times.

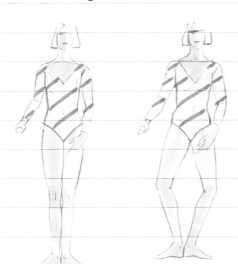

Never force first position – turn out will improve as hips become more mobile

135 GRAND PLIÉ
Standing in first position, as before, with spine well lifted and buttocks tucked under, pass through demi plié position to a turned-out squatting position, lifting heels from floor, for 4 counts. Press heels down and return to starting position for 4 counts. Don't fall forwards. Repeat 3 times.

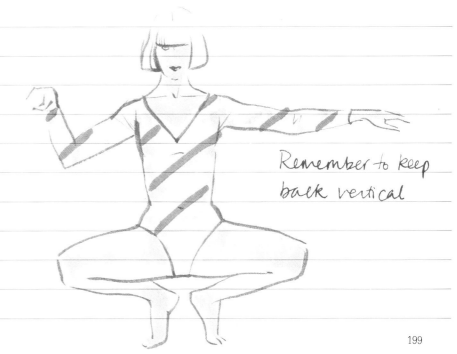

Remember to keep back vertical

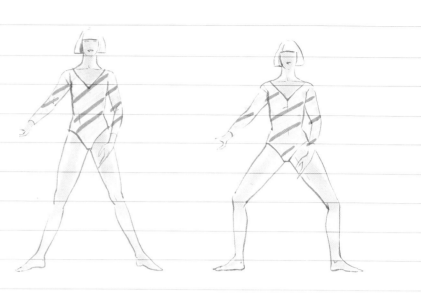

136 DEMI PLIÉ *Stand in second position and bend knees over toes as you go into a demi plié for 2 counts, keeping spine straight, buttocks tucked under and feet flat on floor. Return to starting position for 2 counts. Repeat 3 times.*

137 GRAND PLIÉ

Standing in second position, pass through demi plié and go down as far as you can without lifting heels for 4 counts. Return to starting position for 4 counts. Repeat 3 times.

CAUTION If knees hurt, stop and turn to Therapeutics exercises on page 243.

Pliés, the opening exercises in the ballet class routine, warm up muscles, loosen joints, promote strength and improve balance. Once you have mastered them at the barre, try them in the centre of the room...

138 PETITS BATTEMENTS

Use barre for this progression of exercise 128. As you lift foot off floor rise onto demi-point (ball of supporting foot) and lower gradually as you return to starting position. Repeat to side, to back and to side again keeping back vertical as before. Practise exercise 4 times each side; then try flex/point variation.

The principles of good posture apply as much as ever at the barre. Keep weight evenly balanced, spine lengthened, pelvis centered and buttocks tucked under – especially when doing pliés where benefits to be gained depend on doing them correctly...

_139_ BALANCE _Stand in second position away from barre, with arms at shoulder level. Raise arms gracefully above head, as shown, as you rise up on demi-points, keeping legs fully extended. Slowly lower heels to ground. Repeat 7 times._

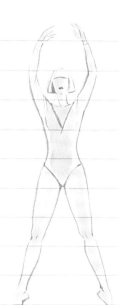

Be careful not to tip forwards as you rise

_140_ WAIST _Place one leg on barre and raise arms above head. Breathe in. As you breathe out, stretch sideways away from barre as far as is comfortable, feeling a good stretch along side for 4 counts. Return to centre for 4 counts and then repeat stretch to other side. Practise 4 times each side._

Height of barre or chair back should be such that raised leg is parallel to ground as here

Not a classical ballet movement but a great stretch on way down, and a good strengthener on way up too . . .

WEEK 23: JAZZ

Easy to recognize, almost impossible to describe, jazz has always escaped strict definition. With individuality and freedom the keynotes, there are as many different styles and interpretations as performers. In some, it's the isolation of rib and hip that's important, in others the swing, in yet others the 'jazzed-up' Latin-American dance steps of the samba and rumba.

In their efforts to break free from the strict, disciplines of classical ballet, both jazz and contemporary dance have remained deliberately loose. You will feel the difference as soon as you start this week's warm-up. Once you have mastered the routine on page 212-17, start improvising. Add a swing in the hips, make the movements more expressive, mix them up to create new combinations or even invent some of your own... That's the essence of jazz.

This week's programme
Preliminaries
32 × several
141 × several
53 × several
142 × 4 each way
143 × 4 each way
144 × 8
123 × 4
101 4 × 5
59 × 16
122
**Active recovery
  cool-down,** see page 161
103, hands clasped
  behind head × 5
52 × several
85, with weight until
  muscles begin to tire
75 × up to 8
Jazz practice, see page
212
**5-minute freestyle
  aerobic sequence
  including 145 and 146,**
  × 8 each side
**Active recovery
  cool-down,** see page 161
43, 44, 45 × several
58

Unlike the highly-organized disciplines of classical ballet and ballet music, which are strictly notated and choreographed down to the last note or step, jazz dance and jazz music rely as much on spontaneity and improvisation as they do on a written score. And there is another difference: in classical music and ballet everything happens on the beat; in jazz the accent of the rhythm is more often syncopated – i.e. more likely to be off the beat than on it.

Hands are very important and often used with palms facing forwards and fingers spread ('jazz palms') to initiate, emphasize or finish a movement.

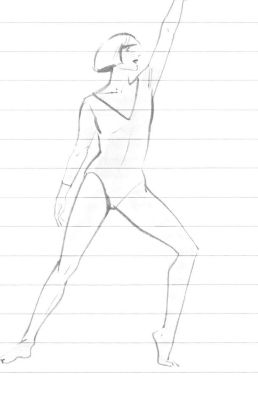

141 **SIDES** *This jazzed-up version of the side lunge and upward stretch (69) works as a good warm-up and will also help you with your timing. Stand with feet 60 cm (2 ft) apart and slightly turned out. Lunge onto right leg lifting right arm to ceiling, palm facing front, for a really good stretch. Repeat to left. Start by stretching to each side for 8 counts, then 4 counts, then 2 counts, then 1 count. Remember to count up to 8 twice through at each stage, so that you are stretching twice to each side to begin with, 8 times to each side to finish. Now run through the exercise again, lifting your heel off the ground but still stretching as far as possible to each side.*

Once you've got the idea, try it to music

142 **HIPS** Stand with feet hip-width apart and parallel. Bend knees and tilt hips up and forwards, then back to centre, then to back. Now try it again but this time move hips forwards and back, passing smoothly through the centre each time.

Starting with hips well centered again, move them to right, to centre, to left and back to centre. Then move them straight through from right to left, passing smoothly through the centre each time.

Now try a square: tilt hips forwards, to right, to back, to left and forwards again before finishing back in the centre. Practise in both directions.

Finish with a circle: tilt hips forwards, then curve them to left, to back, to right and forwards again. Return to the centre and reverse the movement.

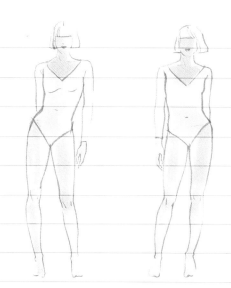

Isolations, one of the signature movements of classical jazz, aim to get ribcage and hips moving independently of each other. At first, only small movements may be possible, but persevere. You will become more supple with practice...

143 **RIBCAGE** Stand well with feet hip-width apart, arms by sides, spine lengthened and ribcage lifted.

Now move ribcage forwards over hips, then to centre, then to back; then, lifting ribcage as before, move it forwards and back, passing smoothly through centre each time.

Lift ribcage again and move it to right, to centre, and to left; then move it to right and left, passing smoothly through centre each time you change.

Now try making a square: lift ribcage and move it forwards, then to left, then back, then to right, then forwards and, finally, back to centre. Try it in other direction too.

Finish with a circle: lift ribcage and move it forwards, then round to right, lthen to back, then round to left, then forwards again before coming back to centre. Try it in both directions.

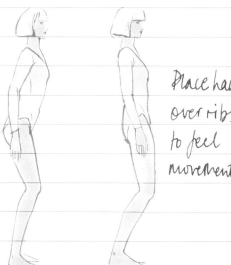

Place hands over ribs to feel movement

144 **BALANCE** Try this jazz version of last week's exercise. Standing in second position, with arms at shoulder level, raise arms upwards so that palms are facing forwards. Now rise up onto balls of feet, keeping legs fully extended, for 2 counts. Lower heels to floor for 2 counts. Practise 8 times. Then repeat whole exercise, raising and lowering heels for 1 count each time.

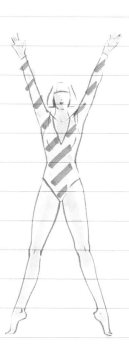

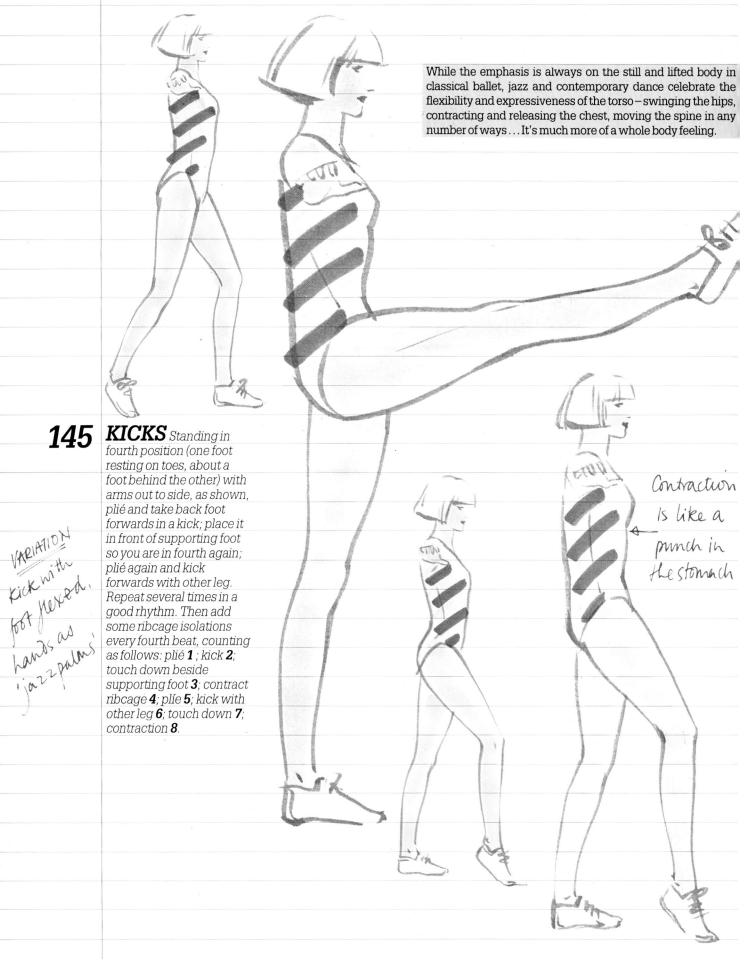

While the emphasis is always on the still and lifted body in classical ballet, jazz and contemporary dance celebrate the flexibility and expressiveness of the torso – swinging the hips, contracting and releasing the chest, moving the spine in any number of ways... It's much more of a whole body feeling.

145 KICKS *Standing in fourth position (one foot resting on toes, about a foot behind the other) with arms out to side, as shown, plié and take back foot forwards in a kick; place it in front of supporting foot so you are in fourth again; plié again and kick forwards with other leg. Repeat several times in a good rhythm. Then add some ribcage isolations every fourth beat, counting as follows: plié **1** ; kick **2**; touch down beside supporting foot **3**; contract ribcage **4**; plié **5**; kick with other leg **6**; touch down **7**; contraction **8**.*

VARIATION
Kick with foot flexed. hands as 'jazz palms'

Contraction is like a punch in the stomach

204

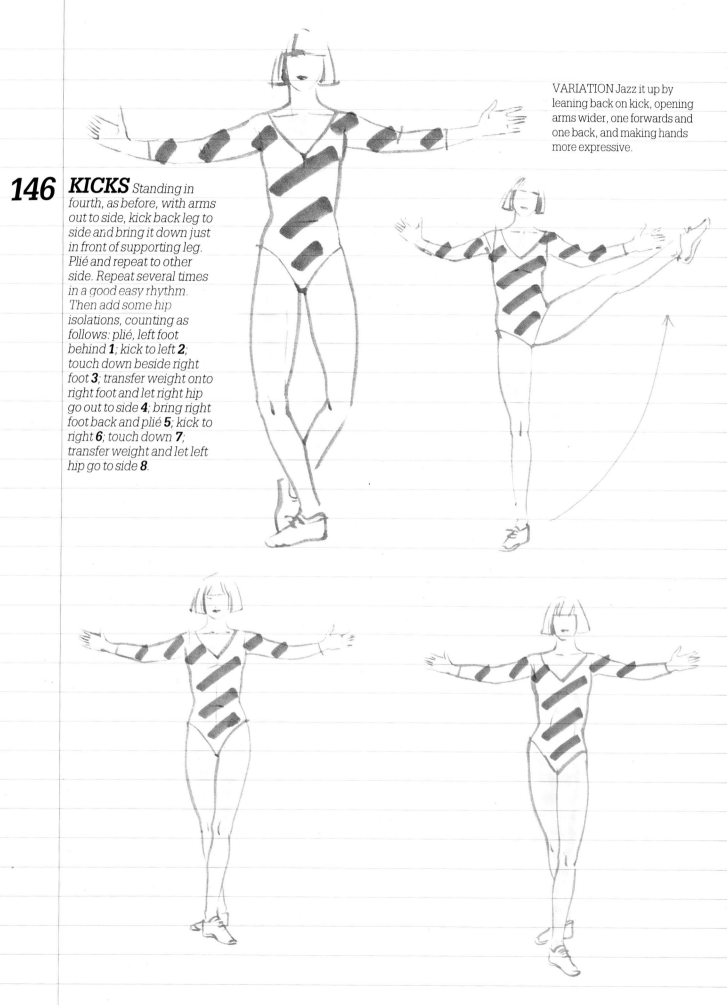

VARIATION Jazz it up by leaning back on kick, opening arms wider, one forwards and one back, and making hands more expressive.

146 | ***KICKS*** *Standing in fourth, as before, with arms out to side, kick back leg to side and bring it down just in front of supporting leg. Plié and repeat to other side. Repeat several times in a good easy rhythm. Then add some hip isolations, counting as follows: plié, left foot behind **1**; kick to left **2**; touch down beside right foot **3**; transfer weight onto right foot and let right hip go out to side **4**; bring right foot back and plié **5**; kick to right **6**; touch down **7**; transfer weight and let left hip go to side **8**.*

WEEK 24: GRADUATION

Week 24, graduating with honours, and you will be feeling really fit – strong, agile, powerful, swift and in altogether better shape than you have probably been for a long time.

   After all this regular exercising, you may now want to have a break, perhaps to take up a new sport or exercise form, such as fencing, yoga or one of the 3 training schedules on pages 218-25. Have the confidence to try anything. Your body is perfectly primed for the challenge.

This week's programme
Preliminaries
116 × 2, breathing well
140 × 4 each side
147 × 3 each side
148 × 4, breathing well
149 × 2 each way
150 × 4 each side
151
Active recovery
   cool-down, see page 1(
84 × several
103, hands behind head
   holding 0.5 kg/(1 lb)
   weight, work up to 5
52 × several
85 with 1 kg/(2 lb) weight
   on each ankle until
   muscles begin to tire
152 × up to 20
6-minute freestyle
   aerobic sequence OR
   Rock and roll/Jazz
   routine
Active recovery cool
   cool-down, see page 1(
39, aiming to rest head
   on legs with back flat
   × 1
43, 44, 45 × several
58
124

147 **CROUCH** *Standing with feet about 60 cm (2 ft) apart, do a small pelvic tilt and lift up onto toes, bringing arms out to balance. Bend knees and twist slowly to side and then round to the back, dropping leading arm to touch far ankle. Return to front equally slowly. Repeat 4 times smoothly to each side.*

BONUS
Excellent for balance

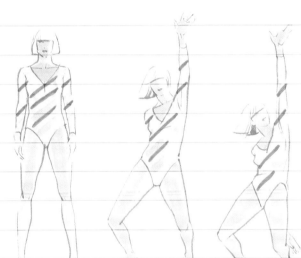

To finish, a super-class to help maintain fitness, and a few more demanding exercises. Try them and, for future weeks, change the programme to incorporate earlier exercises you found helpful. Good luck!

148 **ARMS** *Sitting cross-legged in your non-habitual way (remember week 4, exercise 40?), with spine lengthened and chest lifted, raise arms above head and cross hands so palms are together. Work arms down towards head, pressing palms together and elbows back. Then work them up again. Cross hands the other way and repeat. Practise exercise twice.*

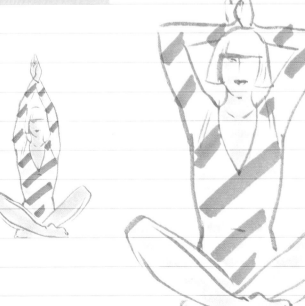

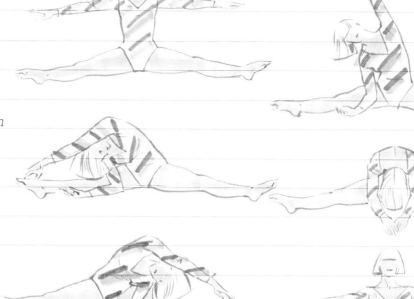

149 WAIST AND LEGS
Sit on floor with legs apart and arms out at shoulder level. Lift right arm up, twist and stretch onto left knee. Keeping back flat, continue round in a circle to right knee. As you come back up, raise right leg, without leaning back, so that it is fully extended and naturally turned out. Release and repeat to other side. Work up to 5 repetitions on each side.

Are you leaning back or over to side when you lift leg? Use a mirror to check or ask someone to watch.

Point foot too, for a different stretch

150 BACKS OF THIGHS
Lie on back. Bend one knee and press it into chest for 7 counts. Then extend leg, keeping knee pulled up, and flex foot. Pull leg back, gently but firmly, breathing out for 4 counts. Repeat with other leg. Do 4 times.

151 SQUATS
Now extend your aerobic sequence to 10 minutes and add these side squats. Squat down, place both hands on floor and stretch one leg out to side. Now hop leg back in to meet the other and then stretch other leg out, keeping both hands on floor all the time.

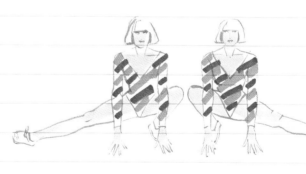

CAUTION Not for weak knees. See Therapeutics section on page 243 instead.

152 UPPER BODY
Lie down on your front, hands just under shoulders. Keeping body long and straight, breathe in. As you breathe out, push yourself up, maintaining line in back. Breathe in and lower, without touching floor, and breathe out and push up again. Start with 5 press-ups and work up to 20 in sets of 5.

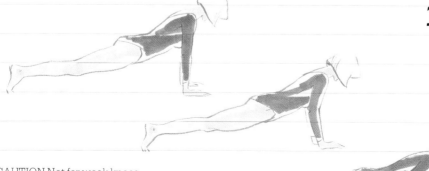

Rock and roll

This rock and roll sequence is divided into six sections. Learn one each day and then put them all together on the seventh for the complete dance routine. The *da capo* musical symbol (:‖) at the end of a musical phrase indicates the end of a section. Once you reach it, go right back to the beginning again and practise that part of the sequence again, until you get the steps right. Then put it to music, using one of the suggestions given.

When you get to the lifts (Day 5), bear in mind that these are extended jumps – your partner should never have to support your full weight. Practise several small lifts before aiming for the height shown here.

Music to practise to

Duke's Place by Duke Ellington
In The Mood by Glen Miller
Swing Brother Swing by Count Basie
Rock Around the Clock by Bill Haley

Glossary

Air step any acrobatic movement involving a jump or a lift.
Charleston exuberant dance step from which many of the later ones evolved, involving flicking feet out to either side (partners use opposite feet).
Hip swings an air step in which the woman swings her legs up to one side, resting her hip on his hip, and then to the other without landing inbetween.
Lindy break series of steps used to finish a dance phrase and prepare for the next, usually involving some sort of air step and twist.
Lindy hop a syncopated kick, travelling across the floor, changing legs between each kick.
Straddle split a floor step performed by the man, who balances on one hand and shoots his legs out from underneath him.
The rock the basic rock and roll step, forwards and back holding hands and then changing places.
Through the trenches a stationary step kicking to front, side, back and side again, finishing by jumping with legs apart and then together.

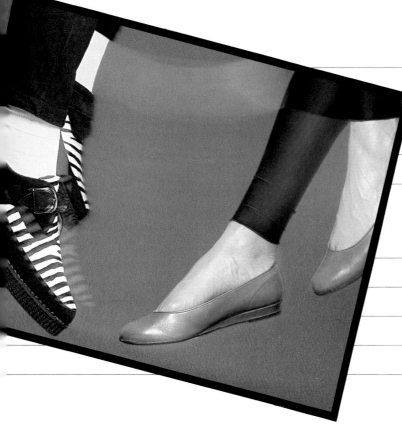

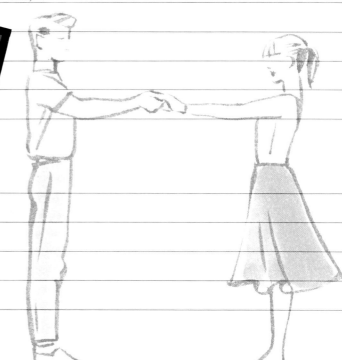

Start facing each other with hands joined, and feet together.

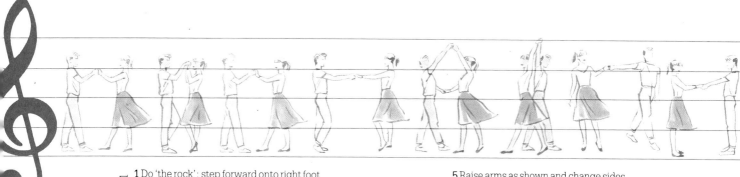

DAY 1
1 Do 'the rock': step forward onto right foot
2 and bring left foot up, lifting heel.
3 Step back with left foot,
4 returning to starting position.

5 Raise arms as shown and change sides
6 by stepping underneath his arm
7 and out to the side, bringing arms down
8 to finish facing each other.

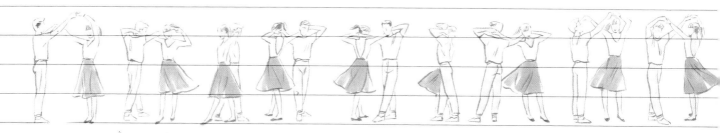

1 Now repeat 'the rock'. Step onto right foot
2 and bring left foot up, lifting heel.
3 Step back with left foot
4 returning to starting position.

5 Raise arms
6 stepping underneath his arm again
7 and to the side. Bring arms down
8 to finish in starting position

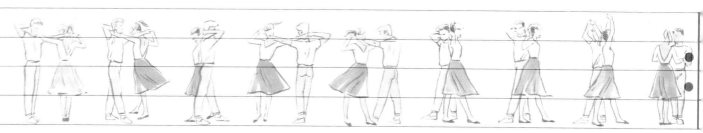

AND Take arms up
1 and, resting them behind head, step round to right
2, 3, 4, 5, 6 for 7 steps, starting with the right foot and

7 bringing arms up on the seventh.
8 Swivel round on the spot to right, through 180 degrees.

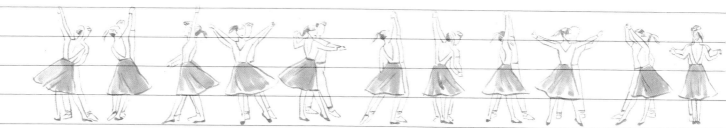

AND Rest arms behind head again
1, 2, 3, 4, 5, 6 and step round to left for 7 steps

7 bringing arms up on the seventh and uncrossing them
8 to finish facing each other.

DAY 2
1,2 Stepping to her right (his left), swing arms up.
3,4 Stepping to left, swing arms up.
5 Turn to left, bringing lower arms through
6 and continue turning, through back-to-back position,
7, 8 until facing each other again.

1, 2 Stepping to left (his right), swing arms up.
3, 4 Stepping to right, swing arms up.
5 Turn to left, bring lower arms through
6 and continue turning, through back-to-back position,
7, 8 until facing each other again.

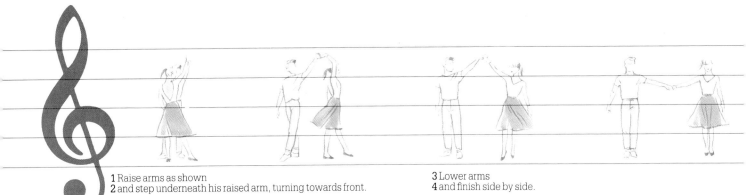

1 Raise arms as shown
2 and step underneath his raised arm, turning towards front.

3 Lower arms
4 and finish side by side.

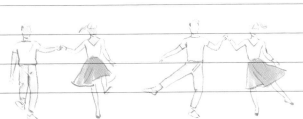

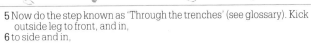

5 Now do the step known as 'Through the trenches' (see glossary). Kick outside leg to front, and in,
6 to side and in,

7 to back, and in,
8 and to side again.

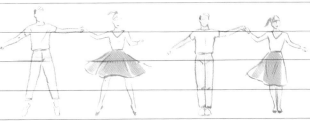

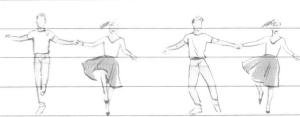

1 Jump feet apart, bending knees,
2 and together again

3 Go 'Through the trenches' again, kicking inside leg to front,
4 to side,

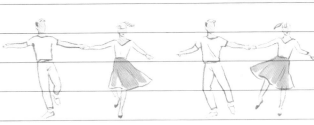

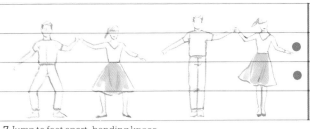

5 to back,
6 and to side again.

7 Jump to feet apart, bending knees
8 and together again.

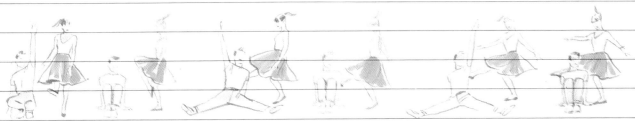

DAY 3

1 Facing front, he crouches down, left arm raised. She does the 'Lindy hop', kicking right foot out.
AND He lowers arm, takes weight onto left hand. She hops onto right foot, starting to travel around him.
2 He raises right arm and does a 'Straddle split'. She kicks left foot out.

3 He lowers arm, brings knees up, takes weight onto right hand. She kicks right foot out.
4 He raises left arm and does a 'Straddle split'. She kicks left foot out.
5 He lowers arm, brings knees up, transfers weight. She kicks right foot out.

210

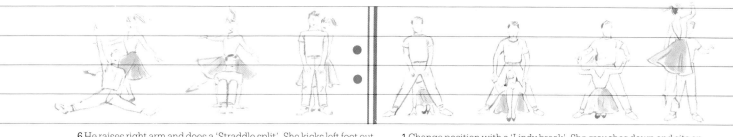

6 He raises right arm and does a 'Straddle split'. She kicks left foot out.
7 He lowers arm, brings knees up, transfers weight. She kicks right foot out.
8 Finish, as shown, with her directly behind him.

DAY 4
1 Change position with a 'Lindy break'. She crouches down and sits on the floor, he reaches for her hands
2 and pulls her through.
3 She squats down and jumps into a turn of 360 degrees,
4 to land in front of him, bending knees.

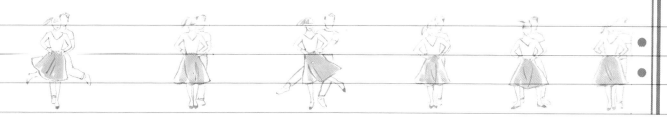

5 With his hands over hers, they do a 'Charleston' – she kicks to right and he kicks to left –
AND and then, touching down,
6 she kicks to left and he kicks to right,

AND and then, touching down,
7 jump feet apart
8 and together again.

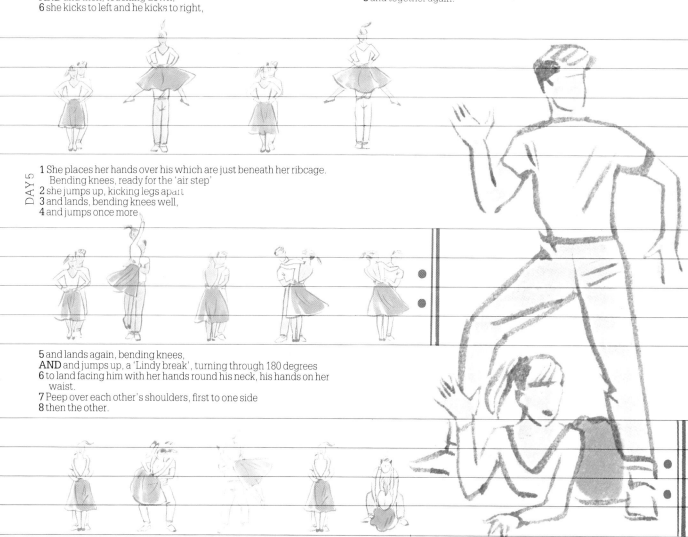

DAY 5
1 She places her hands over his which are just beneath her ribcage. Bending knees, ready for the 'air step'
2 she jumps up, kicking legs apart
3 and lands, bending knees well,
4 and jumps once more

5 and lands again, bending knees,
AND and jumps up, a 'Lindy break', turning through 180 degrees
6 to land facing him with her hands round his neck, his hands on her waist.
7 Peep over each other's shoulders, first to one side
8 then the other.

DAY 6
1 Bending knees,
2 she jumps into a 'Hip swing', swinging her legs to one side so her hip and thigh are resting on his hip
3 and then to the other side, without landing in between.
4 Landing in front of him, she bends knees well

5 and slides through his legs
6, 7, 8 to turn on her front. Both wave hands.

Jazz

This jazz sequence, like the rock and roll one on the previous pages, is divided into six sections – with a *da capo* symbol (:||) at the end of each section. Learn one each day and then put the whole routine together on the seventh.

If unfamiliar with jazz and jazz music, start simply by choosing one of the musical options suggested and tap or clap the beat. Once you feel easy with it, take off the music and work out the steps (preferably wearing jazz or other leather-soled shoes). *Then* put music and steps together. When you get the swing of it, incorporate the variations suggested in the text beneath the pictures. Feel free to improvise, too. Learn more by taking classes. These are now offered at many exercise and dance studios.

Glossary

Battement a kick or leg lift.
Epaulement a shoulder movement in which one shoulder is thrust forward and the other back; always performed *in opposition* (see below) with walking step.
Jazz attitude a striking posture in which leg is lifted and held, bent either forwards or back – a jazz equivalent of the classical arabesque.
Jazz palms hands held flexed at wrist so that palms face forwards.
Lay-back leg kicks forwards as torso leans back – a wide, open movement.
Lunge weight transfer forwards, backwards or to one side, bending knee.
Opposition stationary movement or walking step in which shoulder or arm goes forward with opposite foot.
Plié bended knees, usually in preparation for a movement such as a kick.

Music to practise to

Brazilia by John Klemmer
Tropico by Gato Barbieri
Sanborn by David Sanborn
The Shuffle by Kenny G
Rise by Herb Alpert

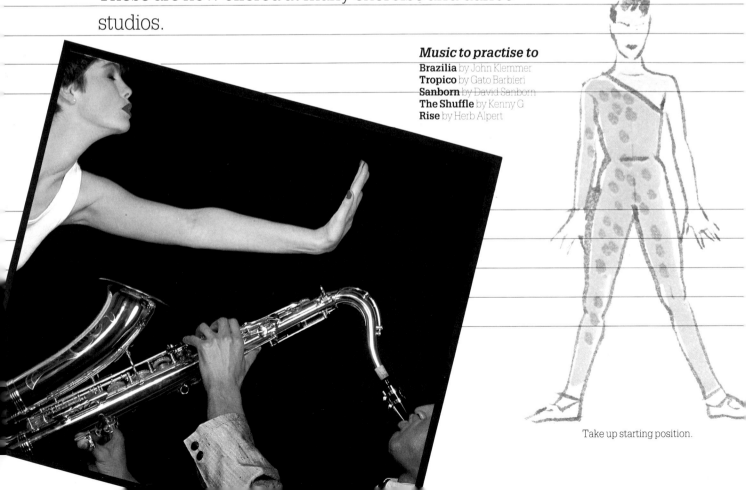

Take up starting position.

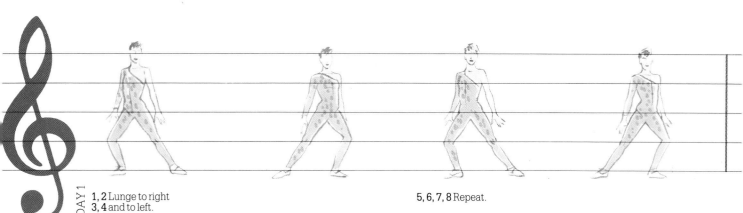

1, 2 Lunge to right
3, 4 and to left.

5, 6, 7, 8 Repeat.

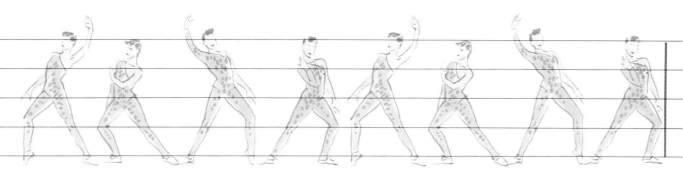

1 Lunge to right, lifting heel,
2 lower heel.
3 Lunge to left, lifting heel
4 lower heel.

5, 6, 7, 8 Repeat.

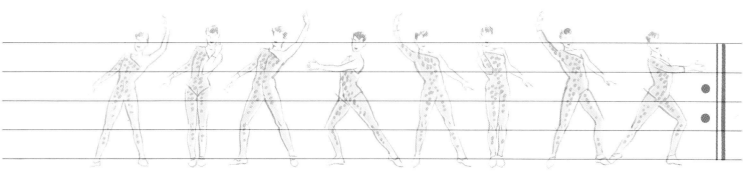

1 Raise left arm and lunge to right, lifting heel
2 and circling arm round in front, lower heel.
3 Raise right arm and lunge to left, lifting heel
4 and circling arm round in front, lower heel.

5, 6, 7, 8 Repeat.

1 Raise left arm and, stepping out with right foot, start circling arm
   above head in lasso action,
2 finishing your circle as you bring in left foot to right foot.
3 Step out to right once more and start to circle upper arm again,
4 this time bringing outstretched arm straight across body, palm facing
   to back, as you bend right knee and lunge forward.

5, 6, 7, 8 Repeat with right arm raised, stepping to left.

213

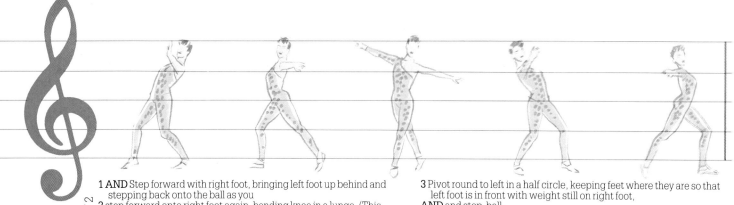

1 AND Step forward with right foot, bringing left foot up behind and stepping back onto the ball as you
2 step forward onto right foot again, bending knee in a lunge. (This movement is easier to do than to read and is called 'step-ball-change'. It has a slight jump at the moment when you transfer the weight from right to left and back to right again, rather like a gallop or a polka step.)

3 Pivot round to left in a half circle, keeping feet where they are so that left foot is in front with weight still on right foot,
AND and step-ball-
4 change with left foot leading, finishing in a lunge with arms to side.

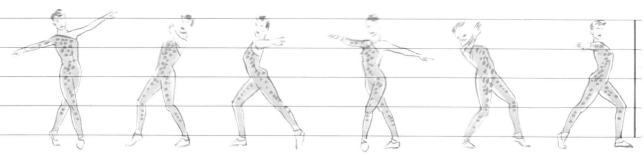

5, 6, 7, 8 Repeat.

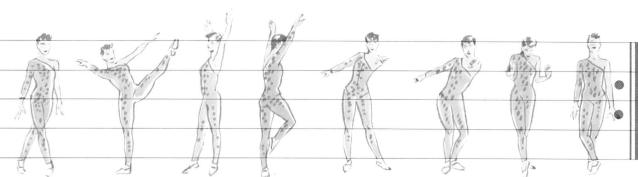

1 Bring arms down and swivel torso to right, so right foot is in front. Take weight onto it
2 and 'Lay-back', kicking leg out to the front, opening arms in a low V.
3 Keeping hands up, return foot to floor, then,
4 transferring weight, bring right toe to left knee and swivel round to right through 360 degrees, lowering arms.

5 Step to side with right foot
6 and swing hip to right, arms in opposition.
7 Contract ribcage (as though punched in stomach), bringing hands up, head down and pointing right foot
8 as you draw it over left foot, bringing hands down, head back

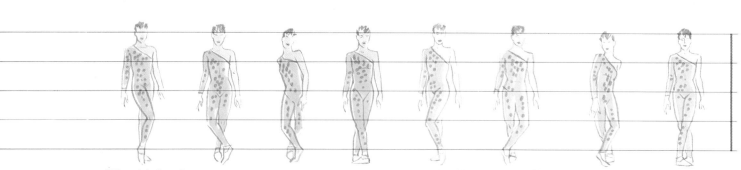

1 Turn right knee in
2 and out again.
3 Plié, pushing left shoulder forwards and across,
4 then return to centre, straightening legs.

5, 6, 7, 8 Repeat, using left knee and right shoulder.

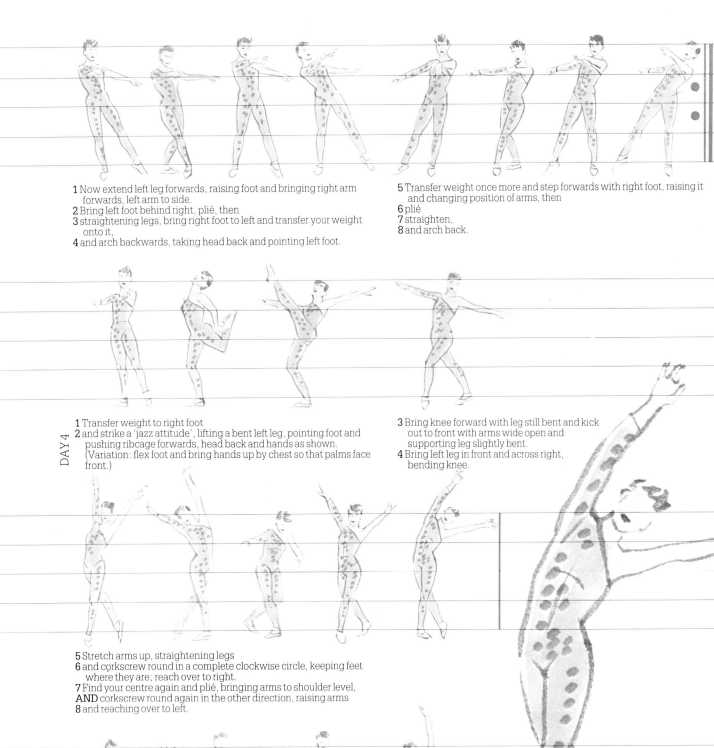

1 Now extend left leg forwards, raising foot and bringing right arm forwards, left arm to side.
2 Bring left foot behind right, plié, then
3 straightening legs, bring right foot to left and transfer your weight onto it,
4 and arch backwards, taking head back and pointing left foot.

5 Transfer weight once more and step forwards with right foot, raising it and changing position of arms, then
6 plié
7 straighten,
8 and arch back.

DAY 4

1 Transfer weight to right foot
2 and strike a 'jazz attitude', lifting a bent left leg, pointing foot and pushing ribcage forwards, head back and hands as shown. (Variation: flex foot and bring hands up by chest so that palms face front.)

3 Bring knee forward with leg still bent and kick out to front with arms wide open and supporting leg slightly bent.
4 Bring left leg in front and across right, bending knee.

5 Stretch arms up, straightening legs
6 and corkscrew round in a complete clockwise circle, keeping feet where they are; reach over to right.
7 Find your centre again and plié, bringing arms to shoulder level,
AND corkscrew round again in the other direction, raising arms
8 and reaching over to left.

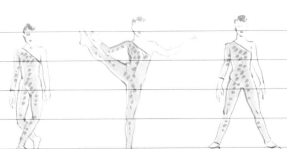

DAY 5

1 Return to centre, straightening up and bringing arms down; plié,
2 and kick right foot to side with both legs straight and foot pointed.
3 Return foot to floor in second position
4 and raise left arm at the same time as you begin to plié.

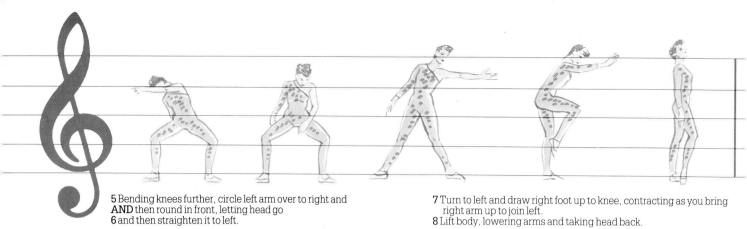

5 Bending knees further, circle left arm over to right and
AND then round in front, letting head go
6 and then straighten it to left.

7 Turn to left and draw right foot up to knee, contracting as you bring
   right arm up to join left.
8 Lift body, lowering arms and taking head back.

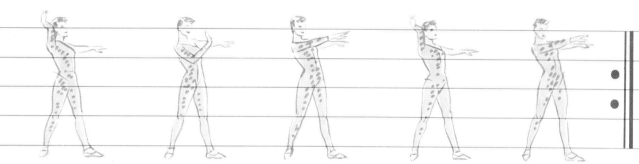

1 Step forwards onto right foot, arms in opposition,
AND and step-ball-change
2 so right foot still leads.

3 Lift left knee, changing arms, then
4 return foot to floor in fourth position.

5 Take right arm behind head,
AND then push flexed hand firmly forwards from shoulder,

6 finishing with arm straight out, palm downwards.
7, 8 Repeat.

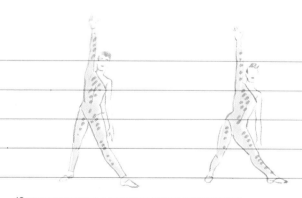

DAY 6 WARM UP WELL BEFORE ATTEMPTING THIS
1, 2 Lower left arm and raise right as you go forwards from hips, sliding
   front foot forwards and bending back leg.

3 Be prepared to take weight onto left hand as you get lower and let
   right knee rest on floor,
4 letting body roll to left to sit down, relaxing right knee if necessary.

Using hand to support weight helps prevent pulled muscles, pain in
hips . . . but only do this when well warmed up and never go further
than feels comfortable.

216

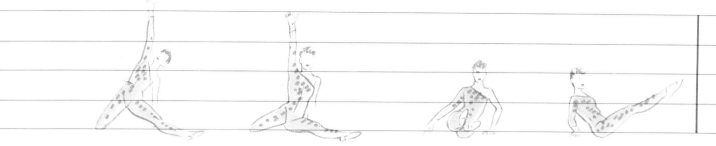

5 Raise right hip, pushing up with left hand and looking up.
6 Return to floor, then

7 take right leg forwards to join left in centre. Lift feet and point them, transferring weight so that it is evenly distributed on sitting bones
8 and swing body and legs round in a half circle to left,

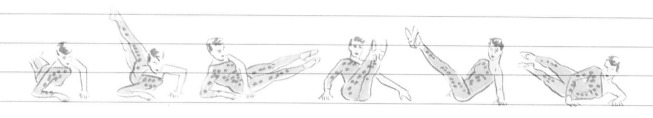

AND 1 bending right knee and letting it rest on floor as you turn onto your front and raise left leg.
2 Push off again and swing round to do the same thing on the other side.

3 so that legs travel round to front, then round to right and behind,
AND 4 bending left knee and letting it rest on floor as you turn onto your front and raise right leg.

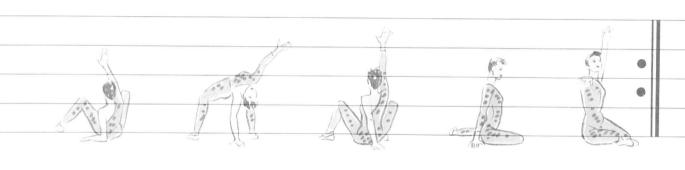

5 Turn body to right so you are sitting with weight on left elbow
6 and push hips up with your left hand, raising right arm and letting head go back.
7 Lower to floor again, keeping right arm raised, then
AND lower arm and let both knees fall to right.
8 Raise left arm up, right arm to side and finish.

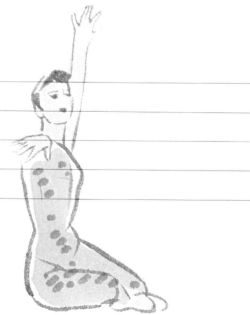

Sports days

Variety is an important part of getting fit. Enjoy sports as well as exercise routines. The key is to choose what you most enjoy, because you will then discover that finding time to exercise ceases to be a problem and becomes a priority – something that you look forward to, enjoy doing and feel good for having done.

The secret is not to expect to continue doing anything for ever – even the most enjoyable activity can pall after a while. Enjoy the challenge of taking up a sport and becoming competent at it, and when you get bored take a break and switch to something new.

On the following pages, you will find training notes and fitness schedules for running, swimming and cycling... basic sports that are reasonably accessible, effective from the fitness point of view and do not require any special expertise, being skills usually learned in childhood.

The schedules are organized in 8 stages: the first is beginner level, the last advanced enough to give heart and lungs substantial aerobic benefits. Start at stage 1 *whatever your level of fitness* and progress stage by stage, graduating only when you feel entirely comfortable with the stage you are on – that means refreshed and energized at the end of a session, not breathless, gasping and nauseous. Aim, ideally, to fit in 3 sessions of your chosen sport a week (or alternate them), but do not try to exercise every day. Rest days are as important as sports days. And remember: these sports days are non-competitive. It's enjoyment that's important, fitness that's the prize.

NB Take your pulse, as directed on page 160, at the start of each new stage as an additional way of monitoring fitness.

RUNNING

RUNNING is simple, easy, accessible, great for mind as well as body, needs little equipment beyond a good pair of training shoes and is one of the most effective ways of getting, and keeping, fit.

RUNNING IS FOR YOU if you are in reasonably good shape before starting.

RUNNING IS NOT FOR YOU if you are very overweight (12.5 kg/2 stone over) as it may place unacceptable strains on heart and joints. Get weight down first, complementing diet with gentle exercise, such as brisk walking or swimming or following the early weeks of the exercise programme. Consult your doctor first if you have problems with heart or high blood pressure, have not exercised for a considerable time or have any doubts about your health.

HOW TO START. Simply get outside for 30 minutes, walking to begin with, then walking/jogging, then jogging and finally running when you feel able. Use the fitness schedule to give you something to aim for, but remember it's not a race: go at your own pace.
Don't run every day; 3 to 4 times a week is quite enough. Rest days will give you a chance to recover energy and help to guard against boredom, keep enthusiasm high.

HOW TO RUN. Sort out your style before you start as postural faults are exaggerated on moving faster. Watch middle-distance (1500-metre) runners on television for an idea of the correct action – legs lifted, upper body still, arms relaxed. Notice, too, that they use the whole of the foot when they run, rolling from heel through to toes. Running on the balls of the feet will not slim thighs or strengthen legs, just tire them unnecessarily. Train on different surfaces – athletic tracks (the best) pavements, parkland, canal towpaths, the beach, up and down hills – and vary the route to help sustain interest.

YOU WILL NEED good quality training shoes. Look for *support* and *cushioning* (at least 2 cm/¾ in on the heel, 1.5 cm/½ in on the sole); *flexibility*, they should bend easily back about a third of the way from the toes; *comfort and fit*, they should feel comfortable right away. Training shoes should never need 'running in'. Also necessary: cotton socks, all-weather tracksuit and jerseys for cold weather, T-shirts, shorts, a good supporting bra and a pedometer (optional).

WARM UP with 10 minutes general stretching. Try yoga sun salutation (116), and general stretches (32, 53, 69). It is particularly important to stretch backs of legs and calves (46, 59 and 39, remembering to hinge forward from hips as you drop down so you feel a stretch along backs of legs).

COOL DOWN by walking the last half-mile home; don't just flake out and stop (see note on page 161). Add a few easy stretches to keep blood flowing to muscles and help guard against stiffness and soreness later.

SUPPLEMENT with mobility exercises for arms (109), shoulders (110) and spine (43, 44, 45); strengtheners for upper body (72, 101) and abdomen (103, 85).

MAKE IT MORE ENJOYABLE: by running with a friend, joining a club, running in the country and on varied surfaces; by taking a pedometer and timing yourself over a given distance or noting down changes in pulse rate, *as instructed on page 160*, and so monitoring progress; by using your imagination – visualize a sail unfurling behind you, a river flowing in the direction you are heading or a breeze blowing – to give you stamina and prevent tiredness taking a hold; by using running time as time off from all the problems and pressures at home – let your attention rest lightly on the moment and feel yourself becoming calmer as your mind becomes quieter.

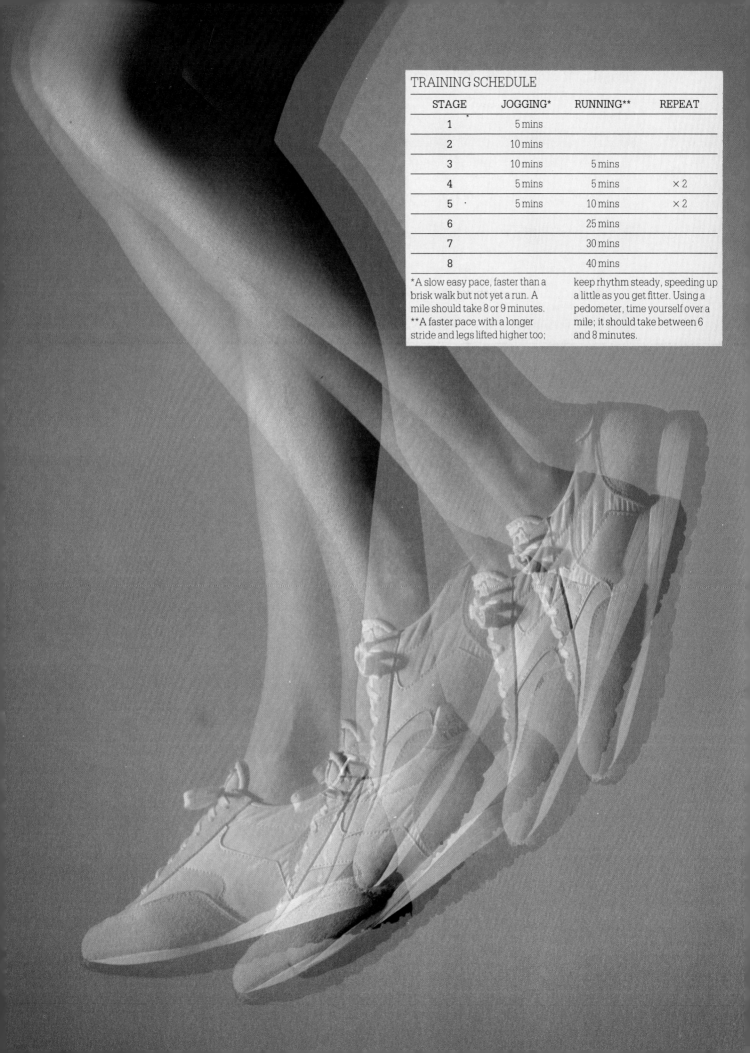

TRAINING SCHEDULE

STAGE	JOGGING*	RUNNING**	REPEAT
1	5 mins		
2	10 mins		
3	10 mins	5 mins	
4	5 mins	5 mins	× 2
5	5 mins	10 mins	× 2
6		25 mins	
7		30 mins	
8		40 mins	

*A slow easy pace, faster than a brisk walk but not yet a run. A mile should take 8 or 9 minutes.
**A faster pace with a longer stride and legs lifted higher too; keep rhythm steady, speeding up a little as you get fitter. Using a pedometer, time yourself over a mile; it should take between 6 and 8 minutes.

CYCLING

CYCLING is fun and marvellous if you find organized exercise classes a waste of time, because it gets you somewhere as it gets you fit. A car would have to do over 1,000 miles to the gallon to be as economical.

CYCLING IS FOR YOU if you are reasonably fit and have no history of back or knee trouble.

CYCLING IS NOT FOR YOU if you have back trouble or weak knees or consider your leg muscles overdeveloped (take your exercise horizontal instead, *see next page*).

HOW TO START. Gently – in quiet lanes and/or side streets, keeping within a reasonable distance of home. Do not cycle in heavy traffic until confident of cycling ability.

HOW TO CYCLE. With your legs, not your back; crucial to prevent back strain due to muscles shortening and tightening . . . Use your feet as you pedal, rotating ankles and not just pumping legs up and down. Change gears for best training effect: use high ones to pedal fast for heart and health benefits and low ones to increase resistance.

YOU WILL NEED a good bicycle with *height of saddle* adjusted so that you can just balance with toes on the ground while sitting on it, at an *angle* that allows you to sit squarely and not tip forwards. Other necessities: gears, back and front lights, reflector strips, repair kit and instruction manual, pump, lock, bell and maps.

WARM UP with some general stretches, particularly for spine (69, 53) and backs of legs (46, 59). Start off with some slow pedalling to loosen joints, get blood flowing freely.

COOL DOWN with easy pedalling and a few general stretches, particularly backs of legs (59), upper back (4) and chest and shoulders (24) to help prevent stiffness.

SUPPLEMENT WITH mobility exercises for arms (109), shoulders (110) and spine (43, 44, 45); strengtheners for upper body (72, 101) and abdomen (103, 85).

MAKE IT MORE ENJOYABLE by joining a club, cycling with a friend, taking your bicycle on holiday or into the countryside, using maps to explore.

TRAINING SCHEDULE

STAGE	LEISURELY CYCLING	BRISK/UPHILL CYCLING	REPEAT
1	15 mins		
2	10 mins	5 mins	
3	10 mins	5 mins	× 2
4	10 mins	10 mins	× 2
5	15 mins	10 mins	× 2
6	15 mins	15 mins	× 2
7	10 mins	20 mins	× 2
8	10 mins	20 mins	× 3

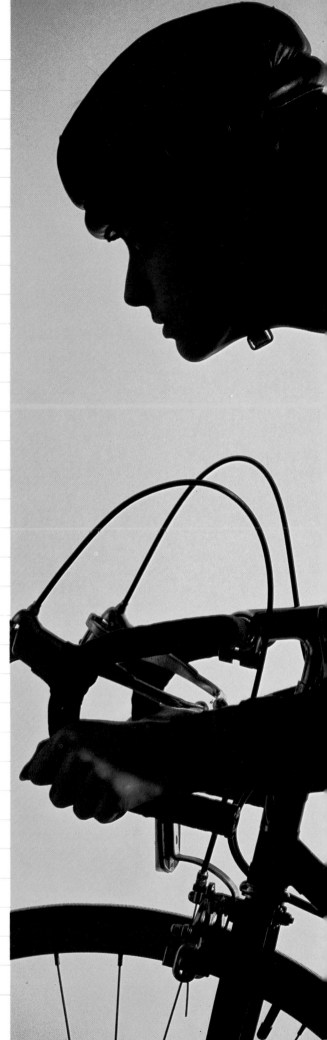

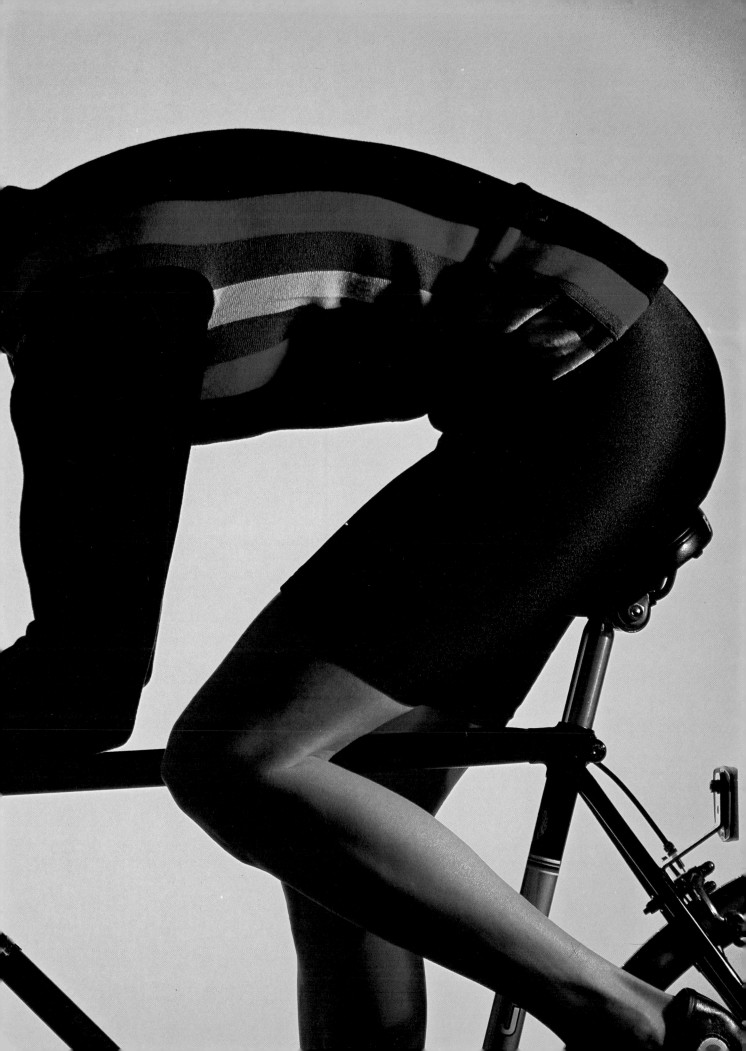

SWIMMING

SWIMMING can be one of the best all-round routes to fitness and relaxing with it. Water removes gravitational pull on bones and joints, so reducing chances of strain or injury, keeps you cool and sweat-free too...

SWIMMING IS FOR YOU if you are very overweight or pregnant, consider your leg muscles overdeveloped, or have joint problems or varicose veins (horizontal position reduces pressure on legs and supporting veins).

SWIMMING IS NOT FOR YOU if you do not have easy access to a pool or have never learned how – though it's never too late to start...

HOW TO START. Purely for pleasure: simply spend about 20 minutes in the pool, and forget about length counting until you feel fit enough to take on the training schedule.

HOW TO SWIM. Lazy breast-stroke or side-stroke up and down the lengths does nothing for heart and lungs, little to tone muscles or promote strength; you must swim fairly vigorously, alternating strokes for best effects. Front crawl gives great aerobic benefits and is a marvellous all-round body conditioner; front butterfly, breast-stroke, back-crawl and back butterfly are all good upper body strengtheners – areas most women do not exercise enough; leg kicks only (back or front holding onto float) streamlines lower body, slimming thighs and firming calves.

YOU WILL NEED a swimming costume cut high at the legs with elasticated straps, a swimcap to protect hair from chlorine or salt, earplugs or goggles if susceptible to ear or eye infections, a float to hold on to for leg-kick-only lengths, towel, hairdrier and warm clothes.

WARM UP with a few minutes general stretching and one or two easy lengths to help stretch muscles and prepare them for more vigorous work.

COOL DOWN with one or two easy lengths and some dry-land stretching.

SUPPLEMENT with some twists for the spine (43, 44, 45); strengtheners for abdomen (103, 85).

TRAINING SCHEDULE

STAGE	SWIMMING	LEG-KICK ONLY	'RESTING' STROKE*	REPEAT
1	2 mins	1 min	2 mins	× 3
2	4 mins	1 min	2 mins	× 3
3	3 mins	1 min	2 mins	× 4
4	4 mins	1 min	2 mins	× 4
5	4 mins	2 mins	2 mins	× 4
6	4 mins	1 min	1 min	× 6
7	5 mins	1 min	1 min	× 6
8	4 mins	1 min	1 min	× 8

Alternate a length of crawl with a length of breastroke; a length of crawl with a length of backstroke, and so on; incorporate butterfly, too, if you can do it.

*A long easy stroke on back or front.

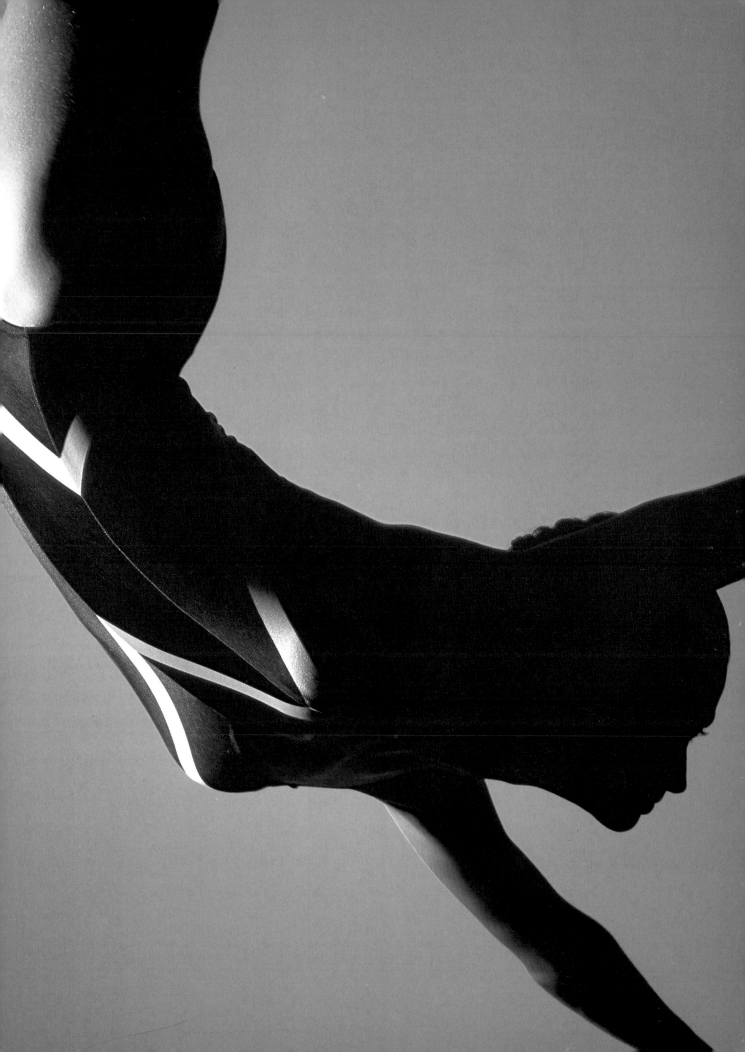

Pre-ski programme

The best guarantee of enjoyment on a skiing holiday is a strong, fit body because skiing makes great demands on muscles and joints. Here is a specially devised pre-ski programme to get you into top physical condition before leaving for the slopes. Give yourself at least 3 weeks to get fit and include an aerobic activity, such as jogging or skipping, to help build up stamina.

WARM UP well first to ease stiffness, lengthen muscles and loosen joints. Suggested sequence: 116, 32, 53, 69, 46 and 39.

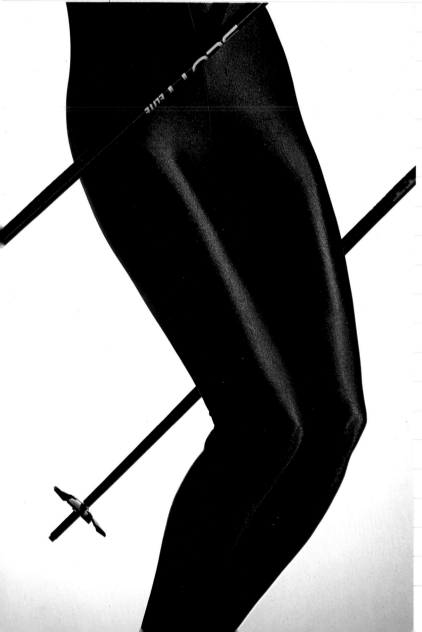

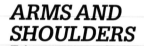

ARMS AND SHOULDERS
Take arms up to shoulder level and make loose fists. Circle them backwards several times, breathing well. Add 0.5 kg/1 lb weights to make this mobility exercise a strengthener too.

THIGHS *Stand with back to wall and gradually bend knees until sitting with thighs parallel to the floor. Stay there until muscles tire, gradually building up holding time to 1½ minutes.*

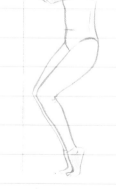

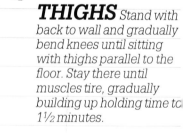

THIGHS *Stand with hands on wall, as shown, and bend knees. Bounce lightly up and down and continue until muscles tire.*

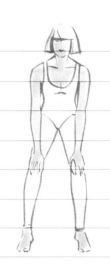
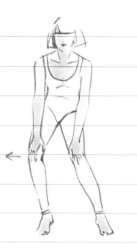
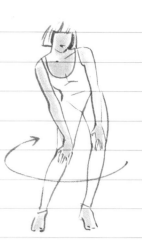

HIPS, KNEES AND ANKLES

Stand with knees slightly bent and feet hip-width apart. Place hands on knees, as shown, and sway from side to side in a good rhythm transferring your weight smoothly. Progress to making circles with your knees in both directions, clockwise and anti-clockwise, and finally try making figures-of-eight.

xcellent oosener ïv hips ınd ankles

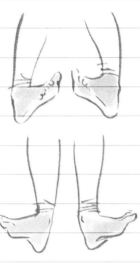

ANKLES *Sit with knees together and heels apart. Bring big toes, together, trying to lift them up as much as possible. Then brush outwards along floor again, pulling little toes upwards and pressing big toes down. Repeat until ankles and calves tire.*
Strong, mobile ankles are important for maintaining balance, absorbing impact.

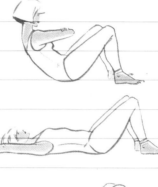

ABDOMEN *Sit with legs bent and feet hip-width apart. Breathe out as you bring chin towards chest, rounding back and lowering yourself backwards, pulling forwards with elbows at same time. Hold at point where you feel abdominal muscles tightening to prevent you falling backwards. Repeat several times.*
Now lie down on the floor and curl up, breathing out and bringing arms in front. Start by holding for 2 seconds and try to build to slow count of 5, but do not attempt to curl up any further than shown. Repeat several times. Progress to hands by your sides, arms folded in front and, finally, fingers interlocked behind head. Repeat exercise to either side to work diagonal abdominal muscles, pulling well across body with top arm each time.

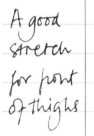
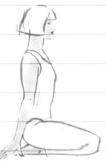

A good stretch for front of thighs

FRONT OF BODY *Sitting on heels, breathe in. As you breathe out, push buttocks upwards. Walk hands back along floor so spine stays lengthened as you arch up, letting head drop gently back. Hold for a few moments, then release.*

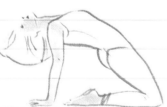

A relaxed body is much less prone to injury

FALLING *Falling is inevitable when skiing. Help overcome your fear of it by practising falling onto a soft sprung surface, letting your body drop and loosen into the movement rather than tensing and resisting it.*

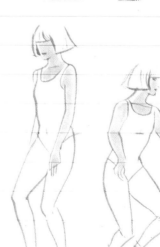
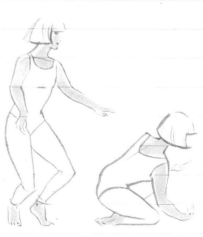

Exercising for childbirth

If keeping yourself fit with the exercises in this book is part of your normal routine, you will find very little change is necessary when you become pregnant. The same is true after the birth, when you should just work gradually from the first week of the programme until you attain your normal level of fitness. There are nevertheless some exercises which you will find particularly helpful and these are set out here.

Best to avoid during pregnancy: sports which involve running or jumping unless already used to them; lying on your front as soon as this becomes uncomfortable; lying on your back if this becomes uncomfortable or makes you feel breathless in late pregnancy; back bends if your back is giving you trouble.

Once used to this, try it away from wall, kneeling on all-fours, lying on back with knees bent (not in late pregnancy if uncomfortable), on your side and any other way you can think of.

BEFORE

PELVIC TILT

This important movement lengthens muscles of lower back and helps keep abdominal muscles strong enough to take weight of growing baby. Start against a wall so you cannot cheat by moving top half as well. Feet should be slightly apart and away from wall and knees slightly bent. Feel back of head, shoulder blades and spine resting against wall and breathe in. As you breathe out, press back of waist into wall so that bottom moves away from it a little. This is a very small movement. Repeat several times slowly with correct breathing.

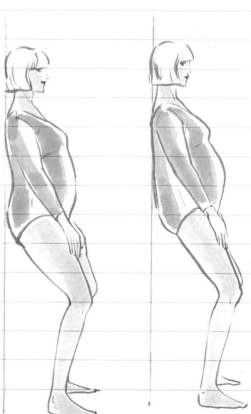

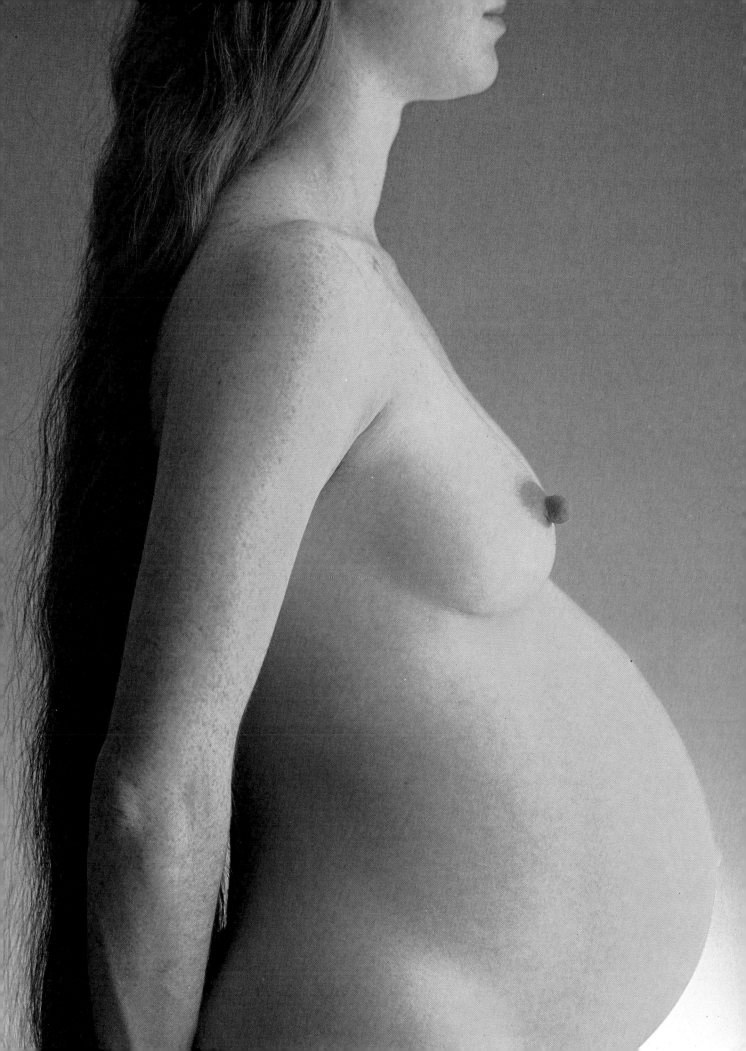

Try this all-fours version during labour. Circling pelvis and rocking whole body back and forth in this position can also help. So try it out regularly well beforehand in case you want to use it on the day.

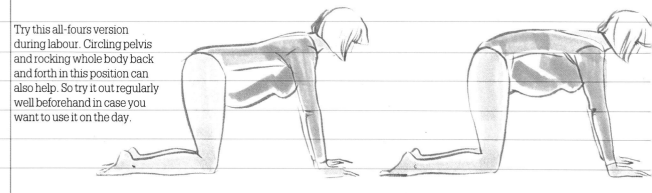

Although it is important to be fit and strong for birth, you should not overstrain yourself during pregnancy (or, indeed, at any time) and that includes forcing yourself to take exercise when you don't feel like it. Listen to your body, and if you feel like taking a great deal of rest, take it – particularly in the first months when you may find you are much more tired than usual. If you stay in tune with your needs and those of your baby, you will find that the day will come when you feel like doing some gentle movements to keep your body strong and supple, ready for the remarkable physical feat of giving birth.

SIDEWAYS PELVIC TILT

Standing with feet apart, lift left hip towards left ribs and then right hip towards right ribs. Repeat several times, transferring smoothly from side to side with a good rhythm, and then try it with knees bent.

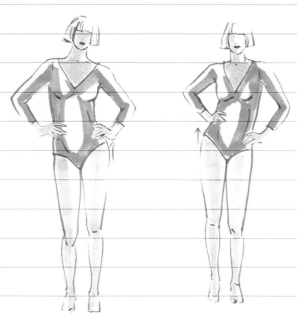

Mobility of the pelvis is essential for comfort during pregnancy and is also very important during labour, especially if you wish to have an active birth when you will be using your body to help you and the baby in every way you can.

PELVIC ROTATIONS *Try*

this kneeling down at first so that you can practise circling pelvis slowly all the way round, clockwise and anti-clockwise, without swaying from thighs. Then enjoy it standing, with knees slightly bent.

Rocking movements are very soothing for you and your baby and you may find them useful in labour

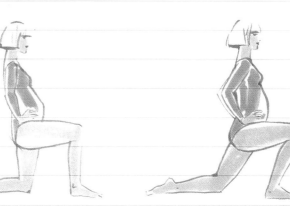

PELVIC ROCKING *Try*

rocking pelvis to and fro in a half-kneeling position, allowing thighs to rock too.

POSTURE CHECK

Starting from your pelvis, check that you are centred and not tipping lower part of pelvis back, shortening and arching your back (this is a very common fault in pregnancy as the bulge grows in front). Check, too, that you are not throwing pelvis too far forwards into pelvic tilt position (this is rarer). Now ask yourself these questions: Is weight evenly distributed between heels and balls of feet with arches well lifted in centre? Are knees at ease and neither pushed too far back nor bent? Is spine lengthened right up to base of skull, so that you feel as though you are being pulled upwards from centre of crown of head? Are shoulders sloping down as far away from ears as possible? Is head balanced easily on neck with chin at about a right angle to throat? Is lower jaw free or is it pressed upwards so that teeth are clenched (practise yawning if it is)? Are arms hanging freely by sides and hands unclenched?

A supple lengthened spine is especially important during pregnancy because it helps prevent the aches and pains that poor posture can cause as you get heavier, particularly backache. It will also help you to make maximum room both for the baby and for your breathing. The ribs are the correct breathing apparatus and, if your spine is lengthened, the whole of your ribcage, which goes nearly down to your waist at the back, will be free to work properly.

Check posture regularly in this way throughout the day

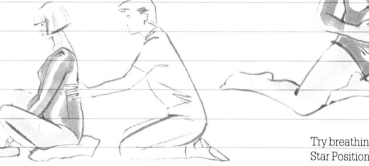

ur partner
ld apply
ntle
ssure as
breathe

Exercising becomes much less of an effort if you make it a part of your daily life. The Star Positions given here can be used whenever you feel like it – not just reserved for a special exercise 'time'. They are excellent preparation for an active birth as they prepare the legs and hips, strengthen and lengthen the back and give you a good chance to practise your breathing. Think of the stretches as active relaxation exercises that will benefit you both while you are pregnant and once labour begins. Use your breathing to help you remain calm throughout...

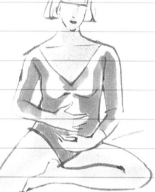

Try breathing this way in the Star Positions, keeping calm and relaxed as you breathe through the stretch.

BREATHING

Sit in any comfortable position where spine is lengthened and ribs are free and concentrate on taking each breath down to the baby and then letting each breath out completely. Think about your baby as you do this. Stroking and circular movements with palms of hands over the bump will be comforting for you both too. Breathe down to the baby at back of body as well, getting a friend to check that you are using whole of ribcage at back by placing hands just above your waist at the back, as shown, and allowing hands to rise and fall with your breathing, so that you can really feel expansion of lower ribs in middle of back.

STAR POSITIONS

FROG POSITION ★

Kneel on a mat or soft surface with toes together and knees apart – eventually aiming to get bottom to touch floor. Now walk hands forwards, with palms on floor, so that you gradually lower body. But try to lengthen out spine completely, placing forehead on a cushion as shown or stretching arms in front if you prefer. Stay there for at least a minute if you can (2 when you get used to it), breathing well and emphasizing out-breath so you stay relaxed.

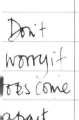

Don't worry if toes come apart a little

You will probably feel an intense stretch in groin area, so use it to practise labour breathing and relaxation.

COBBLER POSE ★

Sit on a cushion or two with knees bent and soles of feet together as close to you as possible. Holding onto feet or ankles, lengthen back, lifting ribs away from hips. At the same time, drop shoulders down away from ears. Hold position, breathing well. Flop, letting back round, and then try again, gradually working towards holding position for up to 2 minutes. Then take hands behind you, lean on them and do a pelvic tilt gently dropping thighs towards floor several times when you feel you can take the stretch.

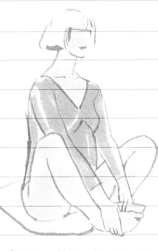

It is a good idea to do this with a partner sitting opposite as shown, so that you get a really good stretch. Breathe and release into it, practising labour breathing and paying full attention to your body. -

Don't worry if you feel very stiff to begin with. As your pregnancy progresses, a hormone will be released which will soften the ligaments and loosen your joints in order to increase the size of the pelvis and so accommodate the growing baby. The later months of pregnancy are therefore an excellent time to work on increasing general mobility. You may find you become so supple that you can put yourself into positions never achieved before.

If you feel a very strong stretch in some of these positions, don't tighten up to protect yourself from it as you may want to do, but breathe through it instead, as if it were a labour contraction, concentrating particularly on the out-breaths. Build up until you can hold the stretch for a full minute. Complete attention is necessary so that you can distinguish between an intense stretch (which will nearly always subside as you accept it and breathe through it, staying relaxed and calm) and acute pain. If you feel acute pain, come out of the position immediately and tell your doctor about it.

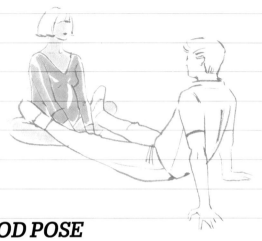

ROD POSE (WITH FORWARD BEND) ★

Still sitting on cushions, stretch legs out in front with knees facing ceiling, insides of feet touching. Place a belt or towel around balls of feet and, gently pulling against it, slowly lengthen up back to vertical, or as near as possible. Hold breathing well and, when you feel you can take more stretch, go forwards from the hips keeping back straight (as exercise 39 in Exercise Programme). Eventually you should be able to rest chest on thighs, head on calves or supported on a towel folded onto calves.

This also helps to relieve cramp in calves

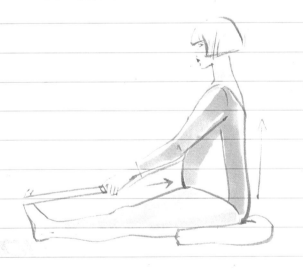

Prepare yourself physically and psychologically for labour by gradually increasing your holding time on the strong stretches given here. Once you can hold them for 2 minutes or more, breathing well, you can be confident in your ability to remain calm and relaxed on the day, for your labour contractions will never last longer than 1¾ minutes. If you find the stretches become less intense as you get more supple, take the positions further until the intensity increases again...

'V' POSITION ★

Sitting with legs apart, press against inside thighs to lift spine up to vertical. Hold as you feel stretch, remembering to think of it like a contraction and breathing through it, staying calm and relaxed.

Do these exercises with back against a wall if they prove too much at first. Eventually your back should be vertical. Check progress from time to time by doing exercise sideways on to a mirror.

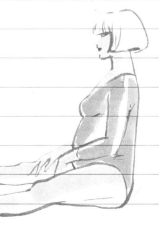

SQUATTING★

This traditional birthing position gives lower back an excellent stretch and also stretches groin area and thighs, so it is very useful both during pregnancy and in preparation for the birth itself. Try it holding onto a chair or other support at first or leaning back against a wall and sliding down. It does not matter if heels don't touch floor, but if they do, it will give calves a useful stretch.

Try pelvic floor exercise in this position. Control is good if you can squeeze and lift pelvic floor with legs so wide apart.

DAILY MAINTENANCE

PELVIC FLOOR *To locate your pelvic floor muscles, test them out while you are passing water (not on an extremely full bladder though, such as first thing in the morning) by stopping flow of urine mid-stream. You should be able to stop it completely with no drips. If you can't, pelvic floor muscles need working on. Lift them up a little (as though stopping urine flow mid-stream), then a little more, more*

again, and finally lift and squeeze upwards as much as you can. Hold for a slow count of 5 and then lower in 3 stages as before. Don't worry if you can't get all stages up or down at first – you will become more precise with practice. Try to do this at least 5 times a day. Lift and squeeze pelvic floor in one quick movement too and repeat several times daily. When you are familiar with exercise, try combining it with pelvic tilt. Use it during love-making too.

The sling of muscle at the bottom of pelvis has a big weight-bearing job to do as pregnancy progresses and is stretched to the limit during childbirth itself.

LEG SWINGS

These will get circulation moving in hips and legs. Try them forwards and back and across and out away from body, holding lightly onto the back of a chair for support.

The first and most essential post-natal exercise so get used to it now

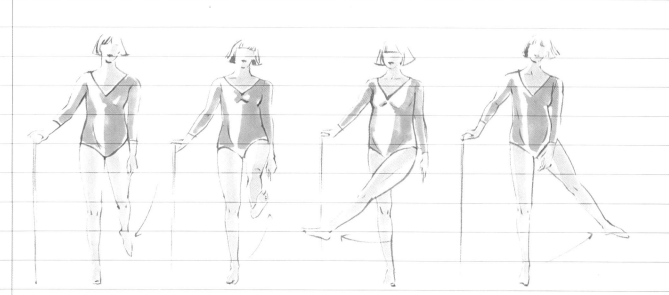

231

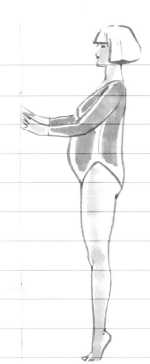

CALF FIRMER

This will also get circulation going. Standing with feet together and fingertips on a support, raise up onto balls of feet, as shown, lower heels half-way to floor and then push up again. Repeat energetically several times until calves begin to tire. Shake legs well.

FRONT OF THIGH FIRMER

Standing as left, lift up onto balls of feet. Do a pelvic tilt and bend knees, let them separate. Do 4 small further bends so front of thighs are working strongly, then straighten legs fully still up on toes. Repeat several times till front of thighs tire. Give legs a good shake-out.

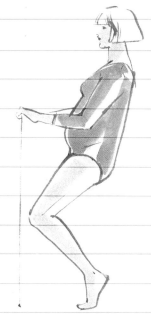

Makes a useful recovery exercise between strong stretches

SIDE STRETCH

Sitting cross-legged, breathe in and stretch one arm up over head. Reach over to opposite side, enjoying stretch and breathing out. Breathe in as you return to centre and then change arms and stretch to other side. Repeat several times.

Walks in the fresh air are marvellous exercise, as is swimming. If you are fit and have been doing yoga for some time, it would be an excellent idea to continue with your classes, avoiding positions such as lying on your tummy or advanced twists when these become uncomfortable. Once you have adjusted your shoulder stand to take your new-found weight, you may find being upside-down a great relief.

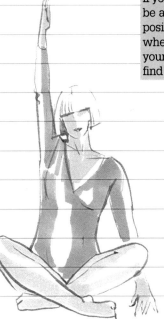

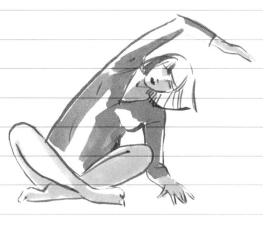

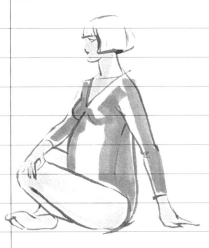

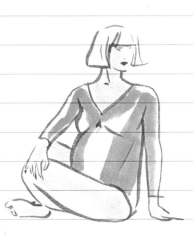

TWIST *Sitting cross-legged, place one hand on opposite knee and press the other into floor behind you to help lift spine as you take a good breath in. As you breathe out, twist gently round towards arm at back and look round gently too. Think of spiralling round on a well-lifted spine as you do this. Hold for a few moments, breathing normally, then repeat to other side.*

COMPLETE RELAXATION

First make sure you are warm enough, covering yourself with a blanket if necessary, and then make yourself comfortable. The position shown here is often the most comfortable in late pregnancy, so try it out and see if you like it (the cushion under the knee is useful for added comfort as is another cushion under tummy). Or try lying on back (providing this is still comfortable) with legs raised on a support about 45 cm (18 ins) above heart; or with a cushion or two under thighs to ease lower back. Whichever position you choose, start by doing a few pelvic tilts to make sure spine is lengthened. Pull shoulders down away from ears. Feel the tension release in the neck and shoulders as you do this. Spread arms a little away from body, quieten your mind by focusing on the rhythm of your breathing and take one or two deep breaths down to the baby. Then let breathing fall into its own rhythm, which will become lighter as you relax more deeply. Check through body to see if anything is tight. Are you holding onto a frown or clenching jaws? Are you tensing hands, tummy muscles, thighs, calves, toes? Let go and feel yourself easing further into floor with each out-breath. Allow yourself to be completely supported. When you have finished, take a few deep breaths, raise arms above head and have a good stretch – then get up SLOWLY. First bend knees, then roll onto side if you are lying on your back.

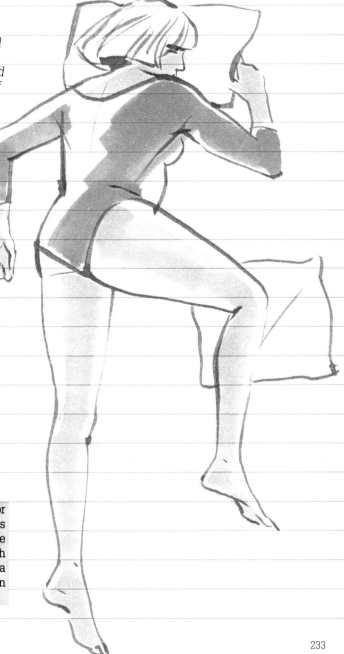

Do a little pelvic tilt to prevent back arching when you raise arms above head into stretch at the end.

Try this routine standing and sitting as well as lying and use it several times a day

AFTER THE BIRTH

The best post-natal tummy exercise is laughter. Add some serious work with the pelvic floor muscles and abdomen and a few movements to keep the circulation going in the legs if you are not yet up and around much and you will have everything you need for the first few days after the birth. After about a week – or as soon as you feel ready, start on the post-natal programme given here. This 5-minute routine should be carried out twice daily and continued for 12 weeks. Once you have had a 3-month check-up, and provided that your doctor agrees you are in good shape, you should be ready to return to the first week of the general programme.

If you have had a Caesarian birth, work your feet and ankles (see feet exercises, opposite) and start lifting and squeezing the pelvic floor muscles as soon as you can. Very soon, you will be able to begin a very gentle tummy exercise – simply pull your tummy in on an out-breath – and add the pelvic tilts as soon as you can. Once you are up and around, you will probably be ready to start the post-natal programme, but check with your doctor first.

If you have had stitches, you may be worried about exercising the pelvic floor. In fact, these exercises will help healing, and cannot possibly harm the stitches.

IMMEDIATELY AFTERWARDS

PELVIC FLOOR LIFTS
The first and most essential post-natal exercise. Do 4 slow and a few quick lifts at least 4 times and continue for at least 3 months, when you can try the test at the end of this section.

The pelvic floor muscles are stretched to the limit during childbirth, so working them is essential if they are to be restored to full strength. Start as soon as possible after the delivery, lifting and squeezing the pelvic floor several times daily and doing a few quick squeezes too. You will now be thankful you practised these in pregnancy for although you may feel practically no sensation at first, you will at least know what to aim for! Keep practising your pelvic floor lifts regularly so that by the time your baby is 3 months old you can lift your pelvic floor up 4 levels and down 3 without any trouble at all.

PELVIC TILTS

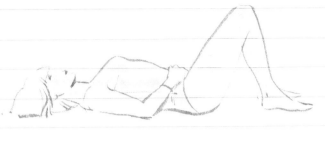

Lie on bed with shoulders down away from ears and spine in a nice straight line, knees bent and feet flat on bed. Place hands on tummy to help you feel what you are doing. Breathe in. As you breathe out, press back of waist firmly into mattress, contracting tummy muscles at the same time. Hold for a few seconds and then breathe in and release. Repeat several times and combine with pelvic floor lifts as soon as you get the idea.

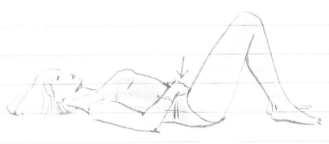

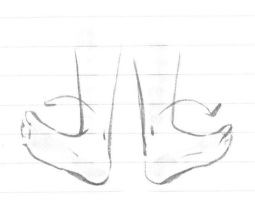

FEET EXERCISES

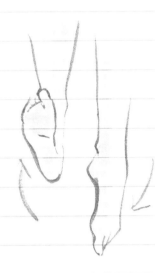

Keep circulation going with feet rotations, clockwise and anti-clockwise, and then try pedalling – first one foot downwards as the other comes up and then both down and up together. Repeat several times throughout the day.

POST-NATAL PROGRAMME

Start a week after the birth or as your physiotherapist advises.

PELVIC FLOOR LIFTS

As previous page.

PELVIC TILTS FOR TIGHTENING TUMMY

As above. Whenever you think of it plus 4 times lying on your back before your afternoon rest and again at night.

Great for tightening tummy
Try squeezing buttocks together

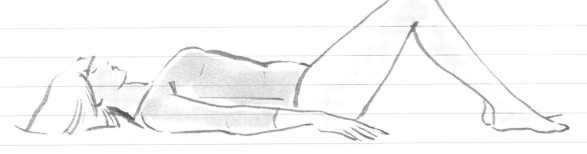

235

STRAIGHT CURL-UPS

Lie on bed with arms at sides, legs bent and feet flat. Breathe in. As you breathe out, lift head and shoulders and pull forwards with hands. (At first, you may only be able to lift head, but persevere.) Breathe in and return to bed. Build up until you can repeat slowly 4 times and then progress by holding curl-up for longer.

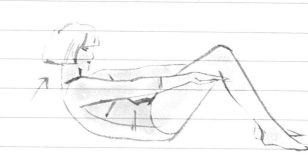

If you feel yourself straining front of neck when you lift head and shoulders, return head to the bed and roll it from side to side a few times or place a cushion or two under head before starting.

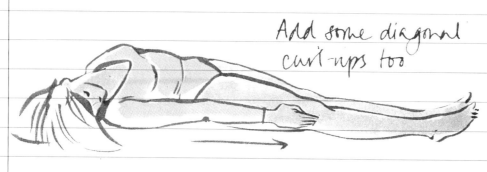

Add some diagonal curl-ups too

CURL-UPS WITH SIDE BENDS

Lie as before, but with arms at sides and hands touching thighs. Breathe in. As you breathe out, lift head and slide right hand down towards outside right knee as far as you can. Then change to left side. Try to repeat twice each side and then rest. Build up to 4 slow repetitions each side.

DIAGONAL CURL-UPS

Lie as before, but with arms about 30 cm (12 ins) away from body. Breathe in. As you breathe out, lift head and take left hand across body to touch right. Lower to bed again and repeat to other side. Try it 4 times slowly on alternating sides.

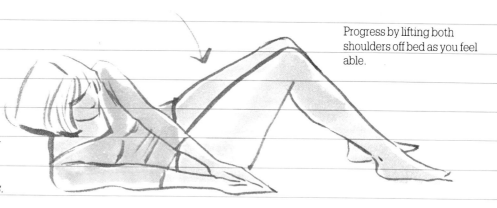

Progress by lifting both shoulders off bed as you feel able.

LEG SLIDES

Lie in a long straight line and slowly bend up one leg and then stretch it out again with foot moving along bed. Repeat with other leg. KEEP BACK PRESSED FIRMLY INTO BED THROUGHOUT. *Repeat several times slowly, and then more quickly, allowing one leg to come up as the other goes down in a pedalling action.*

Increase the number of repetitions on each exercise as the days go by. But don't tire yourself. It is better to do a few several times a day than a large amount all at once.

Place hands under either side of waist to check you are keeping back down.

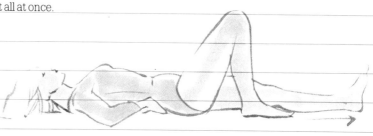

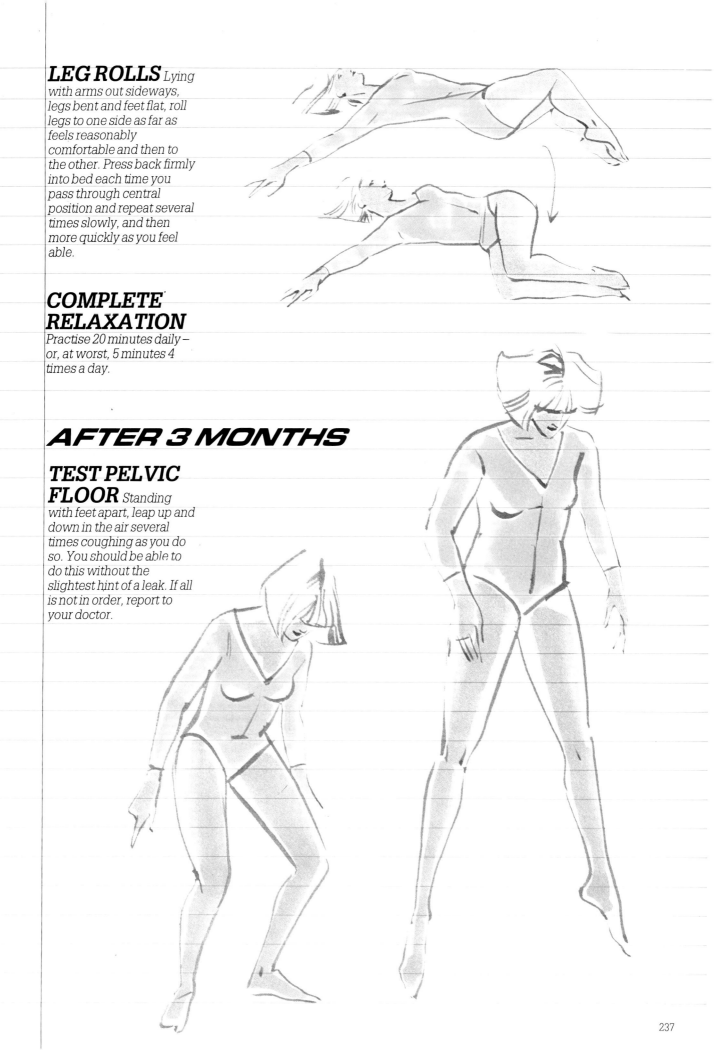

LEG ROLLS Lying
with arms out sideways,
legs bent and feet flat, roll
legs to one side as far as
feels reasonably
comfortable and then to
the other. Press back firmly
into bed each time you
pass through central
position and repeat several
times slowly, and then
more quickly as you feel
able.

COMPLETE RELAXATION
Practise 20 minutes daily –
or, at worst, 5 minutes 4
times a day.

AFTER 3 MONTHS

TEST PELVIC FLOOR Standing
with feet apart, leap up and
down in the air several
times coughing as you do
so. You should be able to
do this without the
slightest hint of a leak. If all
is not in order, report to
your doctor.

Therapeutics

Exercise should ultimately solve problems by making you fitter and healthier, but it often does so by bringing problems to light first. When you start to exercise, you will find that you become more aware of your body, of both its possibilities *and* its limitations. As your range of movement increases, you may become conscious of tensions which you had not noticed before but which were undoubtedly there all along – stiffness in the lower spine, a taut muscle at the side of the neck, less mobility in one hip than the other . . . This inner awareness is the first step to self-help. You must know what is amiss before you can hope to find ways of dealing with it.

The target, then, is to know yourself better than anyone else knows you – and that includes the 'specialists' to whom you might entrust your health. When you take responsibility for your body, you start to feel confident in your own abilities – not least the ability to look after yourself and to find effective ways of making yourself feel better. Massage and movement, you will discover, are two of the best.

This section is divided into three parts. The first part uses massage and movement sequences, the latter largely Feldenkrais-inspired, to help overcome stiffness and loss of mobility in 'problem' areas. Everyone will benefit from them, achieving more freedom and fluidity of movement and so gaining more from their exercising. The second part deals with problems that might occur as a direct result of exercise, such as leg cramps, and gives some practical self-help suggestions. The last part uses movement and massage techniques to help relieve common problems and disorders – much better than reaching for drugs... And, remember, exercise is not only therapeutic but also one of the best ways of safeguarding the good health that you have.

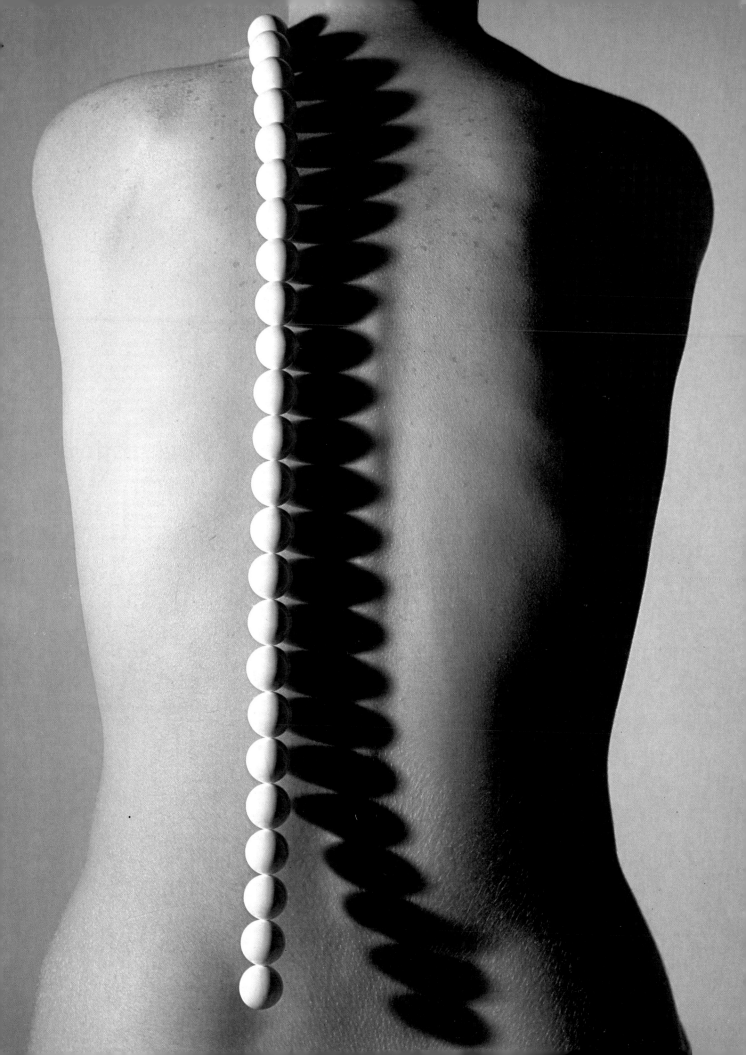

PART 1
NECK AND SHOULDERS

I. *Lie on floor and place hand on forehead. Letting hand lead forehead, turn head to right, back to centre and then slowly over to left. Repeat several times, noting how far head moves and quality of movement. Keeping hand on forehead, let head lead hand as you turn it from side to side several times. Take hand away and repeat several times, slowly and easily, breathing well. Rest.*

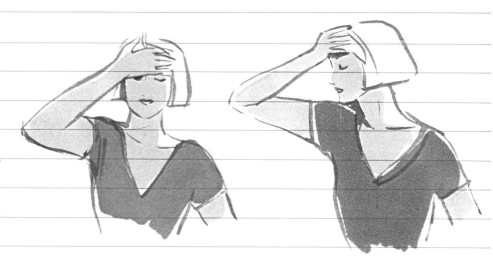

Helps ease tension at back of neck and throat

II. *Roll onto front. Place one hand on top of the other, the first palm down, the second palm up with forehead resting on it. Let this hand lightly lift head up and back so chest and upper back come off floor. Do not force movement, just go as far as is comfortable, noting quality and extent of movement. Repeat several times, then change hands. Rest a moment.*

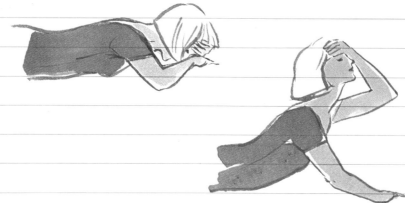

III. *Lie with both hands above forehead, as shown, right cheek on floor. Lift head, keeping right cheek parallel to floor, and move back of head towards right elbow. Pass through centre and move forehead towards left elbow. Rest cheek lightly on floor again and check for signs of* tension. *Are your fists clenched? Your jaws tight? Your eyes staring? Are you frowning? Release these tensions and repeat movement several times, remaining aware of your breathing. Then turn head, so left cheek is resting on floor, and repeat several times. Rest a moment.*

A NOTE ABOUT PAIN. Pain is the body's most basic warning that all is not well. Never ignore it, hoping that it will go away, because it is *always* there for a reason. It might be the way you are doing the exercises and using, or misusing, your body or it might be something much more fundamental. The sooner you find out what is causing it and why, enlisting the help of your doctor if necessary, the closer you will be to taking that pain away permanently.

Loosens shoulders

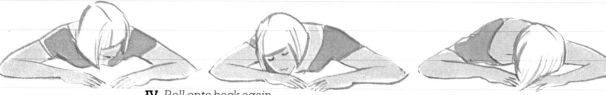

After III, go back to II. Is movement any easier? Once forced feeling goes and muscles relax, movement becomes more fluid...

IV. *Roll onto back again. Turn head to one side and keep it there. Lift opposite shoulder towards ceiling several times, then press it firmly into floor several times. Turn head and repeat on other side. Now go back to* **I.** *Is there any difference?*

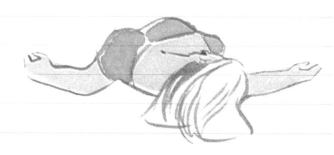

NECK AND SHOULDERS

I. *Place one hand behind the neck so that fingers can feel the muscles along the opposite side. Press index and middle fingers into muscle, rocking head to that side and back to centre as you press and release up and down muscle. Rest a moment.*

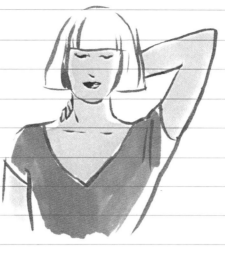

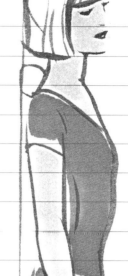

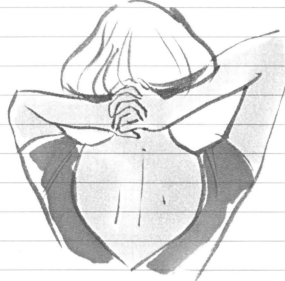

II. *Clasp hands together, interlacing fingers, and massage back, sides and base of neck with heels of hands, pressing firmly and releasing in a gentle rhythm.*

Tension often registers around the base of the neck and shoulders because our natural reaction to stress is to pull in the head and neck. When these muscles tighten up, blood flow to and from the brain may be constricted leading to mental fatigue, headaches and even migraine. Analgesics taken to relieve headache, such as paracetamol (aminocetophen), are often muscle relaxants. They work by reducing tension and so take the pain away. But you can do this for yourself with just massage and gentle exercise.

Help to prevent headaches in the first place with loosening exercises for neck and shoulders and more attention to posture. Your head weighs more than 4.5 kg (10 lb) and should feel *lightly* suspended on your neck, not just dumped on top crushing everything beneath.

III. *Place an orange at back of neck and, gently pressing it between yourself and a wall, roll it around neck, down across shoulders and between shoulder blades, bending and straightening knees, and swaying from side to side. Can you move the orange all the way down to the base of your spine? Enjoy it.*

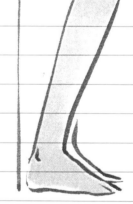

IV. *Place one hand on shoulder and work fingers down towards shoulder blade, pressing them in as far as is comfortable and releasing; then work across shoulder towards arm and back and forth several times. Repeat to other side.*

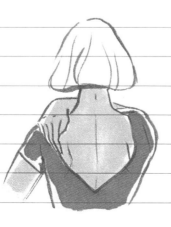

TO BE FREE OF TENSION BE AWARE OF . . .
Shoulders. Where are they? Hanging freely away from your head or clenched up about your ears?
Breathing. One of the first responses to stress is to hold your breath. This reinforces muscular tension and increases anxiety. Remind yourself to breathe OUT.
Basic body needs. When cramped in the same position for too long muscles are bound to protest. Get up and walk around, shake out arms and legs, stretch in any direction that feels good, breathing out to stretch a little more. Then hang over from the hips letting arms and head drop down, releasing back and allowing blood to run to the brain.

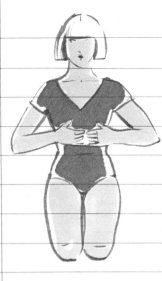

CHEST

Place second, third and fourth fingers of both hands between lower ribs at the front. Breathe in through nose and, as you breathe out, stroke fingers firmly downwards. Repeat several times in a good rhythm, exploring the spaces between your ribs.

Stiffness and tightness in the chest are often indicative of repressed emotion – anger especially and sometimes sadness and grief too. Breathing can help free this area by opening the chest. The pelvic clock exercise (exercise 42 of the main programme) is particularly effective because it encourages you to alternate deep abdominal breathing (6 o'clock) with shallower thoracic breathing (12 o'clock).

SPINE

I. *Lie on floor with knees bent and feet flat. Lift pelvis towards ceiling and then slowly return to floor, unfolding spine vertebra by vertebra. Be aware of your breathing and the quality of the movement. Are you keeping weight evenly on both feet? Repeat several times.*

II. *Lying on floor, with knees bent as before and arms by sides, rock pelvis back and forth between 6 and 12 hands of the pelvic clock, (see page 147). Notice how movement affects position of head and neck.*

III. *Lying as before, raise pelvis towards ceiling again – but not too far. This time visualize two long muscle groups running about 2.5 cm/1 in away from either side of the spine, from the neck to the* coccyx. *Now slowly unroll right-hand side muscles onto floor, making sure waist touches floor before bottom. Notice how pelvis is tilted slightly to that side. Practise several times on same side, then repeat to other side. Which is more agile?*

Identify which side of back is more agile.

IV. *Go back to* **I.** *Can you sense any difference? Is it easier to differentiate between the vertebrae? Does your spine feel more mobile and movement more fluid?*

SPINE

Lie down on floor and place a soft inflated ball the size of a large grapefruit underneath base of head. Now roll your spine over the ball, pushing with feet, so that you feel you are travelling along the top of it. Take ball up and down in this way a few times. Stop and rest. This affects the very deep muscles of the ribcage and spine. So be gentle. Don't overdo it.

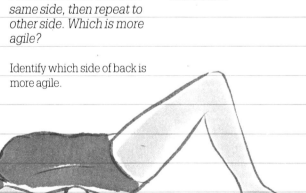

HIPS

I. *Sit as shown. Extend one arm at shoulder level and reach out to side, letting hips move naturally as you go. Return to centre, noticing how hips become level again, and repeat to other side. Repeat several times to each side, rocking gently as you go through centre each time.*

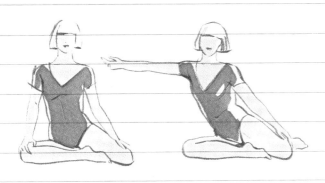

II. *Extend arm to side as before. Now take it round in front of you and over to other side, focusing eyes on hand as it moves so head follows arm naturally round. Then reverse movement and see how far you can go, but don't force it. Repeat several times, then change arms and repeat the exercise.*

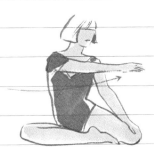

III. *Place one hand on floor beside you. Raise other arm above head and drop head gently back. Return to upright and then lower head and arm as shown. Repeat several times in a good rhythm, noticing what happens to hips and pelvis.*

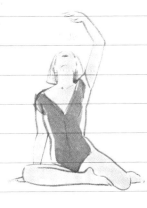

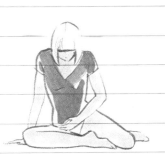

IV. *Place one hand on top of head and tilt it to either side. Notice what happens to hips and pelvis. Repeat a few times, then go back to* **I.** *and* **II.** *Do the movements seem easier? Do you notice an improvement?*

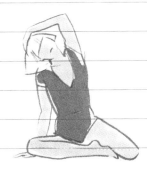

Dancing to Latin or African music is one of the best ways to free the pelvis and loosen the hips because it encourages you to use your body in a sinuous unselfconscious way. Sense movements becoming freer and more fluid as you let yourself go, allowing hips and pelvis to sway and rock and undulate to the rhythms of the music. The best way of freeing the pelvis? Sex!

KNEES

I. *Standing with feet slightly apart, pull up at front of leg so knee feels as though it is being pushed in. Contract firmly several times and repeat several times a day. Many people, women especially, suffer from hyperextension (when knees are pulled back behind the plumbline from hip to arch of foot). This exercise can help to prevent this.*

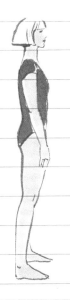

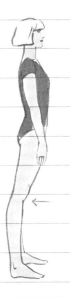

II. *When knee feels stronger, progress to exercise 74 of the main programme, starting without a weight and with thighs well supported on table. Once you can comfortably extend leg, straightening the knee, tie a sock or stocking filled with sand loosely around ankle. Lift slowly and rhythmically up and down several times a day.*

NEVER exercise on a damaged knee; it is a sure way to compound the injury.

When exercising, twisting and rotating movements should come from ankles or hips, not the knee. But if ankles or hips are not sufficiently mobile, the knee may be forced to compensate. Sensations of pain or pulling there, or an apparent lack of flexibility, often reflect stiffness at the joints above and below. Protect your knees by *being aware*. Make sure that they always bend directly over the toes when you exercise, so they are kept in the correct plane and any strain is avoided. If you feel any tension, pressure or twinges of pain, stop working and correct your position. If you find it impossible to do the exercise without straining the knee, leave it for the time being and work instead at increasing mobility at the hips (helpful exercises 42, 111 and 118) and ankles (helpful exercises 17 and 113). If pain persists, consult your doctor.

PART 2
FAINTNESS

Faintness, light-headedness and sometimes even nausea can accompany exercise – especially if it is vigorous. These sensations are all caused by blood being diverted away from brain and stomach to fuel large muscle groups.

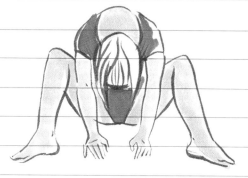

To remedy: *stop what you are doing and let blood flow towards brain by placing head lower than rest of body. Either lie on floor or ground with feet up and supported or sit in a chair or on floor, as shown, with legs wide apart and head and arms hanging down between them.*

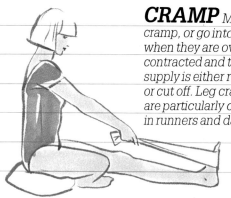

CRAMP
Muscles cramp, or go into spasm, when they are over-contracted and the blood supply is either reduced or cut off. Leg cramps are particularly common in runners and dancers.

STITCH
Stitch, a very sharp pain just below the ribs, is often brought on by unaccustomed exertion – especially running and jumping up and down. Although the exact reason for stitch is not known, it is thought to be caused by lack of oxygen in the respiratory muscles, such as the diaphragm, due to insufficient blood flow. *Stitch is soon relieved by stopping and resting and then recommencing activity very gradually. Some distance runners maintain that very deep breathing can sometimes relieve the discomfort while enabling them to continue to run. Try it and see...*

I. *As cramped muscles are always over-contracted, stretch muscle out first. When in spasm, resistance* is inevitable, so try to enlist the help of someone to hold the leg or arm for you, or use a towel *as shown.*

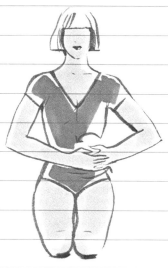

PART 3
HEADACHES

Run through the neck and shoulder loosener sequence first (page 10) and then, if no relief is felt, massage the head itself. Start with forehead.
I. *Close eyes, breathe deeply and check for signs of tension. Release jaw, open brow, let eyes become soft. Place both hands at centre of forehead, just above eyebrows, and stroke firmly outwards. Move up in 3 stages to hairline, and repeat several times.*

II. *Keeping eyes closed, take a few more deep breaths and check again for signs of tension. Now place middle fingers at upper corner of eye just beneath brow, press firmly inwards for count of 5, then release. Repeat this all the way along brow bone to outer corner and then continue underneath the eye. Finish by pressing temples.*
III. *Massage scalp with both hands, working firmly from crown of head backwards.*

STOMACH ACHES
Most digestive problems are caused by stress, manner of eating and diet, in that order. Consider these, especially if you often have digestive problems. Use deep breathing and massage to help increase blood supply to the stomach and ease pain.
I. *Breathe in through nose,* filling lungs with air, letting abdomen expand. Hold for a count of 3, then breathe out through mouth drawing abdomen in. This should be slightly longer than the in-breath. Continue in a good rhythm several times.
II. *Place one hand on top of the other and massage stomach and abdominal area in a clockwise movement.*

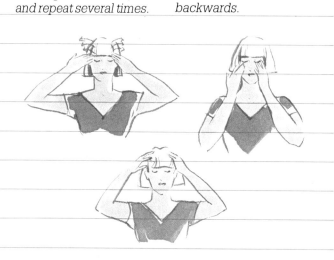

CONSTIPATION

The inverted yoga postures, neck balance (sarvangasana) and plough pose (halasana), can be extremely helpful for digestive problems – relieving abdominal pain and wind and solving constipation especially. In addition, being upside down tends to promote a powerful sense of well-being, clearing the mind and refreshing the system. Practise 5 minutes daily for maximum benefits, but practise with caution: these poses are best learned with the assistance of a professional yoga teacher.

I. Lie flat on floor, with arms by sides. Take a few deep breaths and bend knees in towards chest till you feel thighs pressing against stomach.

II. Raise body up to vertical: move hands down till they are in middle of back and raise hips (only back of head, neck, shoulders and backs of arms up to elbows should now be on floor), stretch legs up and straighten spine. To begin with ask a

NB If neck or throat feel strained, place folded blanket(s) beneath shoulders, and adjust height and position until comfortable.

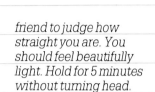

friend to judge how straight you are. You should feel beautifully light. Hold for 5 minutes without turning head.

III. Now, carefully let feet come over head onto floor to plough pose. Let toes rest on floor, keep legs straight and muscles at front of thighs well pulled up. Extend arms as shown.

IV. Cradle knees around head and relax for a moment, before coming out of pose.
To come out: raise legs to ceiling and slowly lower hips, with help of hands, to ground. Keep movement slow and controlled.

If difficult, rest toes on a stool or chair 60cm/2ft away

...t when ...nstruating, ...r on a ...stomach, ...r if you ...ve ...gh blood ...essure

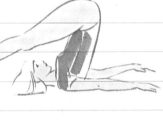

Period Pains

Period pains are caused by strong contractions of the uterine muscles. Tensing up to protect yourself from these contractions makes the pain more intense. Breathing, stretching and curling exercises can help ease pain by encouraging you to relax.

I. Lie down and breathe deeply several times, trying to focus only on the breath as it enters and leaves your body.

II. Raise arms above head, tilt hips to one side and reach up with arms, feeling stretch along side and abdomen. Repeat to other side.

III. Curl up knees into abdomen and stay there, breathing well for a few moments. Then stretch out again. Repeat stretch/curl sequence several times.

IV. Breathe deeply a few more times, releasing areas of tension and feeling heavier and heavier as you become more and more relaxed.

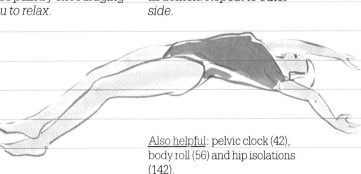

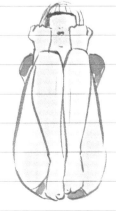

<u>Also helpful</u>: pelvic clock (42), body roll (56) and hip isolations (142).

Index

abdomen: breathing exercises, 139
  co-ordination exercises, 170
  posture exercises, 133
  pre-ski exercises, 225
  relaxation, 152
  shaping exercises, 176
  strength exercises, 156
  test exercises, 172
aches, 244
acupuncture, 183
aerobic exercises, 158-61, 166, 181, 207
air step, 208
alcohol, 24, 51, 58, 72, 76
allergies, 58
almonds: chicken with, 100
  foamy sauce, 85
  trout with, 120
Americana sauce, 96
amino acids, 68
anaesthetic chewing gum, 39
ankles: breathing exercises, 140
  mobility exercises, 182
  posture exercises, 135
  pre-ski exercises, 225
  rock and roll exercises, 191
anorexia nervosa, 18
appetite, 39, 42-3
apples: autumn baked, 96
  baked with blackcurrant sauce, 96
apricot, lamb stuffed with, 108
arms: final exercises, 206
  pre-ski exercises, 224
  shaping exercises, 175
arterial disease, 68
artichokes: salad, 96
  with herb sauce, 84
aubergine: pie, 96
  stuffed, 118
autumn baked apple, 96
avocado, 50
  salad cream, 115
awareness exercises, 144-8, 188

back: awareness exercises, 147, 148
  breathing exercises, 137, 140
  co-ordination exercises, 169, 170
  posture exercises, 130, 131, 134
  stretch exercises, 143
  test exercises, 171, 173
  twist exercises, 150
baked apple with blackcurrant
    sauce, 96
  baked egg, 97
  balance: ballet, 201
  exercises, 164-6
  jazz exercises, 203
  test exercises, 172, 173
ballet exercises, 195-201
bananas, 50
  honey and nut fool with, 97
barbecue lamb, 97
barre work, 199-201
basal rates, metabolism, 34
bass, Chinese steamed, 87
battement, 208
beef: bitkis, 99
  boiled, with horseradish sauce, 90
  carbonnade, 98
  chilli con carne, 101
  cottage pie, 102
  fillet steak with green peppercorns
    and herbs, 104
  goulash, 98

lasagne, 108
steak and kidney casserole, 118
stuffed peppers, 118
Swiss steak, 120
Bender, Arnold, 51
Benson, Herbert, 194
beriberi, 50
Beverley Hills Diet, 50
biceps, 175
binge eating, 18, 43
bitkis, 99
blackcurrant, baked apple with, 96
Blitz diets, 57, 60-3
blood, sugar levels, 42-3, 64
blood pressure, high, 68
blue cheese dressing, 115
Body Mass Index, 15
bowel cancer, 68
braised kidneys, 99
bran, 65
bread, slimming, 50
breakfast menus, 26-7
breast feeding diet, 76-9
breasts, 131, 161, 175
  cancer, 68
breathing: exercises, 136-40
  meditation, 194
  pregnancy, 229
brown fat, 35
bulimia, 18
bulking agents, 42
bust, see breasts
butter, 50
buttocks: co-ordination exercises,
    170
  shaping exercises, 177
  strength exercises, 157

calcium, 65, 76, 77
calories, 24, 50, 51
calves: firmer exercises, 232
  posture exercises, 132
  strength exercises, 154
cancer, 14, 64, 68
cannellini beans: three bean salad,
    120
cannelloni, 99
capers, egg dressing with, 115
carbohydrate: high-carbohydrate
    diet, 60-3
  low-carbohydrate diet, 60
carrots, 50
  potato and onion soup with, 114
  soup, 99
celery: ricotta with herbs and, 92
  soup, 99
cellulite, 46-7
cereals, 64
Charleston, 208
cheese: blue cheese dressing, 115
  ricotta with herbs and celery, 92
  soufflé omelette, 117
  tomato and Mozzarella salad, 82
  wholewheat macaroni with ham
    and, 123
  see also cottage cheese; cream
    cheese
chest: breathing exercises, 138
  therapeutic exercises, 242
  twist exercises, 149
  weights exercises, 162
chewing gum, anaesthetic, 39
chicken: chicken Véronique, 100
  Chinese cabbage salad with, 101
  ginger soup, 82

grilled breasts with watercress, 88
herb chicken, 106
Indian chicken in foil, 106
skewered, 116
sweet and sour, 120
with almonds, 100
  with peach and ginger, 100
childbirth exercises, 226-33
chilli con carne, 101
chin, shaping exercises, 174
Chinese cabbage and chicken salad,
    101
Chinese stuffed peppers, 101
chives: cottage cheese dressing
    with, 115
  jacket potatoes, 107
cider: ham sauce with, 106
  pork chops with, 113
cobbler pose, 230
cod, baked with ginger, 97
colon: action of fibre in, 64
  cancer, 64, 68
compulsive eating, 43
constipation, 64, 76, 245
co-ordination exercises, 167-70
coronary heart disease, 14, 51, 64, 68
cottage cheese: dressing with
    chives, 115
  jacket potatoes, 107
  spinach quiche with, 117
  see also cream cheese; cheese
cottage pie, 102
courgette, pie with tomatoes, 102
crab, hot, 106
cramp, 244
crash diets, 31, 34, 39, 43
cream cheese: jacket potatoes, 107
  spinach roulade, 118
  see also cottage cheese; cheese
crêpes, 102
crouch, 206
cucumber: appetizer, 103
  melon and pear salad with, 111
  soup with mint, 103
  tomatoes stuffed with, 87
  yogurt dressing with, 115
curl-downs, 133
curl-ups, 139, 236
curry: curried mushroom salad, 103
  jacket potatoes, 107
  pork, 113
  vegetable, 121
cycling, 220

dairy foods, 68, 76, 77
decaffeinated coffee, 24
demi plié, 199, 200
developé, 196
developé à la seconde, 197
diabetes, 14, 64
diverticulitis, 64
Dō-in, 183-5
double chins, 174
drinks, 24
  see also alcohol
Durnin, John, 38

ears, 185
eggs, 68
  baked, 97
  caper dressing with, 115
  dressing, 115

grilled breasts with watercress, 88
piperade, 113
  soufflé cheese omelette, 117
elbows, mobility exercises, 179
electric slimming aids, 39
emotion, breathing and, 140
entertaining, 80-93
epaulements, 198, 208
examination exercises, 171-3

failed dieting, 19
faintness, 244
falling, pre-ski exercises, 225
fasting, 58-9
fat: brown, 35
  measurement of, 15
  and weight loss, 38-9
fats: and cancer, 68
  low fat diet, 64-7
feet, 153, 235
Feldenkrais, Moshe, 144
fennel and orange salad, 104
fibre: high fibre diet, 64-7
  sources of, 65
fibre-based bulking agents, 42
fish: corn chowder with, 102
  pie, 104
  stuffed with prawns and lemon,
    104
flageolet beans: three bean salad, 120
folic acid, 72
French dressing, 115
French onion soup, 105
French vegetable quiche, 105
frog position, 229
fruit, 50, 58, 64
fruit salad: fresh, 89
  green, 106
  orange and pear, 111
  red, 115
  winter fruit compote, 123

gallstones, 64
garlic, lamb with rosemary and, 108
Garrow, Dr John, 63
gazpacho, 105
ginger: baked cod with, 97
  baked whole fish with mushrooms
    and, 112
  chicken with peach and, 100
  soup, 82
glycogen, 31, 63
gooseberry fool, 105
goulash, 98
granary bread, 50
grand plié, 199, 200
grapefruit with orange juice, 91
grapes in orange jelly, 83
green fruit salad, 106

habits, 144
haddock: smoked haddock roulade,
    116
  stuffed with prawns and lemon,
    104
halasana, 245
ham: ham and cider sauce, 106
  jacket potatoes, 107
  veal escalope with, 121
  wholewheat macaroni with cheese
    and, 123
hands, jazz exercises, 202
head, 128, 167

headaches, 244
heart disease, 14, 51, 64, 68
herb chicken, 106
herb dressing, 115
herb sauce, 84
herb teas, 24
herring with mustard sauce, 106
high blood pressure, 51, 68
high carbohydrate diet, 60-3
high fibre diet, 64-7
hip swings, 208
hips: awareness exercises, 146
    jazz exercises, 203
    mobility exercises, 181
    pre-ski exercises, 225
    shaping exercises, 177
    stretch exercises, 142
    therapeutic exercises, 243
honey, 50
    banana and nut fool with, 97
hormones, menstrual cycle, 30
horseradish sauce, for beef, 90
hunger, 42-3, 51

Indian chicken in foil, 106
indulgences, 24, 54-5
insulin, 64
Irish stew, 107
iron, 68, 73
isolations, jazz, 203

jazz attitude, 208
jazz exercises, 202-5, 208-17
jazz palms, 208
jelly: orange, with grapes, 83
    raspberry, 84
jogging, 218-19
juice diets, 57, 58-9
jump kicks, 152
jumps: ballet, 198
    strength exercises, 155
    twist exercises, 150
junk food, 20, 51

kebabs, lamb, 108
ketosis, 58
kicks: breathing exercises, 139
    jazz exercises, 204, 205
    relaxation, 152
    strength exercises, 154
    stretch exercises, 143
kidneys: braised, 99
    in red wine, 108
    steak and kidney casserole, 118
Kirlian, 183
knees: bending, 131
    mobility exercises, 182
    therapeutic exercises, 243
Kundalini, 183

lamb: barbecue lamb, 97
    Irish stew, 107
    kebab, 108
    stuffed roast shoulder of, 119
    with apricot stuffing, 108
    with garlic and rosemary, 108
lasagne, 108
    vegetable, 121
laxatives, 43, 64
lay-back, 208
leaps: co-ordination exercises, 169

leek and thyme quiche, 109
legs: awareness exercises, 148
    balance exercises, 165
    breathing exercises, 138
    childbirth exercises, 231
    co-ordination exercises, 170
    final exercises, 207
    post-natal exercises, 236, 237
    posture exercises, 131
    rock and roll exercises, 191
    stretch exercises, 143
    see also kicks
lemon: dressing with mustard, 115
    dressing with tarragon, 115
    fish stuffed with prawns and, 104
    sole with prawns and, 117
lentil soup, 109
light meals, 28-9
Lindy break, 208
Lindy hop, 208
liver: calves' liver with orange
        juice, 92
    provençal, 109
    stroganoff, 110
    wholewheat spaghetti with
        chicken livers, 123
    with orange, 110
loosening exercises, 138
lotus position, 194
low-carbohydrate diets, 60
low fat diet, 64-7
lunge, 133, 208

macaroni, wholewheat, with cheese
        and ham, 123
macrobiotic diets, 68
magnesium, 50, 58, 59
malaise, 58
mantra, 194
margarine, 50
massage, 47, 183-5, 240-1
meat, protein content, 68
meditation, 193-4
Mediterranean seafood, 111
melon, pear and cucumber salad, 11
menstruation, 30
metabolism: ketosis, 58
    metabolic rate, 17, 33, 34-5, 38-9,
        58
    metabolic rate after dieting, 63
Middle Eastern rice, 111
minestrone, 111
mint, cucumber soup with, 103
mobility exercises, 173, 179-82
morning sickness, 72
moxa, 183
multivitamin tablets, 51
muscles, 38-9, 131, 157
mushrooms: baked whole fish with
        ginger and, 112
    curried salad, 103
    prawn and spinach salad with, 89
mustard: lemon dressing with, 115
    sauce, for herring, 106

nausea, in pregnancy, 72
Nautilus, 176
neck: breathing exercises, 137
    loosening exercises, 131
    posture exercises, 128
    therapeutic exercises, 240, 241
neck balance, 245
Neumann, 35

nuts: banana and honey fool with, 97
    brown rice salad with, 99
oestrogen, 30
omelette, soufflé cheese, 117
onion: creamy soup, 102
    French soup, 105
    potato and carrot soup with, 114
opposition, 208
orange: calves' liver with, 92
    fennel salad with, 104
    grapes in orange jelly, 83
    liver with, 110
    peach sorbet with, 113
    pear fruit salad with, 111
    sliced grapefruit with, 91
    tomato soup with, 112
ovarian cancer, 68

padmasana, 194
pain, 240
pancreas, cancer, 68
parsley and thyme stuffing, 120
peach: chicken with ginger and, 100
    sliced with yogurt cream, 87
    sorbet with orange, 113
pear: melon and cucumber salad
        with, 111
    orange fruit salad with, 111
pelvic floor, 189, 231, 234, 235, 237
pelvic rotations, 228
pelvic tilt, 226, 228
pelvis, 188, 189
    awareness exercises, 147
    childbirth exercises, 228
    clock, 147
    co-ordination exercises, 167
    posture exercises, 128
pepperoni, 113
peppers: Chinese stuffed, 101
    grilled salad, 87
    pepperoni, 113
    piperade, 113
    stuffed, with tomato sauce, 118
period pains, 245
petits battements, 196, 200
pheasant, ginger soup, 82
phytate, 65
piperade, 113
pizza: quick, 114
    wholewheat pan, 123
plaice, stuffed with prawns and
        lemon, 104
pliés, 199, 200, 208
plough pole, 245
pork: casserole, 113
    chop with cider, 113
    curry, 113
    fillets with prunes, 114
post-natal exercises, 234-7
posture: barre work, 200
    exercises, 128-35
    pregnancy, 229
potassium, 43, 58, 59, 72
potato: carrot and onion soup with,
        114
    jacket, 107
prawns: fish stuffed with
        lemon and, 104
    jacket potatoes, 107
    sole with lemon and, 117
    spinach and mushroom salad with,
        89
pregnancy: diet, 72-5
    exercises, 76, 226-33

press-ups, 175
    wall, 139
progesterone, 30
prostate, cancer, 68
protein, sources, 68
prunes, pork fillets with, 114
pulse, 160, 172

quiche: French vegetable, 105
    leek and thyme, 109
    ratatouille tartlets, 114
    smoked salmon, 116
    spinach and cottage cheese, 117
quick pizza, 114

raspberry jellies, 84
ratatouille, 114
ratatouille tartlets, 114
red fruit salad, 115
red kidney beans: smoked trout salad
        with, 116
    three bean salad, 120
red mullet, baked with ginger and
        mushrooms, 112
refined foods, 50, 51, 58
refined sugar, 64
Reich, Wilhelm, 188
relaxation, 140, 149, 150-3
    pregnancy, 233
    retire, ballet, 198
rib cage, jazz exercises, 203
riboflavin, 68
rice: Middle Eastern, 111
    salad with nuts, 99
ricotta with herbs and celery, 92
rock and roll exercises, 190-2, 208-11
rod pose, 230
rolls, relaxation, 152
rosemary, lamb with garlic and, 108
running, 148, 218-19

salad dressings, 115
    see also sauces
salads: artichoke, 96
    brown rice and nuts, 99
    Chinese cabbage and chicken, 101
    crunchy, 102
    curried mushrooms, 103
    fennel and orange, 104
    grilled pepper salad, 87
    Mediterranean seafood, 111
    melon, pear and cucumber, 111
    mixed red and green, 84
    prawn, spinach and mushroom, 89
    smoked trout, 90
    smoked trout and bean, 116
    three bean, 120
    tomato and Mozzarella, 82
    vegetable, 122
salmon: poached steak, 113
    smoked salmon quiche, 116
salmon trout, Chinese steamed, 87
salt, 46-7, 51, 76
sarvangasana, 245
sauces: Americana, 96
    blackcurrant, 96
    foamy almond, 85
    ham and cider, 106
    herb, 84
    horseradish, 90
    mustard, 106
    tomato and basil, 123

white, 123
see also salad dressings
scales, 30
scallops: ceviche, 88
scampi provençal, 115
seafood: Mediterranean, 111
   Mediterranean salad, 111
   see also fish; prawns
sequence, aerobic exercises, 160
set ranges, weight, 17
sexuality, 188-9
Shaitsu, 183
shaping exercises, 174-8
shoes, posture and, 132
shoulders: awareness exercises,
   146
   mobility exercises, 180
   posture exercises, 128, 130
   pre-ski exercises, 224
   stretch exercises, 142
   therapeutic exercises, 240, 241
   weights exercises, 162
sides: childbirth exercises, 232
   jazz exercises, 202
   shaping exercises, 175
   posture exercises, 130
   test exercises, 171
skewered chicken, 116
ski-ing exercises, 224-5
slimming products, 42-3
smoking, 72, 76
sodium, 58, 59, 72
sole: poached goujons with tarragon,
   82
   sole Florentine, 116
   with herbs and wine, 117
   with lemon and prawns, 117
sorbet: peach and orange, 113
   strawberry, 118
soufflé, spinach, 118
soup: carrot, 99
   celery, 99
   corn and fish chowder, 102
   creamy onion, 102
   cucumber and mint, 103
   French onion, 105
   gazpacho, 105
   ginger, 82
   lentil, 109
   minestrone, 111
   orange and tomato, 112
   potato, carrot and onion, 114
   watercress, 122

spaghetti, wholewheat: with
   chicken livers, 123
   with tomato and basil sauce, 123
special diets, 56-79
spinach: cannelloni, 99
   cottage cheese quiche with, 117
   prawn and mushroom salad 89
   roulade, 118
   soufflé, 118
   veal Italienne, 121
spine: awareness exercises, 146
   mobility exercises, 182
   posture exercises, 128
   therapeutic exercises, 242
sport, 218-25
spring onions: jacket potatoes, 107
squat jump, 155
squatting, 207, 231
steak and kidney casserole, 118
stiffness, 143
stitch, 244
stomach aches, 244
straddle split, 208
strawberry sorbet, 118
strength exercises, 154-7
stress, 17, 143
stress-induced eating, 18
stretch exercises, 141-3, 186-7
stuffed aubergine, 118
stuffed peppers with tomato sauce,
   118
stuffed roast shoulder of lamb, 119
stuffed veal, 119
stuffing: thyme and parsley, 120
sugar, levels in blood, 42-3, 64
sun salutation, 186-7
sunlight, vitamin D, 68
sweet and sour chicken, 120
sweet corn: corn and fish chowder,
   102
   jacket potatoes, 107
sweets, slimming products, 42-3
swimming, 222
Swiss steak, 120

tarragon, lemon dressing with, 115
teas, herbal, 24
tendu, 196
tension, 131, 241
terrine, vegetable, 92
therapeutic exercises, 238-45
thiamin, 50, 68

thighs: aerobic exercises, 158
   breathing exercises, 138
   childbirth exercises, 232
   final exercises, 207
   posture exercises, 132, 133
   pre-ski exercises, 224
   rock and roll exercises, 192
   shaping exercises, 178
   strength exercises, 156, 157
   test exercises, 172
   weights exercises, 163
Thousand Island dressing, 115
three bean salad, 120
through the trenches, 208
thyme: leek quiche with, 109
   stuffing with parsley, 120
tisanes, 24
tomato: Americana sauce, 96
   courgette pie with, 102
   dressing, 115
   gazpacho, 105
   Mozzarella salad with, 82
   soup with orange, 112
   stuffed peppers with tomato
      sauce, 118
   stuffed with cucumber, 87
   wholewheat spaghetti with
      tomato and basil sauce, 123
training shoes, 218
triceps, 175
trout: poached, 84
smoked trout and bean salad, 116
   salad, 90
   with almonds, 120
tuna: jacket potatoes, 107
twist exercises, 149-50, 232

under-nutrition, 50, 51
upper body: breathing exercises, 139
   final exercises, 207
   posture exercises, 130
   shaping exercises, 175
   test exercises, 172
'V' position, 230
varicose veins, 64
veal: escalope with ham, 121
   Italienne, 121
   stuffed, 119
vegans, 68
vegetables: curry, 121
   fibre, 64
   French vegetable quiche, 105

juices, 58
lasagne, 121
protein content, 68
salad, 122
terrine, 92
vegetarian diet, 68-71
vitamin A, 64
vitamin B, 50
vitamin B (thiamin), 50, 68, 72
vitamin B2, 68
vitamin B12, 68
vitamin C, 68, 73
vitamin D, 68
vitamin tablets, 51
volatile fatty acids (VFAs), 64
vomiting, in pregnancy, 72

waists, 176
   ballet exercises, 201
   breathing exercises, 138
   final exercises, 207
   posture exercises, 132
   rock and roll exercises, 190, 192
   stretch exercises, 142
   twist exercises, 150
wall press-ups, 139
warm down, 135
warm-up: ballet, 195
   cycling, 220
   running, 218
   stretch exercises, 141
   swimming, 222
watercress: grilled chicken breasts
   with, 88
   soup, 122
weight: optimum weight, 14-17
   set ranges, 17
   tables, 14-15
weight balance, posture exercises,
   128
weight loss, crash diets, 31
weight training machines, 176
weights, 162-3
white sauce, 123
winter fruit compote, 123
wrist exercises, 140

yoga, 186-7, 245
yogurt, 50
   cucumber dressing with, 115
   sliced peaches with, 87

ACKNOWLEDGEMENTS

The following pictures were taken specially for Octopus Books

Christian Von Albensleben 69; Sandra Lousada 4-5, 227; Butch Martin 219, 220-1, 224; Tom Wool 1, 2-3, 126-7, 197, 208, 212; Charlie Stebbings 8-9, 13, 22-3, 25, 27, 32-3, 36-7, 40-1, 44-5, 48-9, 52-3, 55, 56-7, 59, 61, 65, 73, 77, 80-1, 82-3, 85, 86, 88-9, 90-1, 93, 94-5, 96-7, 98, 100-1, 103, 104-5, 106-7, 108-9, 110, 112, 114, 116-7, 119, 120-1, 122, 124-5.

The following pictures were supplied courtesy of Vogue:
(Jonathan Lennard) 159, 180; (Butch Martin) 105, 223, 239; (Tom Wool) 137, 144, 189.